RXpert SERIES
Student's Companion

ADVANCED ORGANIC CHEMISTRY - I

Rxpert SERIES
Student's Companion

ADVANCED ORGANIC CHEMISTRY - I

Y. V. D. Nageswar
M.Sc., PhD
Professor
Former Chief Scientist,
Indian Institute of Chemical Technology
(CSIR-IICT), Hyderabad India.

Pooja Chawla
M Pharm. PhD
Professor
University Institute of Pharmaceutical Sciences and Research.
Baba Farid University of Health Sciences Faridkot
Punjab India.

PharmaMed Press
An imprint of BSP Books Pvt. Ltd.
4-4-309/316, Giriraj Lane,
Sultan Bazar, Hyderabad - 500 001.

Advanced Organic Chemistry - I
by **Y. V. D. Nageswar and Pooja Chawla**

Published by:

PharmaMed Press™

An imprint of BSP Books Pvt. Ltd.
4-4-309/316, Giriraj Lane, Sultan Bazar, Hyderabad - 500 001.
Phone: 040-23445688
e-mail: info@pharmamedpress.com
www.pharmamedpress.com/pharmamedpress.net

ISBN: 978-93-49562-32-5 (Hardback)

Preface

Advanced Organic Chemistry – I brings together the entire M.Pharm 1st year Organic Chemistry syllabus in one comprehensive volume. Designed as both a complete reference for students and a practical guide for faculty, it presents essential concepts, reactions, and applications in a clear and structured manner. The content is drawn from a wide range of authoritative Organic Chemistry textbooks, ensuring accuracy, depth, and relevance to both academic study and research.

The book is organized into five chapters:

Chapter 1 introduces the fundamental aspects of Organic Chemistry, including nomenclature of organic compounds, and key concepts such as inductive effect, electromeric effect, mesomeric effect, hyperconjugation, bond fission, and reactive intermediates like carbonium ions, carbanions, free radicals, carbenes, and nitrenes. It also outlines various types of organic reactions with examples.

Chapter 2 presents fifteen important name reactions, complete with mechanisms and examples.

Chapter 3 describes several protecting groups used in organic transformations, illustrated with examples.

Chapter 4 covers selected name reactions employed in the synthesis of heterocyclic compounds, along with the synthesis of a broad range of representative drugs.

Chapter 5 explains the principles, applications, advantages, and limitations of the synthon approach and retrosynthesis in organic synthesis, and provides guidelines for molecular dissection.

Beyond fulfilling syllabus requirements, this book is designed to encourage postgraduate students to engage with current research trends. Each chapter includes multiple reactions illustrated with examples, making it a valuable resource for both students and faculty members. Literature references have been selectively included for further reading.

During the preparation of this work, we have consulted many outstanding Organic Chemistry textbooks. We express our sincere gratitude to the authors of these works, whose contributions have guided and inspired generations of students and teachers worldwide.

All reactions reproduced from the literature have been redrawn and cited with their respective references. We gratefully acknowledge the original researchers, scientists, and publishers whose work is quoted in this book.

Finally, we extend our deep appreciation to Mr. Anil Shah, Mr. Nikunjesh Shah, Director, PharmaMed Press; Mr. Naresh Davergave, Production Manager and the entire supporting team, whose cooperation and encouragement have been invaluable in bringing this book to completion.

-Authors

Contents

CHAPTER 1

Basic Aspects of Organic Chemistry

The chemistry of organic substances is known as organic chemistry. Carbonaceous resources such as coal, natural gas, and petroleum, as well as plants, are the main natural sources of organic compounds. The unique feature of organic substances is that they have a considerably higher number of carbon-containing compounds than non-carbon-containing molecules. These substances may be big and intricate. It is also possible for the arrangement of carbon atoms to be complex. Aside from that, biology and medicine depend heavily on organic chemistry. It serves as the foundation for technological advancement and is crucial to many businesses.

Agrochemicals, plastics, dyes, pigments, textiles, biochemicals, medications, vitamins, and many more materials are all made possible by organic chemistry, which is also essential to human life. Although prehistoric cultures were aware of numerous organic substances, such as sugar, lipids, starches, indigo, and alcohol, modern organic chemistry was founded in the 18th century when natural products were isolated from a variety of natural sources. From natural sources, Scheele separated malic acid, tartaric acid, and citric acid. He also created lactic acid, oxalic acid, and glycerol. The phrase "organic compounds" was created by Berzelius to describe substances that came from plants and animals. He stated that the area of chemistry that deals with organic chemicals is called organic chemistry. The branch of chemistry known as inorganic chemistry studies compounds derived from minerals. Vital Force Theory believes that organic chemicals were made from nature by the operation of vital force, inherent in living cells. With the synthesis of urea from ammonium cyanate by Wöhler in 1828, the era of synthetic organic chemistry started.

The important features of organic compounds:

1. The carbon atoms can bind to each other carbon atoms by stable covalent bonds; these can form chains, branched chains or rings. These are also capable of forming complex molecules. This kind of self-linking is called Catenation.
2. These are non-ionic in nature.
3. These form bonds to a limited number of other elements like H2, halogens, oxygen, nitrogen, sulfur, selenium, silicon, phosphorus, boron, etc.
4. These can form isomers.
5. These are generally insoluble in water but soluble in organic solvents.
6. These are highly volatile and flammable.
7. These have characteristic odor and color.
8. These have low melting point and boiling point.

9. These can be classified based on various functional groups which attribute special properties particular to that class.

Classification of organic compounds:

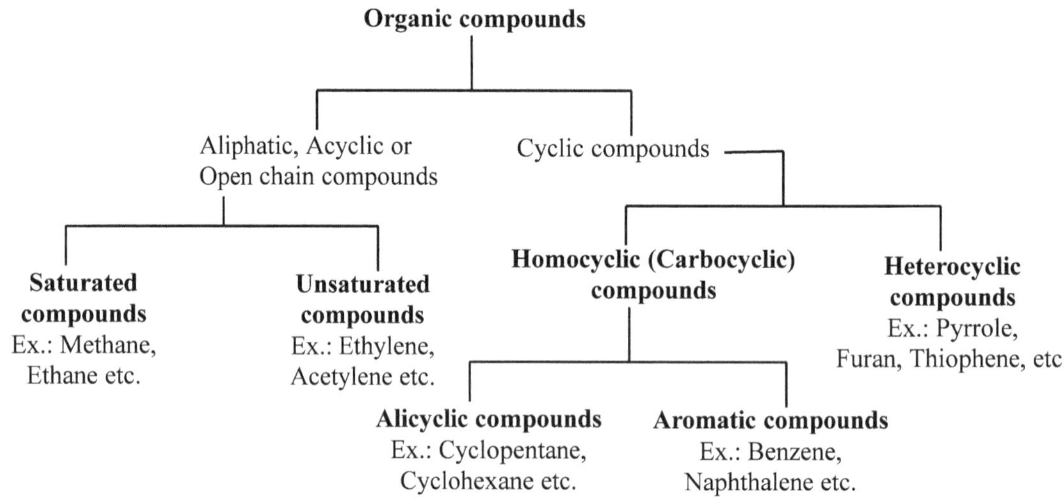

Types of bonds:

Three types of bonds are known:

a) Ionic or Electrovalent Bond:

The bond is formed due to the electrostatic attraction between the reacting oppositely charged ions. The electrons are completely transferred to the other reacting ion. Ex.: NaCl, KCl.

b) Covalent Bond:

Here the bond is formed due to the mutual sharing of electrons between two reacting species. Ex.: CH_4, C_2H_6.

c) Coordinate Covalent Bond:

It is formed by the donation of a pair of electrons to other deficient reacting species. Ex.: $NH^{+}4$, O3.

General properties of Inorganic and Organic compounds:

S. No.	Inorganic compounds	Organic compounds
1.	These are ionic molecules	These are covalent molecules
2.	These undergo ionic reactions	These undergo covalent bonding and related to molecules
3.	Isomerism is not exhibited	These molecules show isomerism
4.	These exist as acids, bases and salts	These are classified depending on the functional group like alcohols, amines, aldehydes, ketones, carboxylic acids, esters, amides etc.
5.	These exhibit high melting point and boiling point	These have low melting point and boiling point
6.	These are generally colorless and odourless	These possess characteristic color and odour
7.	These are generally water soluble	These are generally water insoluble, but soluble in organic solvents
8.	These have less volatility and flammability	These are highly volatile and flammable

Sources of organic compounds:

These can be obtained both from natural and synthetic sources. From nature, these can be isolated from plants and animals.

Important applications of organic compounds in daily life:

We depend every day on many organic compounds for our use. Apart from several complex molecules like amino acids, peptides, proteins, DNA, RNA, enzymes, lipids and hormones, Compounds, play a significant role in keeping us in good health

Foods: Glucose, Sucrose, Starch, Fats, Proteins, Vitamins, etc.

Clothes: Cotton, Wool, Silk, Nylon, Terylene, etc.

Fuels: Coal, Kerosene, Petrol, Diesel

Dyes: Indigo, Congo-Red, Malachite Green, etc.

Rubbers, Polymers, Plastics: Bakelite, Melamine, Teflon, Polyethylene, Polypropylene, Polystyrene, Polyvinyl chloride, etc.

Paints, Varnishes, Enamels:

Agrochemicals, Pesticides, Pheromones and Fertilizers: Urea, DDT, Malathion, Boric acid, Acephate, Diazinon, Glyphosate, Gammaxene, etc.

Stationery: Inks, Papers, etc.

Refrigerants:

Cosmetics and Perfumes: Parabens, Phthalates, Lanolin, Triclosan, Hydroquinone, Ammonium lauryl sulphate, Propylene glycol, Isopropanol, Phenoxyethanol, Vanillin, Camphor, etc.

Medicines: Aspirin, Penicillin, Sulfonamide, Streptomycin, Cortisone, Cephalosporin, Penams, Propranolol, Tetracyclines, etc.

Disinfectants: Ethyl Alcohol, Chlorine compounds, Formaldehyde, Peracetic acid, Phenols, *ortho*-phthalaldehyde, Glutaraldehyde, Iodophors, etc.

Explosives: TNT, Picric acid, Nitroglycerin, etc.

Composition of organic compounds:

The principal elements present in organic compounds, in general, are carbon, hydrogen, oxygen, nitrogen, sulfur, fluorine, chlorine, bromine, iodine, phosphorus, boron, etc.

Structure of organic molecules:

Tetracovalency of Carbon: The atomic number of carbon is six. C = $1s^2, 2s^2, 2p^2$.

Ground state = $1s^2, 2s^2, 2p_x^1, 2p_y^1, 2p_z^0$. Excited state = $1s^2, 2s^1, 2p_x^1, 2p_y^1, 2p_z^1$. Carbon can complete octet by sharing one electron each with four atoms with mono-valency such as hydrogen. Ex.: CH_4; One important characteristic of carbon is that it can form covalent bonds with other carbon atoms. Catenation is the name given to this characteristic. This characteristic leads to the formulation of both straight and branched carbon chains. It may also create cyclic formations that resemble rings. Many naturally occurring compounds, often known as natural products, are examples of the complex molecules that carbon may make. Synthetic substances are molecules or compounds that humans have created in a lab. Covalent bonds are formed when the electron of one bonding atom fills the half-filled orbital of another atom. They may alternatively be described as the increasing overlapping of bonding or combining atomic orbitals. The original orbitals merge to form new molecular or hybrid orbitals, and this merging is known as hybridization. The effective overlap takes place when (a) Two combining orbitals are half-filled, (b) When both bonding orbitals approach closer with proper alignment, (c) When the electrons of bonding orbitals move in opposite direction (spin). Greater is the overlap, greater is the energy released and higher is the bond strength, lower is the bond length.

Type of bond	Bond energies (kcal/mol)	Bond length (Å)
H-H	103.2	0.74
C-H	98.7	1.12
C-C	83.0	1.54
C-N	148.1	1.47
C-O	84.0	1.43
C-Cl	83.0	1.77

Types of covalent bonds:

Covalent bond can be formed by the s-s overlap and s-p overlap, p-p overlap (linear or sidewise). These overlaps form different molecular orbitals with shapes and energies. Two main types of molecular orbitals are formed depending on directional dispositions. Two types of covalent bonds are formed σ-sigma and π-pi bonds.

Sigma bond (σ): When the overlapping bonding orbitals form a molecular orbital, which is symmetrically distributed along the nuclear axis, the bond is called σ-sigma bond. These are formed by overlap of (a) 2-s orbitals or (b) one s- and one p-orbital or (c) one p-orbital and one p-orbital-overlap in linear direction. Ex.: H_2 (s-s); H-F (s-p); F_2 (p-p).

Pi bond (π): Lateral or sideways overlap of bonding p-orbitals of two atoms results in pi-(π) bond formation. Such bond is weaker than sigma bond and there is no free rotation of atom about the nuclear axis, the rotation about the bond axis of a π bond will be restricted. Ex.: O_2- $1s^2$, $2s^2$, $2p_x^2$, $2p_y^1$, $2p_z^1$ (one σ bond and one π bond); N_2- $1s^2$, $2s^2$, $2p_x^1$, $2p_y^1$, $2p_z^1$ (one σ bond and two π bonds).

With four half-filled atomic orbitals ready to overlap carbon can form 4 sigma bonds such as in CH_4 resulting in 1 s-s, 3 s-p bonds. As the experimental data indicate that all four bonds are equivalent, the concept of hybridization explains that all the bonding atomic orbitals merge and redistribute. Their energy and shape, forming entirely "new", symmetrically four equivalent sp3 orbitals. The hybrid orbitals are equal in number to merging atomic orbitals. The orbitals have two electrons with opposite spin. The hybridization can be explained based on tetra covalency of carbon.

Types of Hybrid Orbitals:

Mixing orbitals	Hybrid orbitals	Types of hybridization	Shape	Bond angle	Example
1s and 1p	2-sp	sp	Linear	180°	—C≡C—
1s and 2p	3-sp^2	sp^2	Trigonal	120°	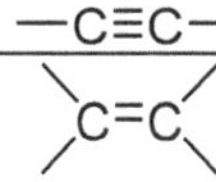 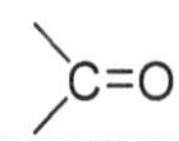
1s and 3p	4-sp^3	sp^3	Tetrahedral	109°28'	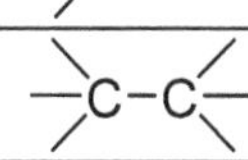

In ethylene molecule two sp^2 hybridized carbon atoms form one sigma-bond by head-on overlap of two sp^2 orbitals and the remaining two sp^2 hybrid orbitals of carbon form two sigma bonds with two hydrogen atoms. The unhybridized $2p_z$ orbitals of two carbons form sidewise overlap forming π bond- a part of C=C bond. Similarly, in acetylene molecule, 2sp orbitals of two carbons each form a sigma bond between two carbons. The remaining sp orbital overlap with s orbital of hydrogen atom. The two unhybridized 2py, 2pz orbitals of two carbon atoms form sideways overlap resulting in two π bonds – part of C≡C.

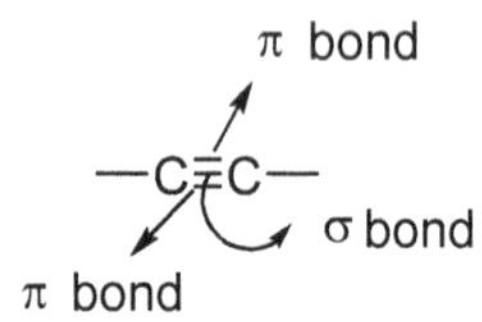

The resonance can be defined as the concept of delocalization of electrons across multiple conventional Lewis structures to form a more stable hybrid structure with lower energy. The amount of difference of energy between the real conjugated molecule and hypothetical resonance structures is called resonance energy.

Bond angle: It is the angle between the direction of two covalent bonds.

Bond energy: It is the average value of all bonds' dissociation energies of a molecule.

Bond order: Number of covalent bonds in the molecule H2=1; O2=2; N_2=3"

Bond dissociation energy: It is the amount of energy required to break a particular bond in a polyatomic molecule in the gaseous state into free radicals or neutral fragments in the gaseous state.

Hybridization: Linus Pauling in 1931 defined hybridization as the combination inter-mixing of atomic orbitals or slightly different energies to form a new set of equivalent orbitals of equivalent energies and shapes.

The important criteria for hybridization are:

a) The orbitals undergoing hybridization must have nearly equal energy.
b) Valence shell orbitals are to be hybridized.
c) Both filled or partly filled orbitals can participate in hybridization.
d) The hybridized orbitals are equivalent in shape and energies.
e) These hybridized orbitals can form stable bonds.
f) The number of resultant hybrid orbitals after hybridization is equal to the number of orbitals undergoing hybridization.
g) The hybridized orbitals direct into characteristic geometric patterns to have minimum repulsion between electron pairs and to have a stable arrangement.

Nomenclature of organic compounds:

The following are some of the important rules for naming the organic compounds under IUPAC system:

1. Longest chain rule: In the given compound, the longest carbon chain of the molecule is identified and named as the derivative of that alkane.
2. Lower number of substituent rules: While numbering the longest chain, the number should start from the end so as to give the lowest number to the substituent.
3. Arrangement of prefixes: In a given compound, when more than two groups are there, these groups are numbered in alphabetical order. When the same group is present more than one time, they are prefixed as di, tri, tetra, etc.

4. Lowest number for the functional group: Double or triple bonds are also considered as functional groups. Violating rule 2, when a functional group is also present, numbering is to be done so as to give first preference to the functional group.
5. The order of preferences in numbering: 1) Principal functional groups, 2) double bond or triple bond, 3) Substituent groups or atoms. Among these, the priority order is: a) carboxylic acid, b) acid derivatives, c) aldehydes, d) nitriles, e) ketones, f) alcohols, g) amines, h) ethers, i) olefins, j) acetylenes.

   Some functional groups are mentioned as prefixes and some as suffixes.
6. Writing for compounds having more than one functional group: when more functional groups are present, the names are combined in endings, or the important functional group is mentioned as a a substituent.
7. Considering groups of one kind of a single molecule as same and numbering as well as naming are preferentially given.
8. Selected chain to include maximum number of functional groups. This can sometimes violate longest chain rule (rule 1).

Steps in writing IUPAC name of a given compound:

a) Locate largest chain, write functional group including multiple bonds.

b) Select the root word for the carbon chain according to the number of carbons present.

c) Number the longest possible chain from the end nearest to the functional group.

d) Depending on the carbon chain, carbon bonds are given suffixes like ane, ene, yne.

e) Add suffixes or prefixes with numerals indicating the number and position of all important attachments to the main chain, placing the numerals before the functional group or unsaturation.

f) Add hyphens to connect numbers and letters to connect prefixes with the main compound name.

g) Commas are used to separate the individual numbers.

h) Parentheses and square brackets are used to demarcate certain locants.

Organic reactions are chemical reactions taking place between organic compounds. Basically, these are: 1. Addition reactions, 2. Elimination reactions, 3. Substitution reactions, 4. Rearrangement reactions. Apart from these photochemical, pericyclic and redox reactions are also familiar in organic synthesis. These play significant role in the preparation of simple to complex organic molecules. Many name reactions are known by their inventors' names and are applicable both in basic and industrial research as well as manufacturing sectors. These make use of various organic and inorganic reagents. Polar reactions are characterized by the movement of electron pairs from sources like nucleophiles or lone pairs to electrophiles. Radical reactions are known by single electron transfers or movements and participated by radicals. These reactions may proceed by chain or non-chain processes. Pericyclic reactions are concerted reactions involving cyclic rearrangement of atoms/groups and redistribution of chemical bonds, as well as a cyclic transition state. These require continuous overlap of participating orbitals and are governed by orbital symmetry considerations. Generally, organic reaction can be represented by

Organic molecule or substrate + Attacking reagent

↓

Transition state or Transitionary Intermediate

↓

Products or Byproducts

Substrate is the reactant that contains carbon atoms some of whose bonds with other atoms are broken and some new bonds are formed due to the reaction between substrate molecule and attacking reagent. Organic reaction mechanism depicts the total steps involved in breaking of bonds and making of bonds, resulting in the formation of product molecules. Through the transitionary intermediates, including the details of electron movements, are explained. The reaction is made possible by the displacement of bonding electrons, resulting in polarity in the reacting molecules due to electron displacement effects. Four important effects are generally observed in the organic molecules.

1. **Inductive Effect:** It can be defined as the local change in the electron density due to the electron donating or electron withdrawing groups attached in the molecule. It results in the permanent dipole in the bond (sigma bond). This permanent effect of polarity caused by minor displacement of electrons can be a -I effect or a +I effect depending on the polarity of the substituent attached to the parent carbon chain.

When a halogen atom is attached to a carbon atom as in an alkyl halide, the shared electrons between the C-X bond are moved or displaced towards the more electronegative X atom (Cl, Br, I). The positive charge is relayed towards down the chain. This is known as -I effect. In case of electron releasing (Y) substituent attached to carbon, negative charge is relayed down the chain. This is known as +I effect. Both these -I and +I effect decrease slowly from α, β, γ-carbon atoms. The effect falls rapidly in the carbon chain as the distance from the functional group increases.

C ⟶ X

(-I effect)

C ⟶ C ⟶ C ⟶ X

δ+++ δ++ δ+ δ-

C ⟵ X

(-I effect)

C ⟵ C ⟵ C ⟵ Y

δ--- δ-- δ- δ+

a) -I effect groups (electron attracting)

$-NO_2 > F > CO_2H > Cl > Br > I > OH > C_6H_5$

b) +I effect groups (electron releasing or donating)

$(CH_3)_3C- > (CH_3)_2-CH- > CH_3CH_2- > CH_3-$ or $3^o > 2^o > 1^o$

tert-butyl > Isopropyl > Ethyl > Methyl

2. **Electromeric Effect:** It is the temporary molecular polarizability caused by the intramolecular electron displacement in the substrate molecule by the shift of an electron pair from one atom to another under the influence of an electrophilic reagent, usually when a double bond or triple bond is expose dually when a double bond or triple bond is exposed.

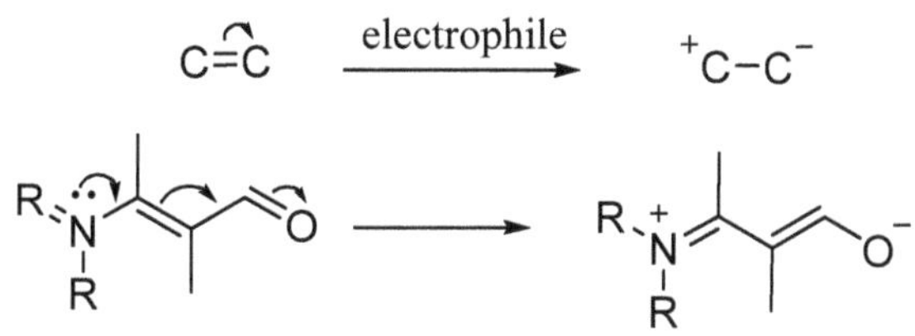

3. **Mesomeric Effect:** When an electron withdrawing or electron releasing group is conjugated with a π-bond or a set of alternatively positioned σ or π bonds, the electron displacement is transmitted through the π electrons in the chain of the substrate molecule. π-electrons get delocalized as a consequence of mesomeric effect, resulting in a number of resonance structures of the molecule.

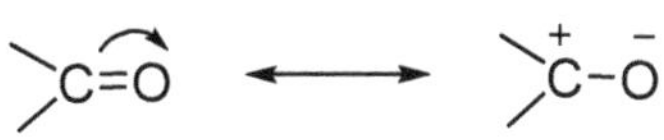

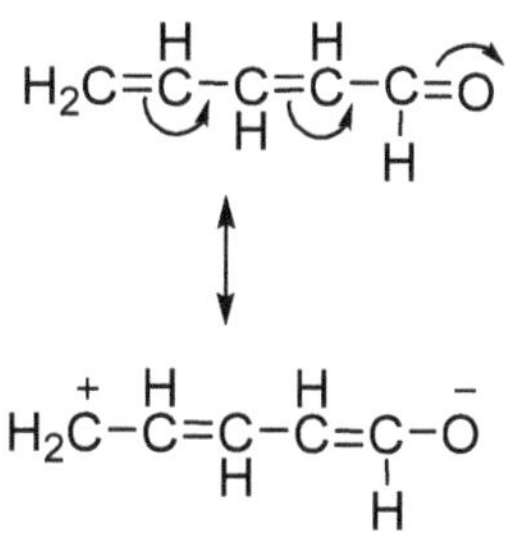

Just like the inductive effect, the mesomeric effect can also be shown as a +M effect or a -M effect, depending on the electron displacement direction. Greater the degree of delocalization, greater is the stability.

+M effect: direction of electrons away from the group. Ex.: -OH; -OR; $-NH_2$; -SR

-M effect: direction of electrons towards the group. Ex.: -C(O)-; $-NO_2$; -CN; $-SO_3H$

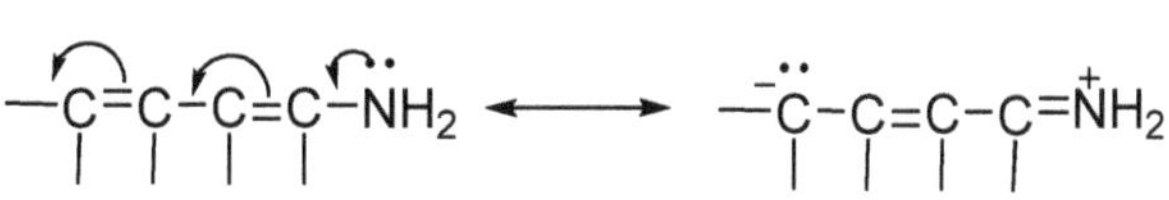

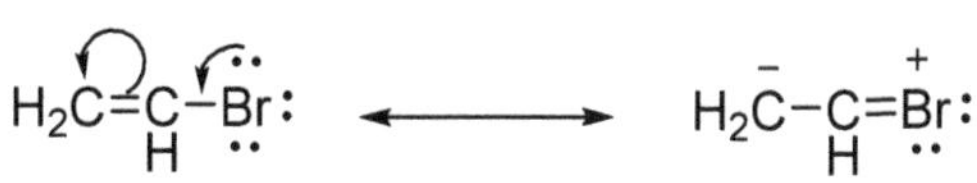

Both these electromeric effects and mesomeric effects are combinedly known as resonance effects.

4. **Hyperconjugation:** It is the delocalization of electrons with the participation of bonds of primarily σ character. This is also known as no-bond resonance or σ-conjugation. It involves the electrons of σ-orbitals such as those of C-C or C-H bonds; increased electrons delocalization due to hyperconjugation increases the stability of the system in the substrate molecule. It affects bond lengths, dipole moments, heat of formation of molecules, as well as the stability of carbocations According to Baker and Nathan, the hyperconjugation effect takes place through the interaction of σ electrons of C-H with π electrons of C=C.

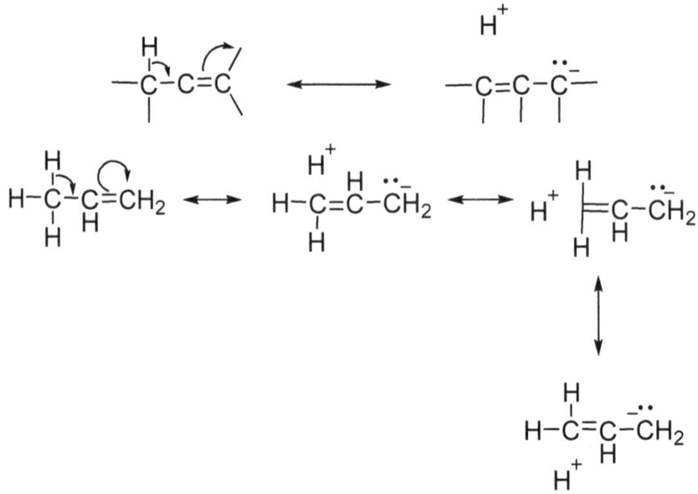

The hyperconjugative effect depends on the number of C-H bonds at the α-carbon to the unsaturated system. It would be maximum with a CH3 group at the α-position, followed by an isopropyl group. As there is no C-H bond at the α-position, a tert-butyl group shows zero effect. The order of release of electrons for the alkyl group is as follows:

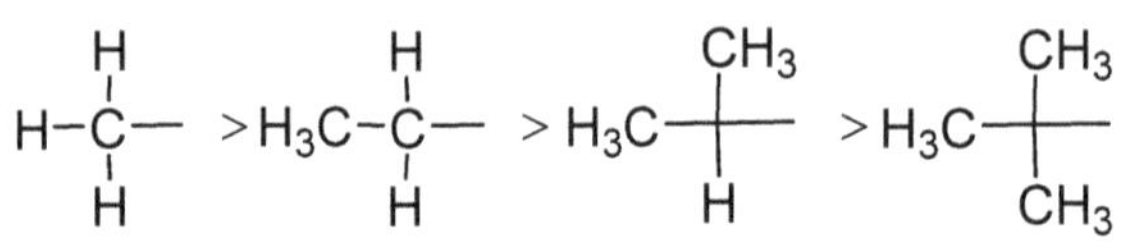

methyl primary secondary tertiary

Bond Fission:

A covalent bond is formed due to the sharing of a pair of electrons. Bond fission separates these two atoms. The process can take place in two ways. When each electron of the shared pair is taken away by each atom symmetrically it is called homolytic fission or homolysis. Such single-electron species are called free radicals, and these are not charged. These are transitory and react immediately to gain stability, by pairing up with another electron of the available species.

$$A:B \longrightarrow A\cdot + B\cdot$$

Molecule → Free radicals

$$Cl:Cl \xrightarrow[\text{light or heat}]{} Cl\cdot + Cl\cdot$$

Chlorine free radicals

When a covalent bond breaks in such a way that both the bonding electrons go to only one of the bonded atoms, forming one negatively charged and one positively charged species, determined by the electronegativities of the two atoms. The process is called heterolytic fission. It is most common in organic reactions conducted in solution phase. The progress of this process depends on the nature of the solvent. Polar solvents and ionic catalysts contribute significantly for the progress of the heterolytic fission of covalent bonds. The energy required to break the bond is partly taken from the energy of solution of the ions generated.

$$A:B \longrightarrow A^{\ominus} + B^{\oplus}$$

Molecule → Anion + Cation

Reactive intermediates:

1. **Carbocation:** It can be defined as the ion containing positively charged carbon species. As the carbon of a carbocation has only 6 electrons (six). It is very reactive and unstable. It will have a tendency to gain an octet. It will be ready to react with any species that can donate a pair of electrons. It is a flat structure with all three bonds in one plane. Bonding is 120° between all three bonds.

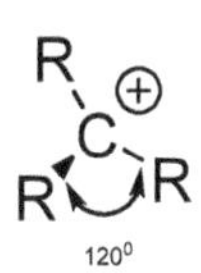

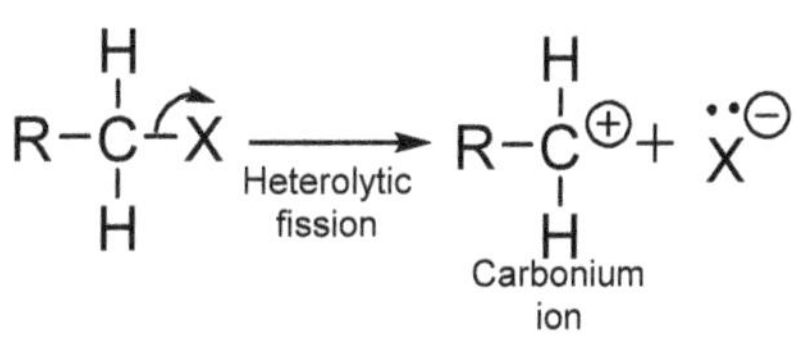

Ex. $\overset{\oplus}{C}H_3$, $CH_3\overset{\oplus}{C}H_2$, $(CH_3)_2\overset{\oplus}{C}H$, $(CH_3)_3C^{\oplus}$

Primary, Primary, Secondary, Tertiary

Ex. $\overset{\oplus}{C}H_3$ Methyl carbonium ion

$CH_3\overset{\oplus}{C}H_2$ Ethyl carbonium ion

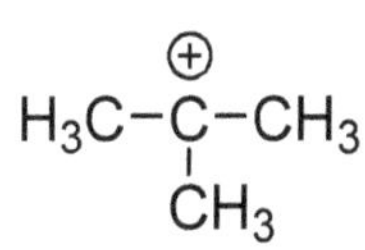

tert-butyl carbonium ion

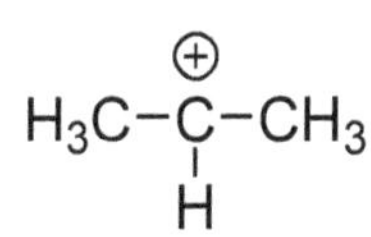

Isopropyl carbonium ion

The stability of carbonium ion follows-

Tertiary carbonium ion > Secondary carbonium ion > Primary carbonium ion

Electron-withdrawing groups such as -NO2, -C(O)- attached to the carbon reduce the carbocation stability by withdrawing electrons through the connecting bond and enhancing the positive charge on the carbon. Electron donating groups (+I effect) release electrons through the connecting bond and make the carbonium ion more stable.

Allyl carbonium ion hybrid

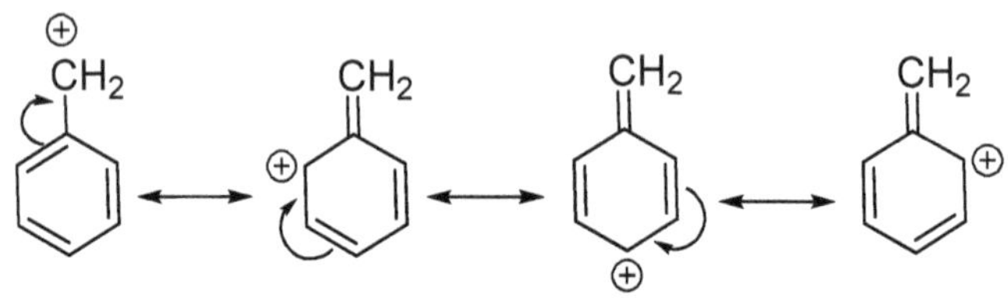

Benzyl carbonium ion hybrid

Allyl and benzyl carbocation hybrids are stabilized by resonance and are depicted by canonical structures. These are more stable than an isopropyl carbocation due to the resonance effect. Resonance, hyperconjugation, and inductive effects influence the carbocation stability.

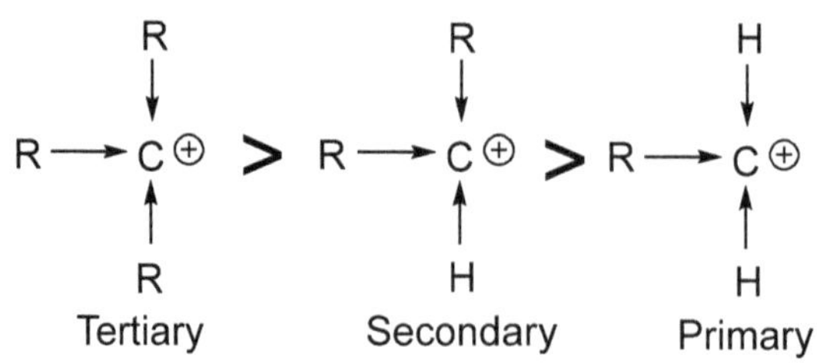

Formation of Carbocations:

1. Direct ionization of alkyl and aryl halides in polar medium

a)

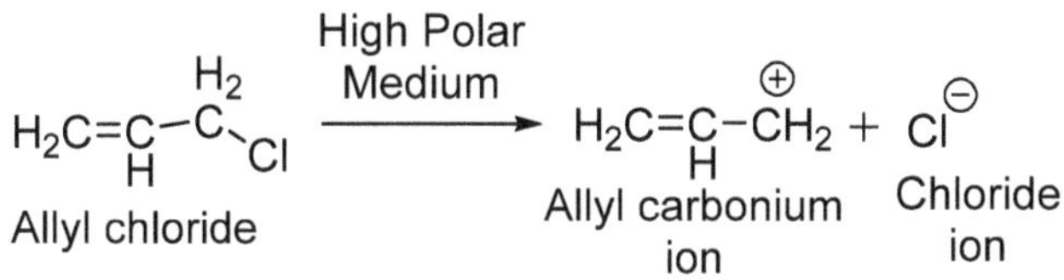

b)

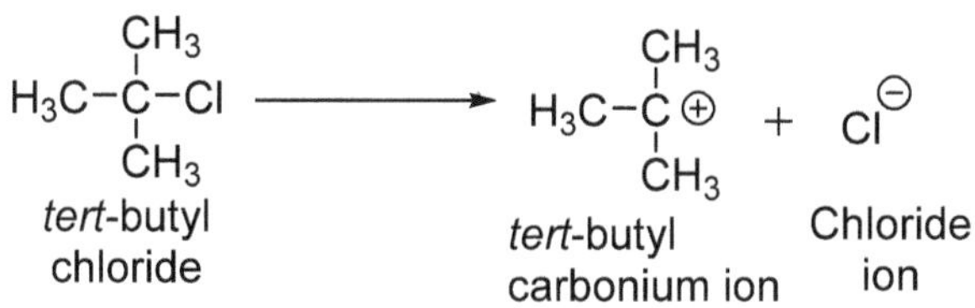

c)

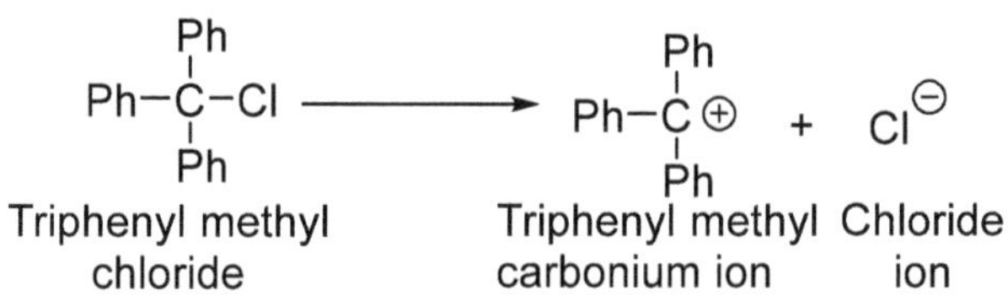

2. By the decomposition of diazonium salts

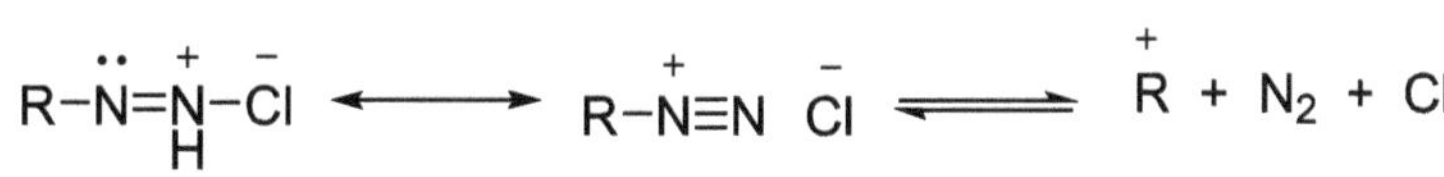

3. By the protonation of alkyl or aryl halides in the presence of Lewis acid or proton donating solvent

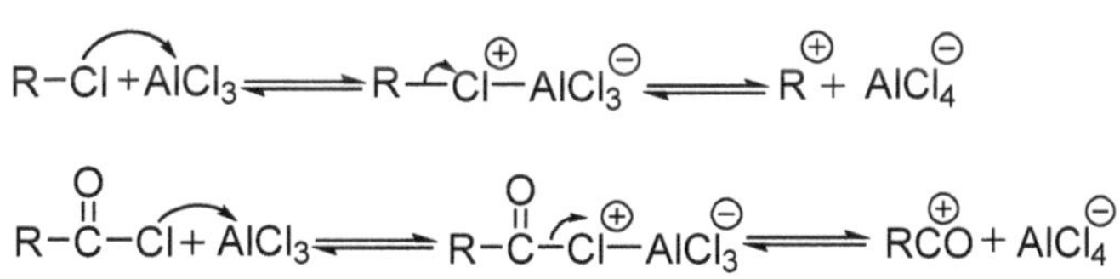

4. By the protonation of unsaturated compounds such as alkenes carbonyl compounds and nitriles in the presence of a Lewis acid or proton donating solvent

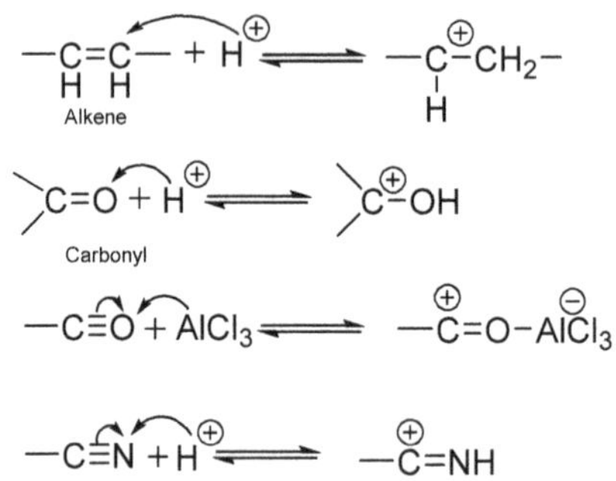

5. By the deprotonation of an atom with lone pair of electrons in the presence of an acid

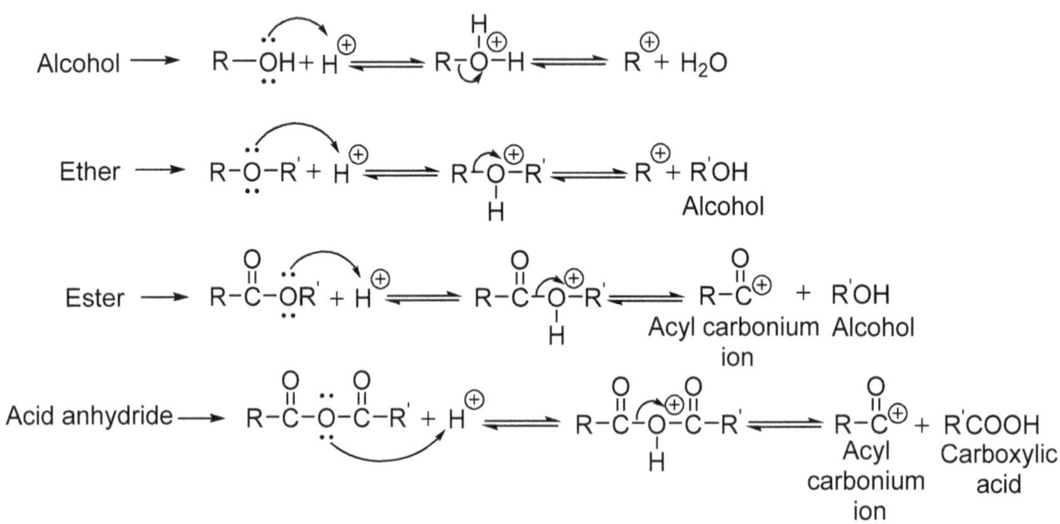

Reactions of Carbocations:

Carbonium ions react or participate in the following reactions:

a) It may lose a proton to form an alkene

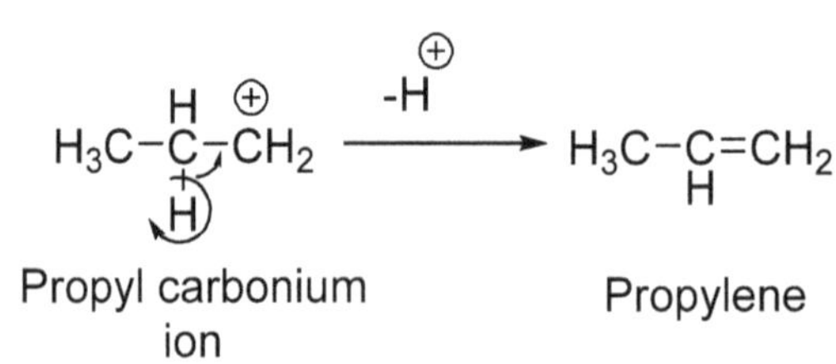

b) Carbocation may combine with nucleophiles by accepting a pair of electrons and forming a bond. Nucleophiles such as H2O, NH3, or available anions such as X-, OH-, CN- may react with carbocations

i)

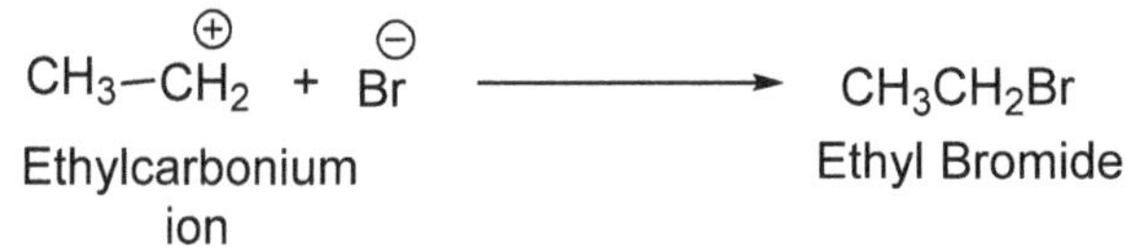

ii)

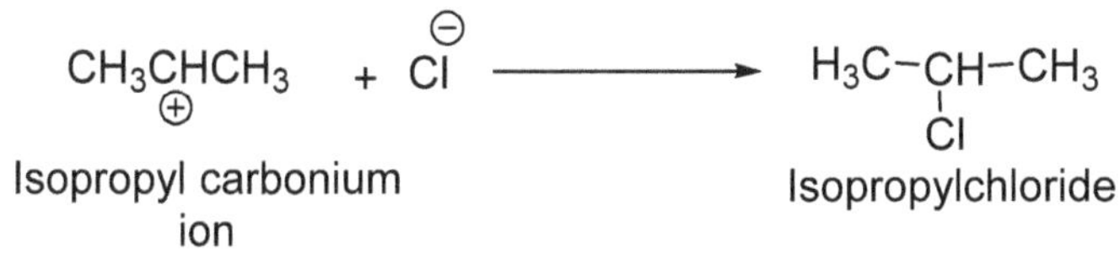

iii)

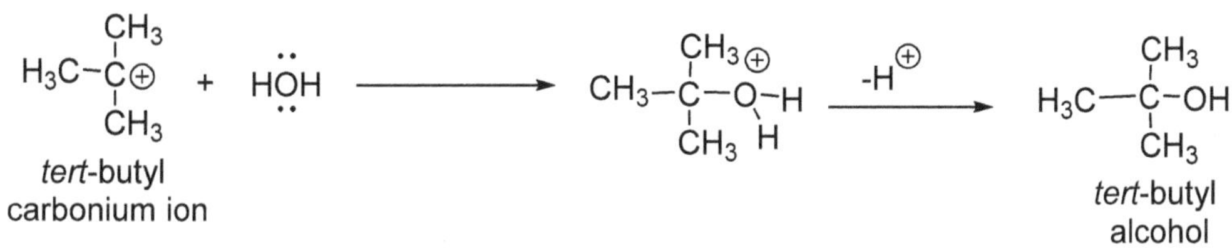

iv)

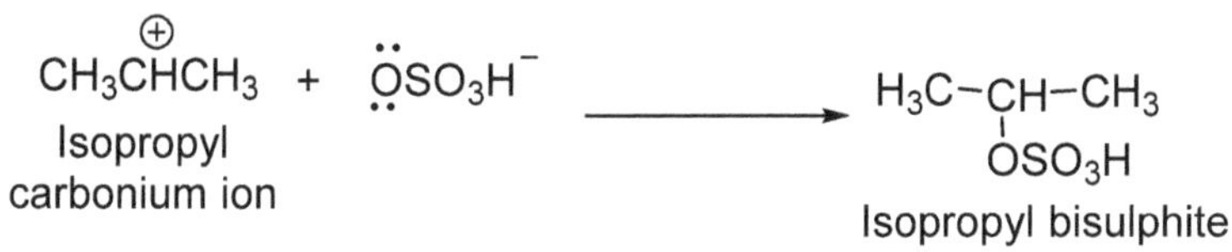

c) Addition to an Olefin

The carbocation adds to an alkene forming a bigger carbocation.

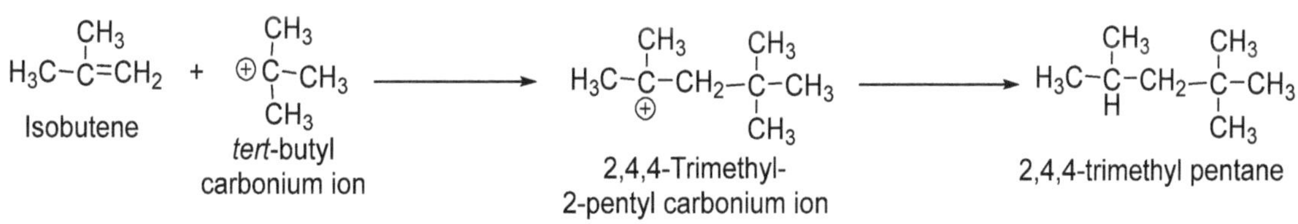

d) Molecular rearrangements

A carbocation can undergo rearrangements to produce more stable molecular species. Stability of the carbocation follows the order.

tertiary > secondary > primary

3° > 2° > 1°

These rearrangements take place by the migration of a hydrogen atom (hydride shift) or an alkyl group (alkyl shift), with a pair of bonding electrons. These rearrangements are known as 1,2-shifts.

1,2- Hydride Shift :

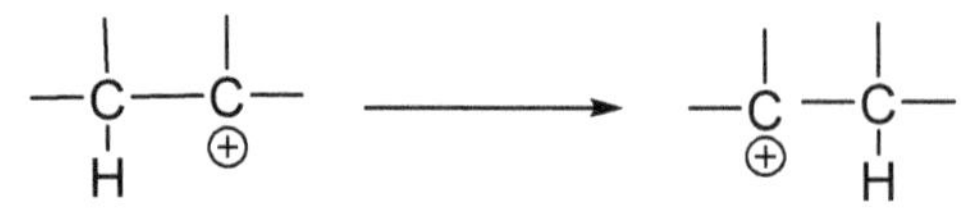

1,2- Alkyl Shift :

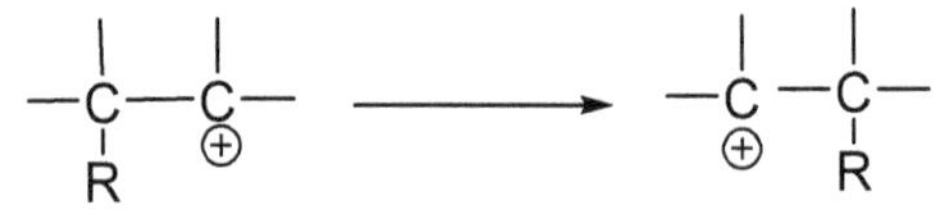

2. Carbanions

Carbanions are defined as negatively charged species containing a carbon atom with three bonds along with an unshared pair of electrons.

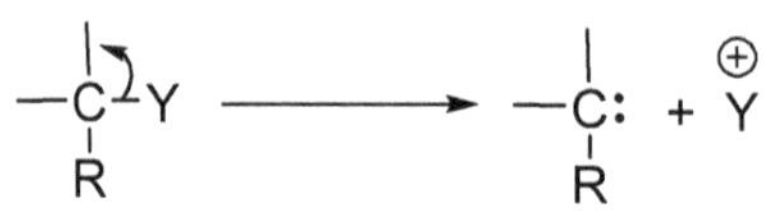

Y = Less electronegative atom than carbon

$$R-CH_2-X + \ddot{B} \longrightarrow R-\overset{\ominus}{C}HX + BH$$

These are formed as electron rich fragments from heterolytic fission. These are highly reactive intermediates and react readily with electrophiles. Even though these are unstable, they can be stabilized by the attached electron-attracting groups like carbonyl and nitrile groups. However, the presence of electron-releasing groups such as alkyl groups increases the negative charge on the carbon atom, making the carbanion unstable.

$H_3C-\overset{\ominus}{C}H_2$ ethyl carbanion

$H_3C-\overset{\ominus}{C}H-CH_3$ Isopropyl carbanion

Carbanions can also be stabilized by means of resonance. Ex.: Benzyl carbanion.

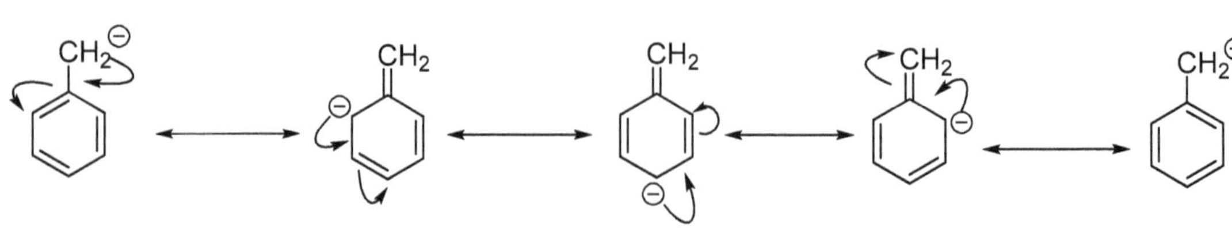

The carbanion carbon atom is sp3 hybridized. It has a pyramidal shape. In this, three sp3 hybrid orbitals form three covalent bonds with other atoms, and the fourth sp3 orbital contains an unshared pair of electrons. But when the carbanion is in conjugation, it is planar with sp2 hybridization.

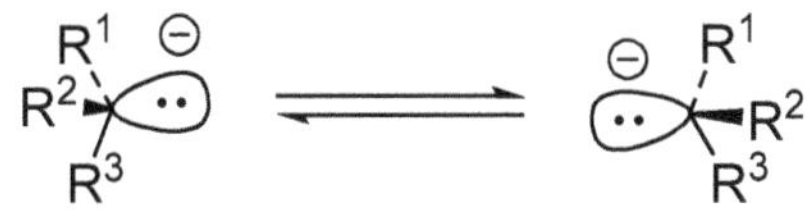

Formation of Carbanion:

1. By the ionization of an α-hydrogen: In the case of carbonyl compounds, the α-hydrogens are acidic, and the negative charge generated on the α-carbon caused by the loss of a proton is stabilized by the carbonyl group, just as in the case of carboxylic acids.

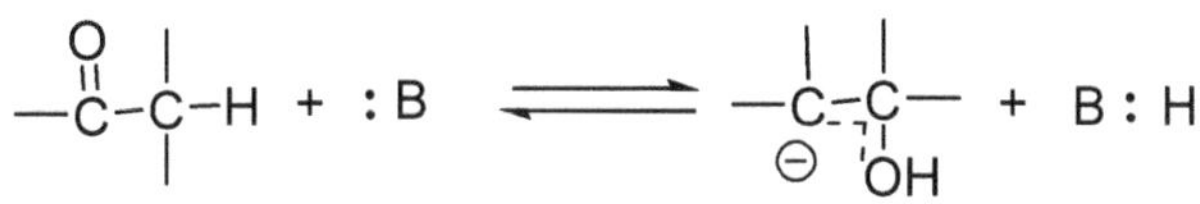

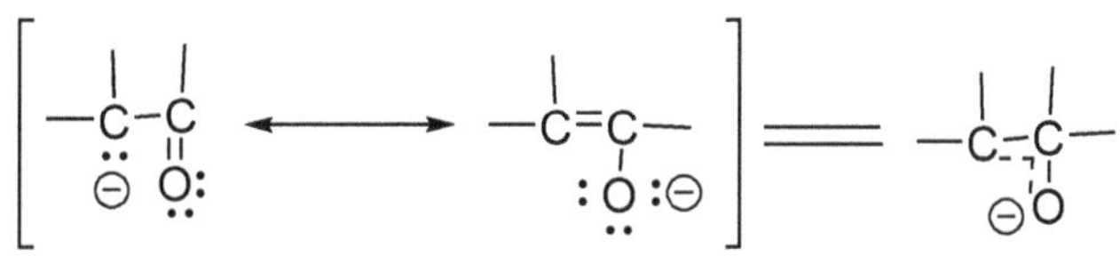

Example:

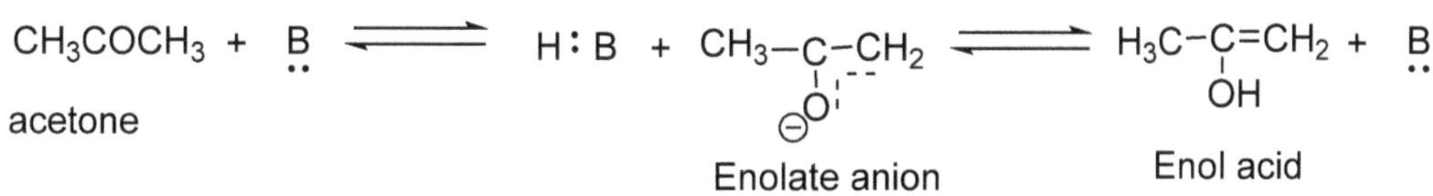

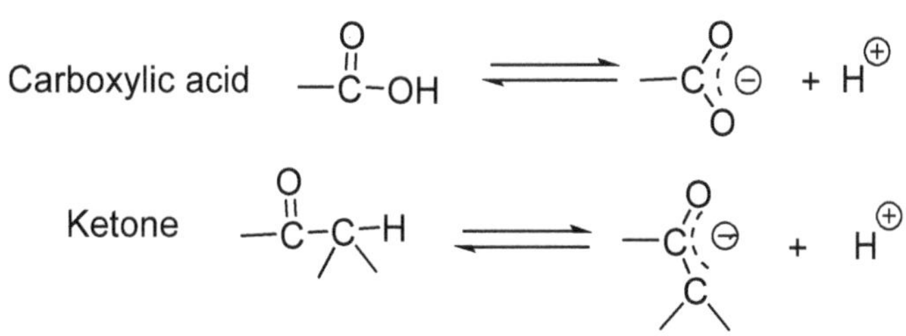

Reactions of carbanions:

Carbanions are electron-rich and act as potential nucleophiles. These actively participate in many addition and substitution reactions.

1. Addition reactions (Nucleophilic addition to carbonyl compounds)

a) Aldol condensation

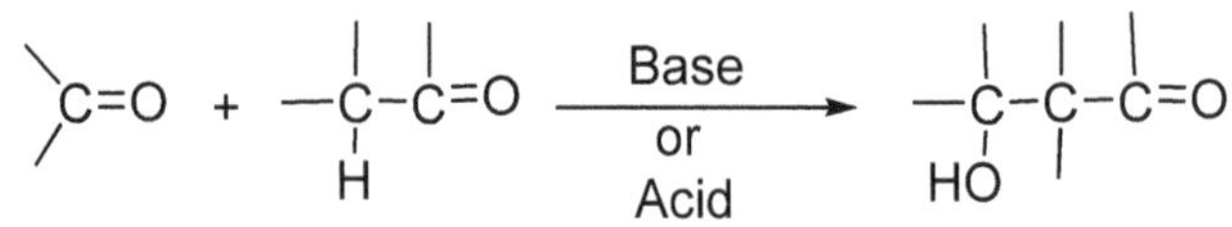

Compounds containing carbonyl groups like aldehydes, ketones, anhydrides, and esters can be used. The abstraction of α-hydrogen from carbonyl groups can be performed by the use of different bases like NaOH, NaOEt, CH_3COONa, amines, etc.

Examples:

a) Aldol reaction

$$\underset{\text{acetaldehyde}}{CH_3CHO + CH_3CHO} \xrightarrow{OH^{\ominus}} \underset{\text{3-OH-butanal}}{CH_3CHOHCH_2CHO} \xrightarrow[\text{Heat}]{NaHSO_4} \underset{\text{crotonaldehyde or 2-butenal}}{H_3CHC{=}CH{-}CHO} + H_2O$$

Crossed aldol condensation between two different aldehydes

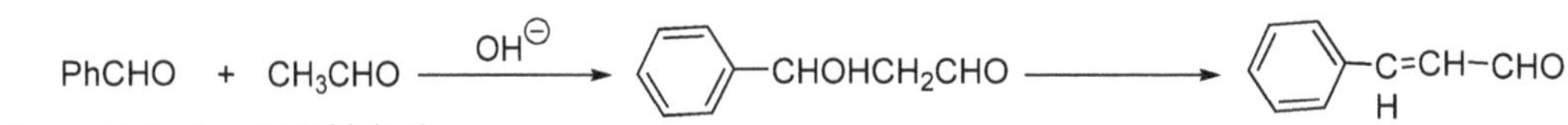

Benzaldehyde acetaldehyde

Cinnamaldehyde

b) Perkin reaction

$$\underset{\text{Benzaldehyde}}{PhCHO} + \underset{\text{Acetic anhydride}}{(CH_3CO)_2O} \xrightarrow{CH_3CO_2Na} \underset{\text{Cinnamic acid}}{PhHC{=}CH{-}CO_2H}$$

c) Knoevenagel condensation

$$PhCHO + CH_2(CO_2Et)_2 \xrightarrow[\text{2° amine}]{} PhHC{=}C(CO_2Et)_2$$

d) Claisen reaction

$$\underset{\text{Ethylacetate}}{2CH_3CO_2Et} \longrightarrow \underset{\text{Ethyl acetoacetate}}{CH_3COCH_2CO_2Et}$$

Crossed Claisen condensation with different Carbonyl Compounds

$$HCO_2Et + CH_3CO_2Et \xrightarrow{OEt^{\ominus}} HCOCH_2CO_2Et + EtOH$$

Ethylformylacetate

e) Dieckmann reaction

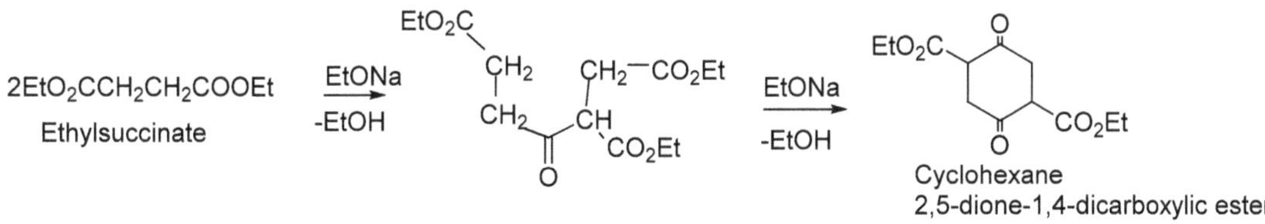

f) Cope reaction

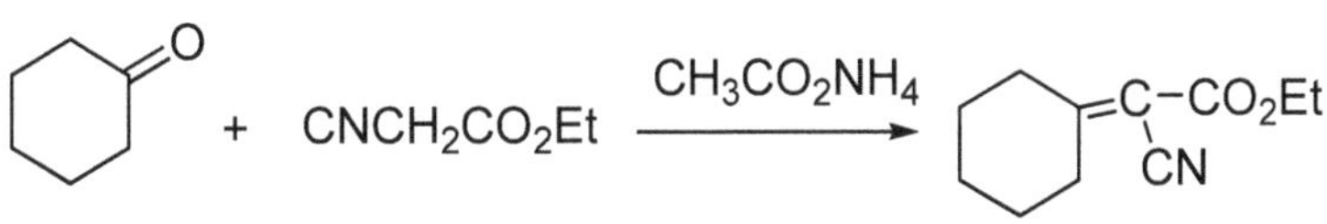

g) Addition of Grignard reagent

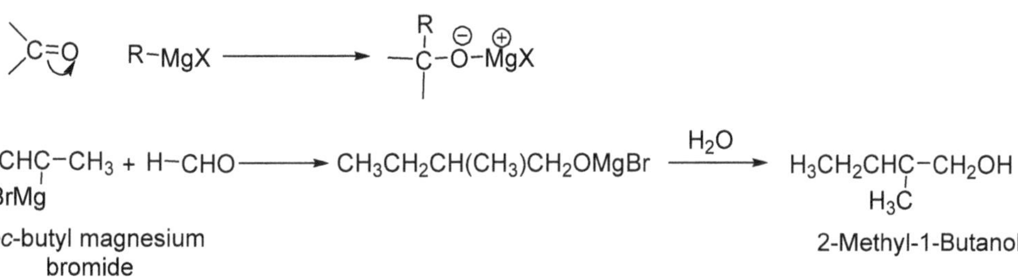

h) Michael addition

Addition of carbanion to α, β-unsaturated carbonyl compounds

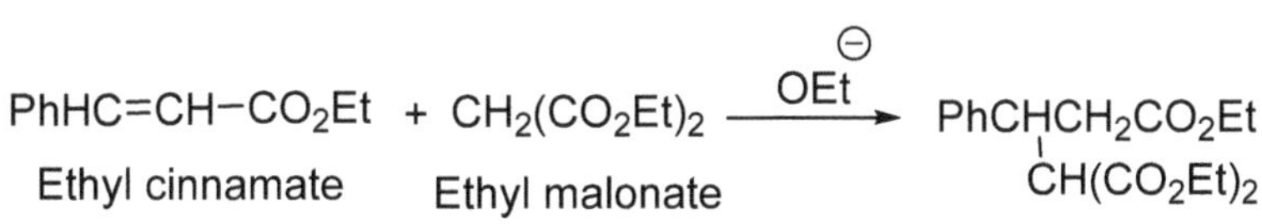

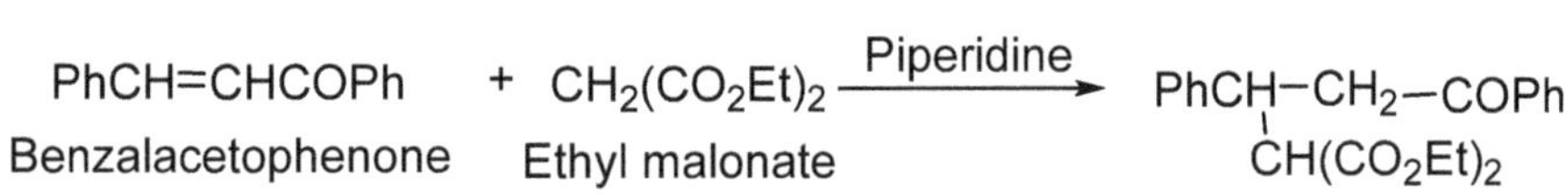

i) Reformatsky reaction – Preparation of β-OH esters

When an α-bromo ester is treated with metallic zinc in the presence of an aldehyde or ketone, a β-OH ester is formed.

$$\underset{\text{Benzaldehyde}}{PhCHO} + \underset{\text{Ethyl-}\alpha\text{-bromo propionate}}{BrCH(CH_3)CO_2Et} \xrightarrow[\text{ether}]{Zn} \xrightarrow[H^+]{H_2O} \underset{\text{Ethyl-}\beta\text{-OH-}\beta\text{-Ph-}\alpha\text{-Me-propionate}}{Ph{-}CHOHCH(CH_3)CO_2Et}$$

j) Wittig reaction

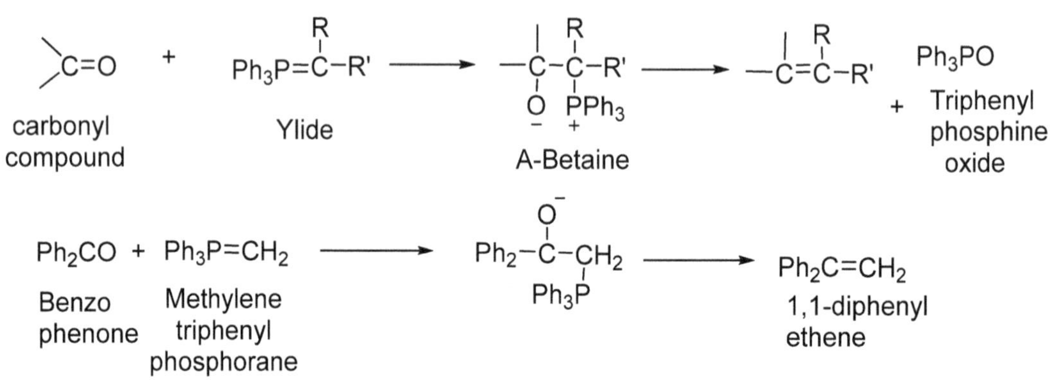

2. Substitution reactions

a) Halogenation of ketones

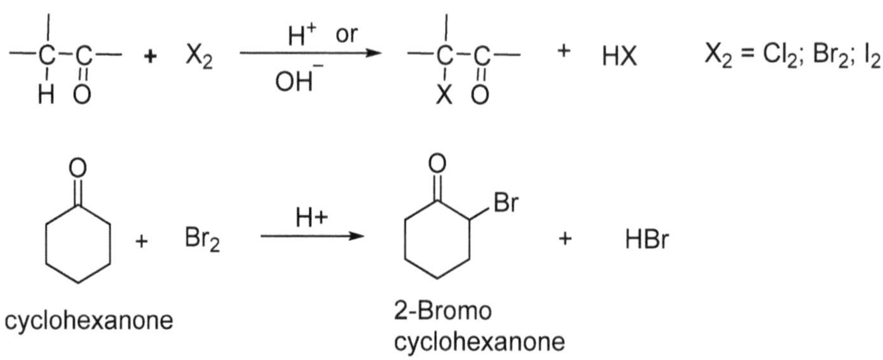

b) Acetoacetic ester; synthesis of ketones

In this reaction, a hydrogen atom is replaced by an alkyl group.

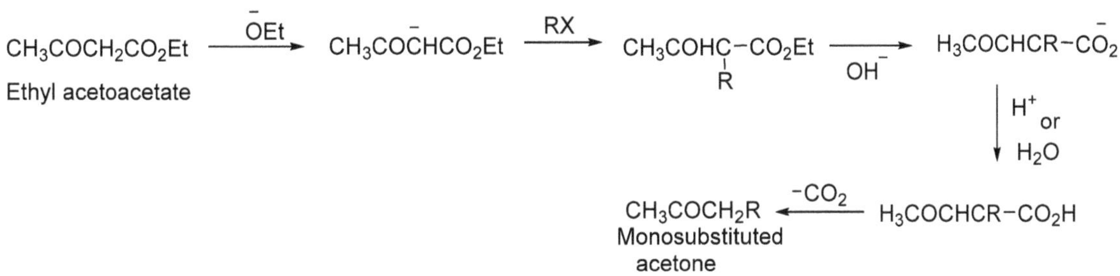

c) Malonic ester; synthesis of carboxylic acids

The synthesis provides acetic acid derivatives in which one or two hydrogens are replaced by the alkyl groups.

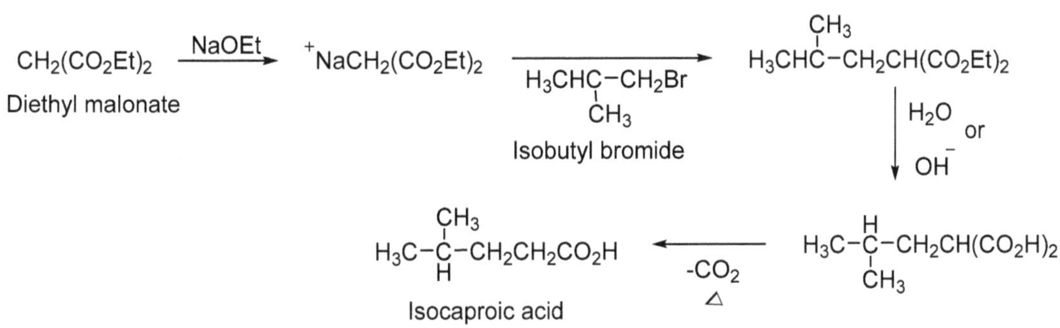

d) Synthesis of acetylides

A A carbon-carbon triple bond is an important building block in organic synthesis. The acidity of a terminal alkyne allows easy conversion of the triple bond to a metal acetylide. It is allowed to be introduced easily into molecules.

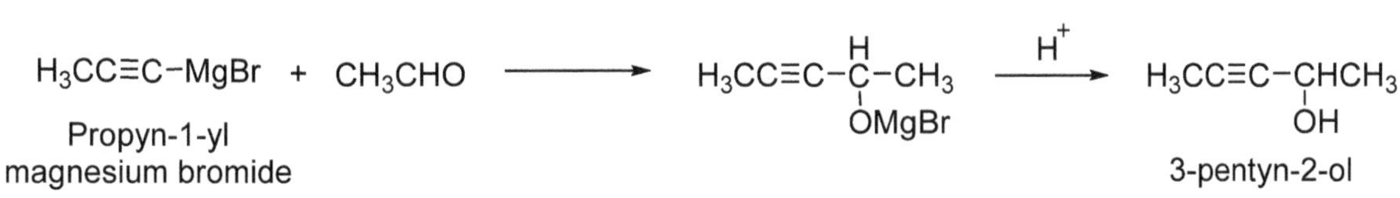

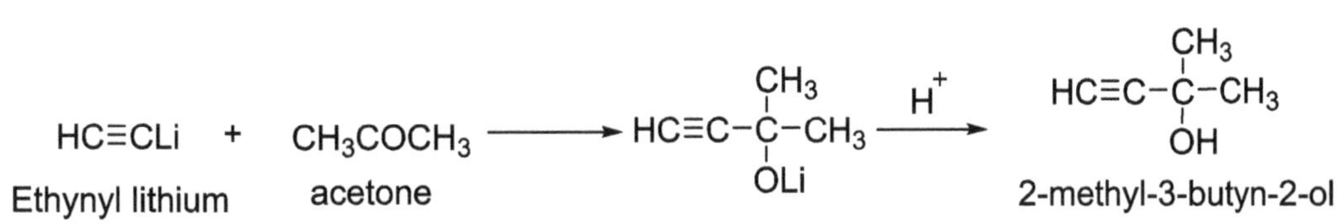

e) **Coupling of alkyl halides with organometallic compounds:** The alkyl group in organometallic compounds can be primary, secondary, or tertiary. Primary halides give good yields.

$$\underset{\text{Methyl bromide}}{CH_3Br} \longrightarrow \underset{\text{Methyl lithium}}{CH_3Li} \xrightarrow{CuI} \underset{\text{Lithium dimethyl copper}}{(CH_3)_2CuLi} \xrightarrow[\text{iodide}]{n\text{-octyl}} \underset{n\text{-nonane}}{CH_3(CH_2)_7CH_3}$$

3. Free radicals

Free radicals can be defined as an atom or a group of atoms having an odd or unpaired electron and acting as neutral species. In the example below, a chlorine molecule underwent homolysis to form a chlorine radical, with cleavage in a symmetrical manner. Homolytic cleavage takes place when both bonded atoms have similar electronegativities. Ease of formation of free radicals and also stability of free radicals follows the order-

$$\text{allyl} > 3° > 2° > 1° > \dot{C}H_3 > \text{Vinyl}$$

Formation of free radicals:

1) By Homolysis:

$$\underset{\text{chlorine molecule}}{Cl_2} \xrightarrow[\text{light}]{\text{heat or}} \underset{\text{chlorine radical}}{2\dot{Cl}}$$

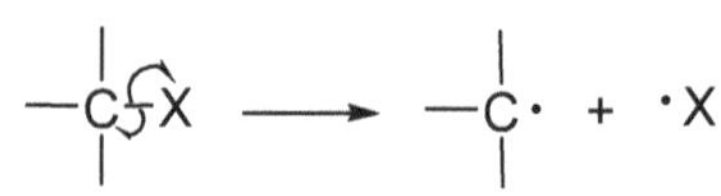

2) By abstraction

$$CH_4 + {}^{\bullet}Cl \longrightarrow HCl + \underset{\text{Methyl radical}}{CH_3^{\bullet}}$$

In the above equation, it is shown that Cl° abstracts hydrogen atom with an electron to form HCl and a methyl radical.

Ease of abstraction follows an order-

$$\text{allylic} > 3° > 2° > 1° > CH_4 > \text{Vinylic}$$

3) **By addition:** In the presence of peroxides, HBr adds to alkenes followed by the peroxide initiated free radical reaction. This is also known as peroxide effect or Kharasch effect. The mechanism is as follows-

i) $\text{peroxides} \longrightarrow \text{radical}^{\bullet}$

ii) $\text{radical}^{\bullet} \xrightarrow{HBr} \text{rad}:H + Br^{\bullet}$

iii 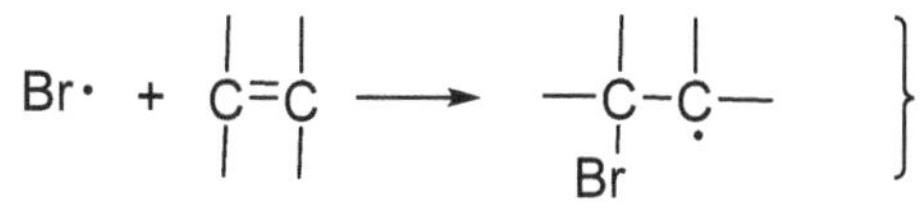 chain initiation

iv 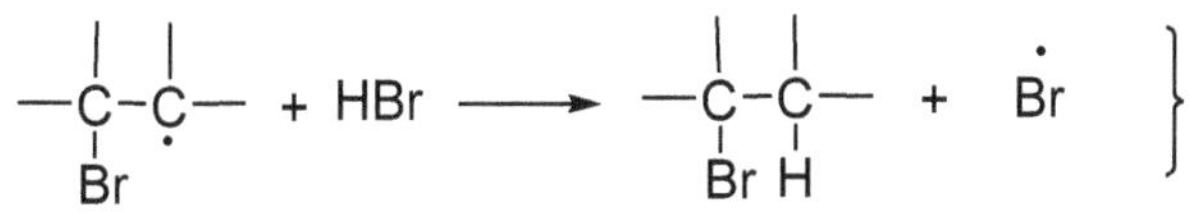 chain propagation

4) **By photochemical fission:** Electromagnetic radiation causes bond fission, forming free radicals. Ex: Cl_2, Br_2, peroxides, acetone etc.

5) **Thermal fission:** Pyrolysis of organic compounds result in free radical formation. Heating of lead tetraethyl leads to free radical formation.

$$(C_2H_5)_4Pb \longrightarrow Pb + \text{Ethane} + Me^{\cdot}$$

Organic peroxides undergo decomposition to give free radicals. Methyl free radical is obtained when azomethane is decomposed at 570K.

6) **Oxidation or reduction of inorganic ions and metals form free radicals:** Oxidation of ferrous ion with H2O2 in the presence of Fenton's reagent and Kolbe electrolysis of an aqueous solution of an alkali salt of a fatty acid are some examples.

Reactions of free radicals: Generally, free radicals undergo a) Combination i.e., dimerization of two free radicals to yield bigger products, b) Abstraction- Abstraction of an atom from saturated organic compounds, c) Fragmentation- Some types of free radicals undergo fission resulting in a radical or non-radical fragments, d) Addition- Some free radicals add on to multiple bonds like double or triple bonds, e) Substitution reactions- Cycloalkanes undergo chiefly free radical substitution reactions.

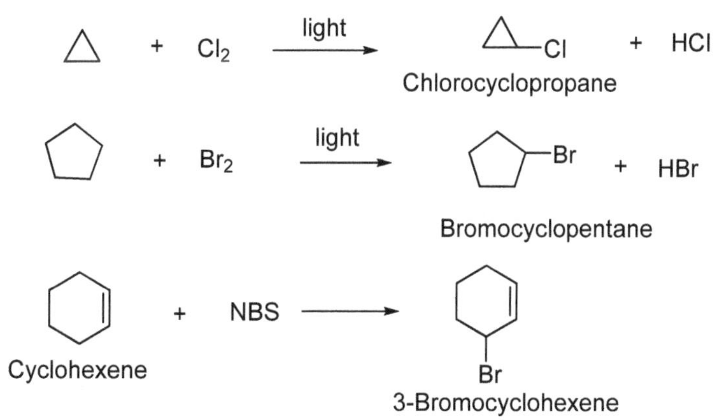

$$H_2C=\overset{H}{C}-H \xrightarrow[Cl^{\cdot}]{} H_2C=CH\text{-}Cl$$

vinyl chloride

Tert-butyl peroxide is a stable and easy to handle liquid. It is a good source of free radicals.

$$(CH_3)_3COOC(CH_3)_3 \xrightarrow[\text{Heat or light}]{} 2(CH_3)_3CO^{\bullet} \xrightarrow[CCl_4,\ 130^{\circ}C]{\text{Isobutane}} \textit{tert}\text{-butylchloride} + CHCl_3$$

Free radical substitution leads to allylic rearrangements in alkenes.

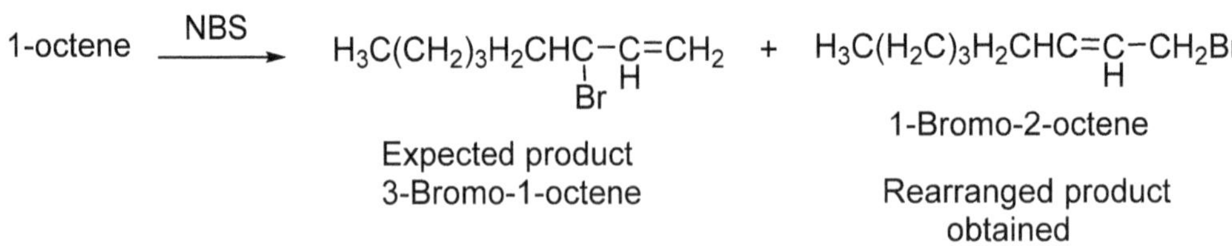

In conjugated alkenyl benzenes such as 1-phenyl propene, bromination in the absence of peroxides goes to the benzylic carbon, and in the presence of peroxides, bromide is attached to the carbon adjacent to the benzylic carbon.

$$PhHC{=}CHCH_3 \xrightarrow[2.\,Br^{\ominus}]{1.\,HBr} PhCHBrCH_2CH_3$$

$$PhHC{=}CHCH_3 \xrightarrow[\text{Peroxide}]{Br^{\bullet}} Ph\dot{C}HCHBrCH_3 \xrightarrow{HBr} PhCH_2CHBrCH_3$$

Structure of free radical: In carbon free radical, three sigma bonds are formed with three sp^2 hybrid orbitals and the odd electron is in the half-filled p orbital which exists above and below the plane of sigma bonds. These highly reactive species are generally named after the parent alkyl group or by their systematic names. These are obtained by the homolytic fission of alkanes. A decrease in the dissociation energy of the bond increases the stability of the free radical.

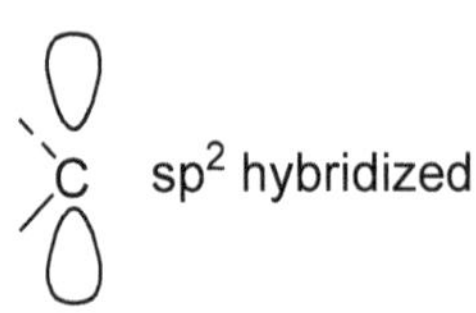

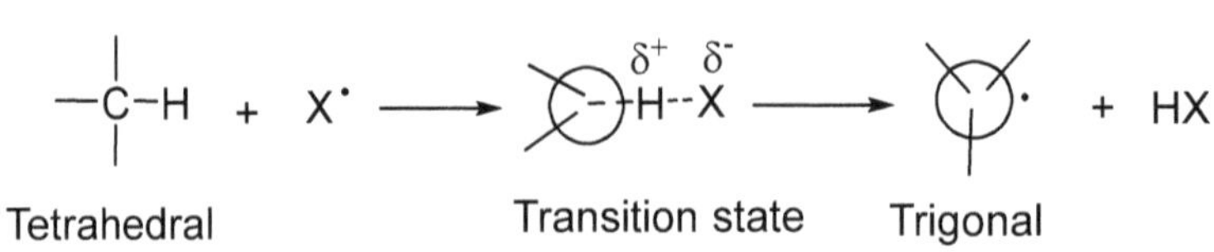

4. Carbene:

Carbenes are neutral carbon species with two bonds and two electrons. These behave as electrophiles in order to complete the octet state and gain the stability. Two states of carbenes known to exist are-

a) **Singlet state:** In this, both the electrons are present in the same orbital and move in anti-parallel and opposite spins.

b) **Triplet state:** In this, the two electrons stay in two different orbitals with parallel spins.

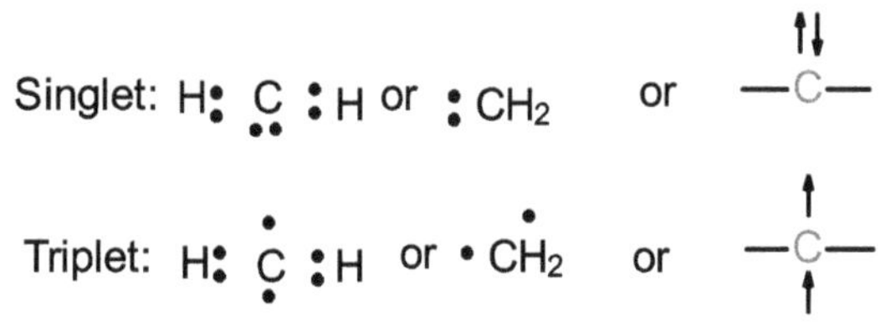

Formation of carbenes:

1) By the pyrolysis or photolysis of aliphatic diazo compounds or ketenes

a) $H_2C=\overset{+}{N}=\overset{-}{N}$ (Diazo methane) ⟶ $:CH_2$ (carbene) + N_2

b) N_2HC-CO_2Et ⟶ $H\ddot{C}-CO_2Et$ (carbethoxy carbene) + N_2

c) $R-\overset{O}{\overset{\|}{C}}-CHN_2$ (Acyl diazomethane) ⟶ $RCO\ddot{C}H$ (Acyl carbene) + N_2

d) $H_2C=C=O$ (Ketene) ⟶ $:CH_2$ (carbene) + CO

e) $R-C=C=O$ ⟶ $\ddot{C}R_2$ (carbene) + CO

2) Reaction of poly halogen compounds with base

a) $$\underset{\text{dichloro methane}}{CH_2Cl_2} + LiR \xrightarrow[-RH]{} [LiCHCl_2] \xrightarrow[-LiCl]{} \underset{\text{chloro carbene}}{:CHCl}$$

b) $$\underset{\textit{tert}\text{-butoxide ion}}{(CH_3)_3C\bar{O}} + CHCl_3 \rightleftharpoons \underset{\textit{tert}\text{-butanol}}{(CH_3)_3COH} + :\bar{C}Cl_3$$

$$:\bar{C}Cl_3 \longrightarrow \underset{\text{dichloro carbene}}{:CCl_2} + \bar{Cl}$$

Reaction of carbenes:

1) Addition to alkenes (Cycloaddition)

Singlet methylene undergoes cyclopropane stereospecific cycloaddition and triplet methylene undergoes non-stereospecific cycloaddition.

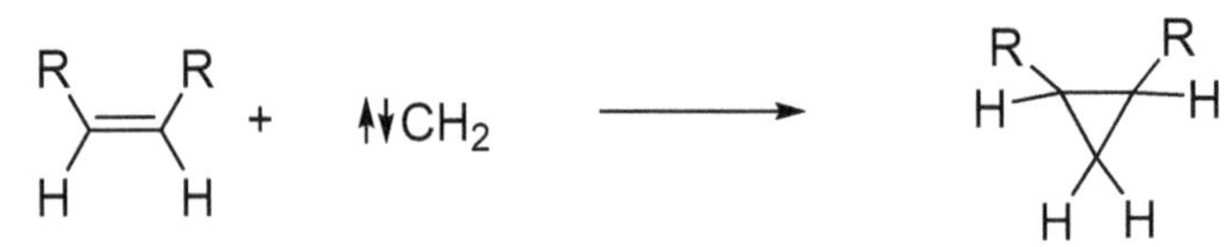

Cis-Olefin Singlet carbene

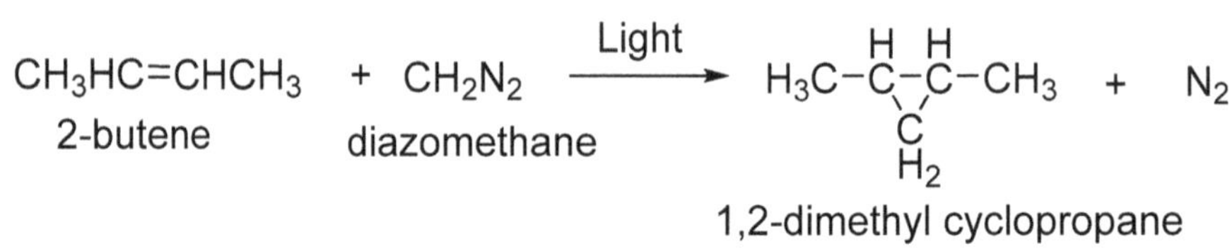

Addition of dihalocarbenes like singlet methylene is also stereospecific reaction.

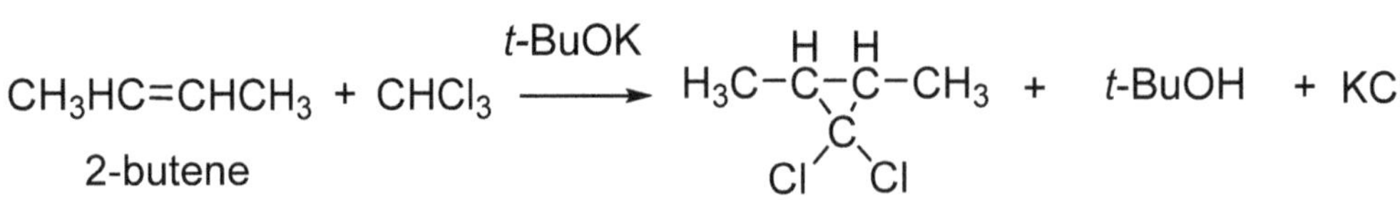

1,1-dichloro-2,3-dimethylcyclopropane

2) Ring expansion reactions

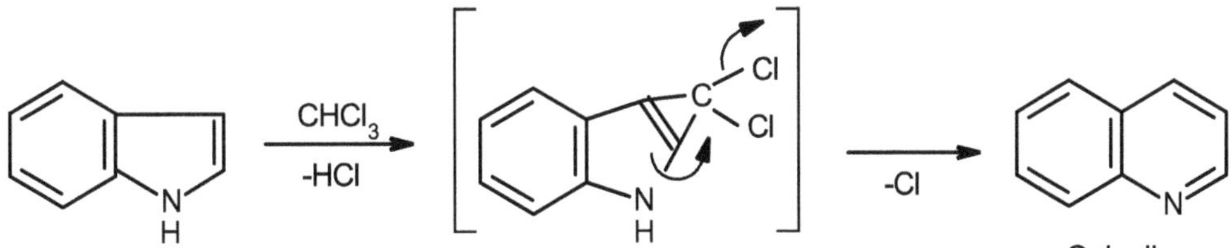

Indole

Quinoline

3) Insertion reactions

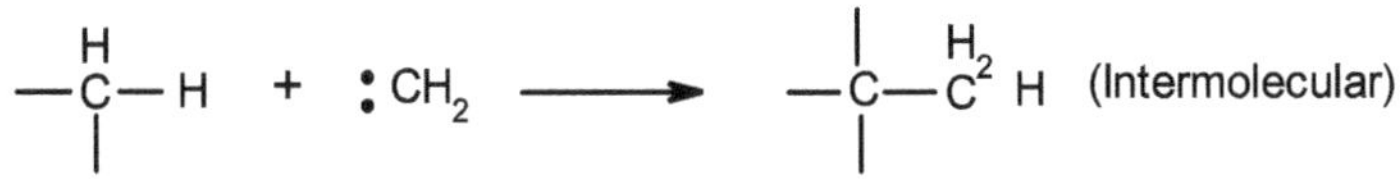

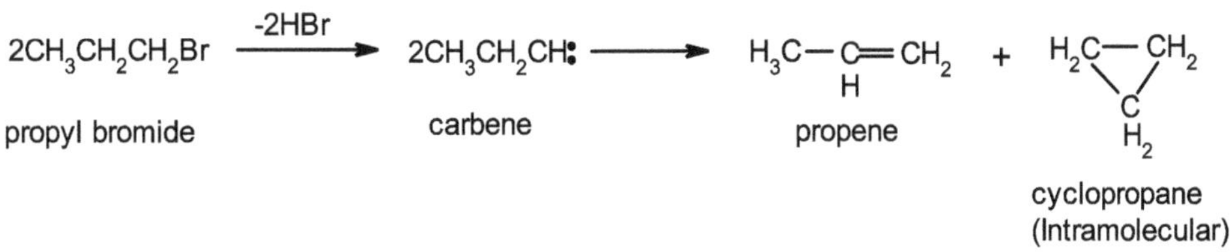

Applications- some examples:

1. Carbylamine reaction

$$PhNH_2 + CHCl_3 + 3KOH \xrightarrow[\Delta]{} Ph-\overset{\oplus}{N}\equiv\overset{\ominus}{C} + 3KCl + 3H_2O$$

2. Reimer-Tiemann reaction

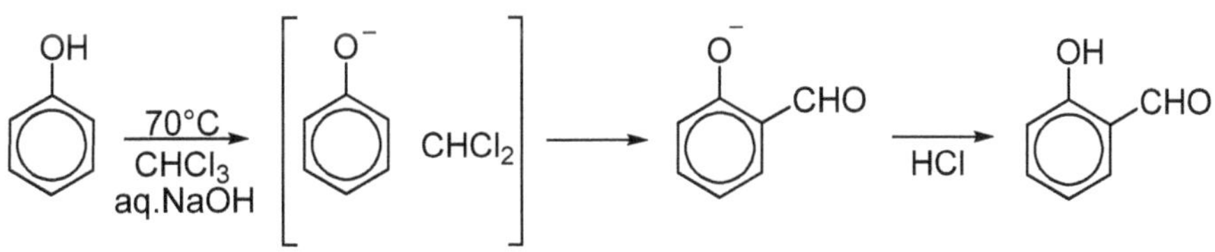

$$OH^- + CHCl_3 \rightleftharpoons H_2O + :\bar{C}Cl_3 \longrightarrow Cl^- + :CCl_2$$

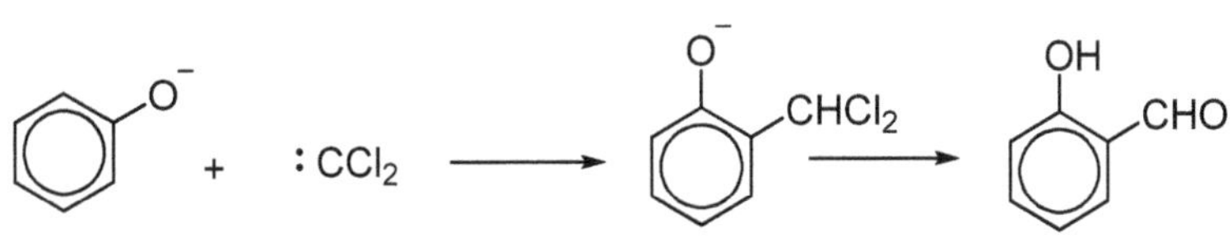

3. Synthesis of alkanes
4. Synthesis of spiro compounds
5. Wittig reaction

5. **Nitrenes:** Nitrenes are nitrogen-containing, electron-deficient species with a sextet of electrons. These are highly reactive and tend to complete octet to get stabilization.

Formation of Nitrenes:

1. Photolysis of N_3H

$$N_3H \xrightarrow{h\nu} N_2 + \ddot{N}H$$

2. Generation of alkylated acyl nitrenes by the photolysis of isocyanates and acyl azides.

$$R-N=C=O \xrightarrow{h\nu} CO + R-\ddot{N}:$$

alkyl nitrene

$$R-\overset{H}{N}-OSO_2Ar \xrightarrow[-BH]{\ddot{B}} R-\bar{N}-OSO_2Ar \longrightarrow R\ddot{N}: + \bar{O}SO_2Ar$$

alkyl nitrene

$$R-\overset{O}{\overset{\|}{C}}-N_3 \xrightarrow{h\nu} N_2 + RCO\ddot{N}:$$

acyl azide, acyl nitrene

Reactions involving nitrenes:

1. Abstraction of hydrogen

This process can be observed in the preparation of pyrrolidines and piperidines.

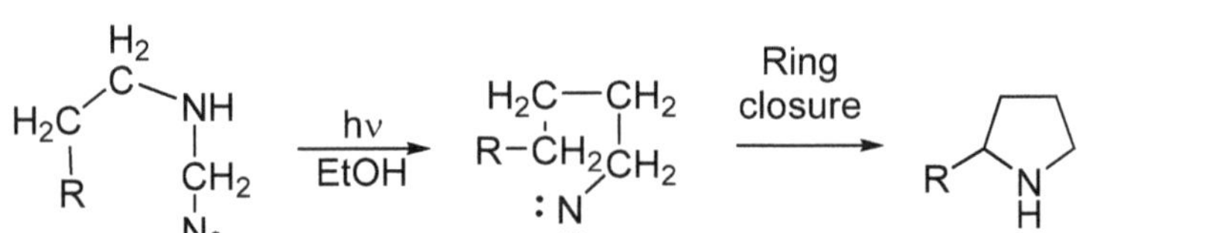

Pyrrolidine derivatives

2. Addition to Olefins: These add to olefins

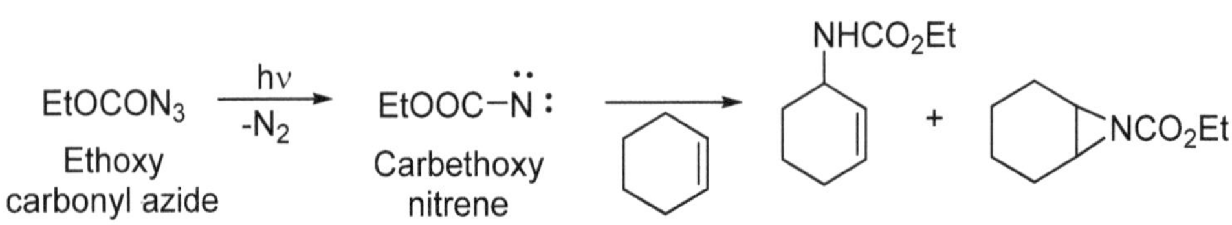

3. Ring enlargement reactions

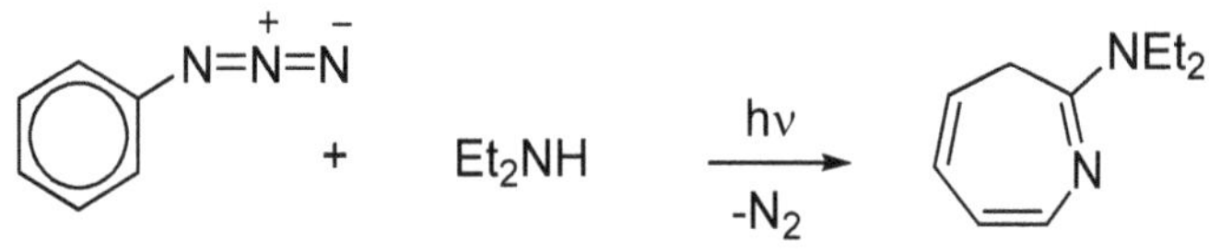

Phenyl azide diethylamine Azepine

4. Combination of two nitrenes

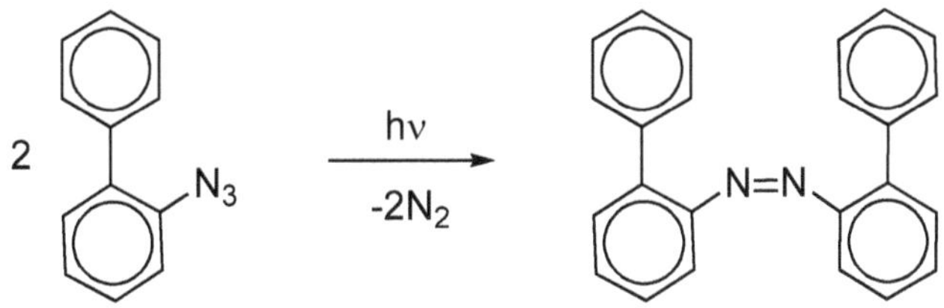

2-azido biphenyl 2,2-azido biphenyl

5. Rearrangement of reactions involving nitrenes

Rearrangements *via* migration to electron deficient nitrogen on treatment with base gets converted to amines *via* nitrene intermediate.

a) Hoffmann rearrangement: Primary amides on treatment with hypohalites result in primary amines with one less carbon via isocyanates involving a nitrene intermediate.

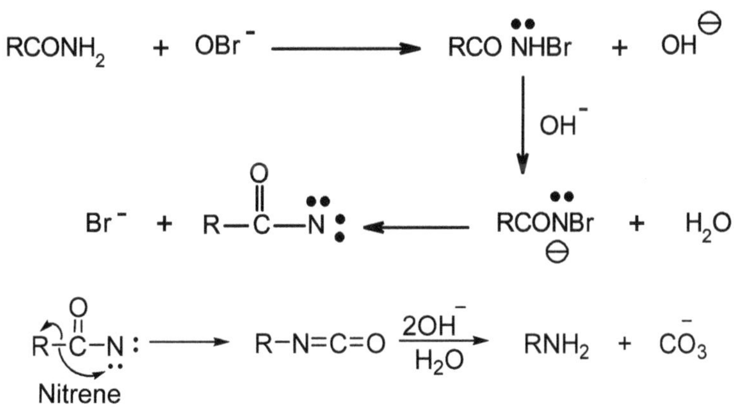

R-migration is like SN^2 and involves a 1,2-shift as an intramolecular rearrangement. It proceeds with complete retention of configuration at the chiral center of the migrating group. Here, the loss of Br and the migration of R in N-bromamide anion are concerted. Mostly, Br_2 is used in the reaction for *N*-bromamide formation. It is also known as Hoffmann bromamide reaction.

Examples:

a)

$$RCONH_2 + Br_2 + 4NaOH \longrightarrow RNH_2 + 2NaBr + Na_2CO_3 + 2H_2O$$

(R= aliphatic, aromatic, heterocyclic)

b)

$$\underset{\text{Caproamide}}{CH_3(CH_2)_4CONH_2} \xrightarrow[\text{KOBr}]{} \underset{n\text{-pentylamine}}{H_3C(H_2C)_4{-}NH_2}$$

c)

$$\underset{\text{Urea}}{H_2NCONH_2} \xrightarrow[\text{Br}_2\text{ / KOH}]{} \underset{\text{Hydrazine}}{NH_2NH_2}$$

d)

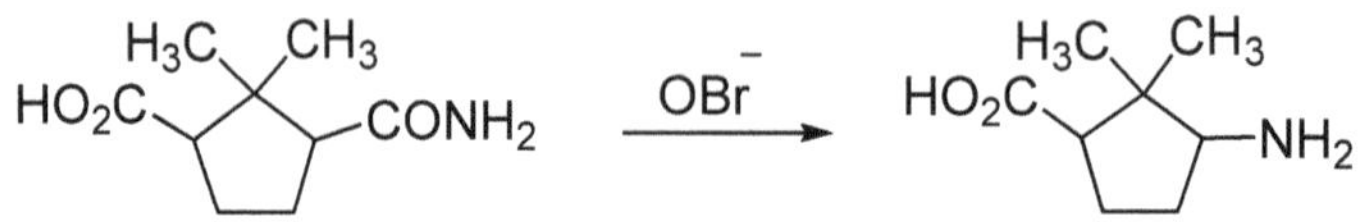

e)

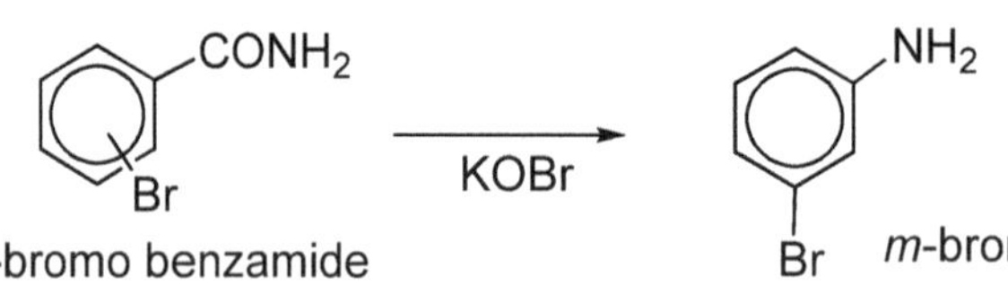

m-bromo benzamide *m*-bromoaniline

f)

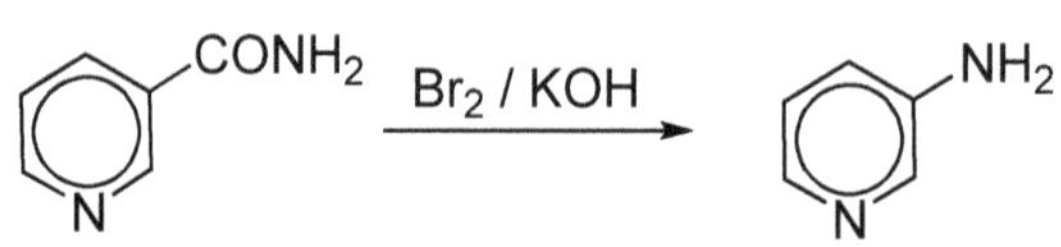

Nicotinamide β-aminopyridine

g)

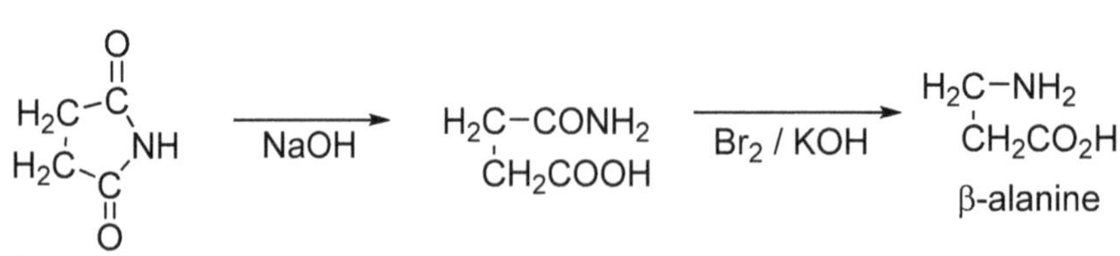

Succinimide

h)

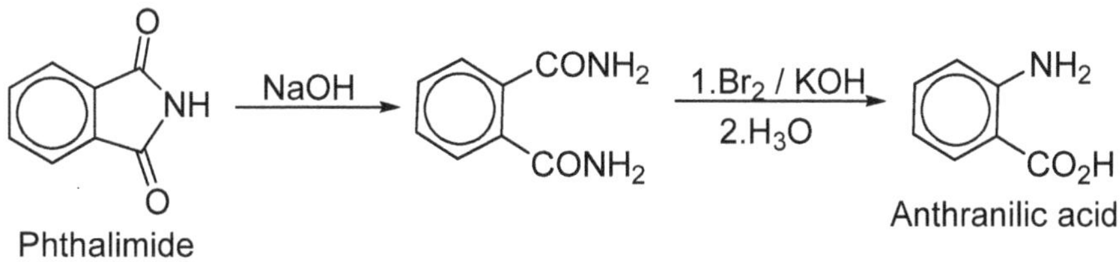

i)

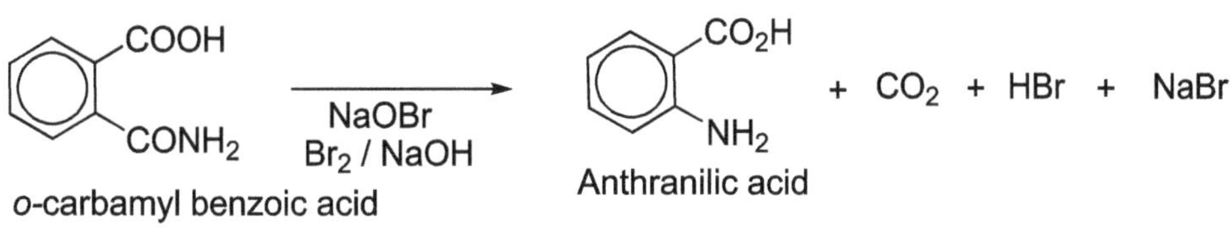

b) Curtius reaction or Curtius rearrangement

The decomposition of acylazides in inert solvent to isocyanate is called Curtius rearrangement. If the reaction is conducted in an aqueous medium or alcohol, isocyanate forms an amine or urethane, or if an amine is present, it forms substituted urea. The reaction involves the formation of electron-deficient nitrogen species with the loss of N_2. All the steps are concerted.

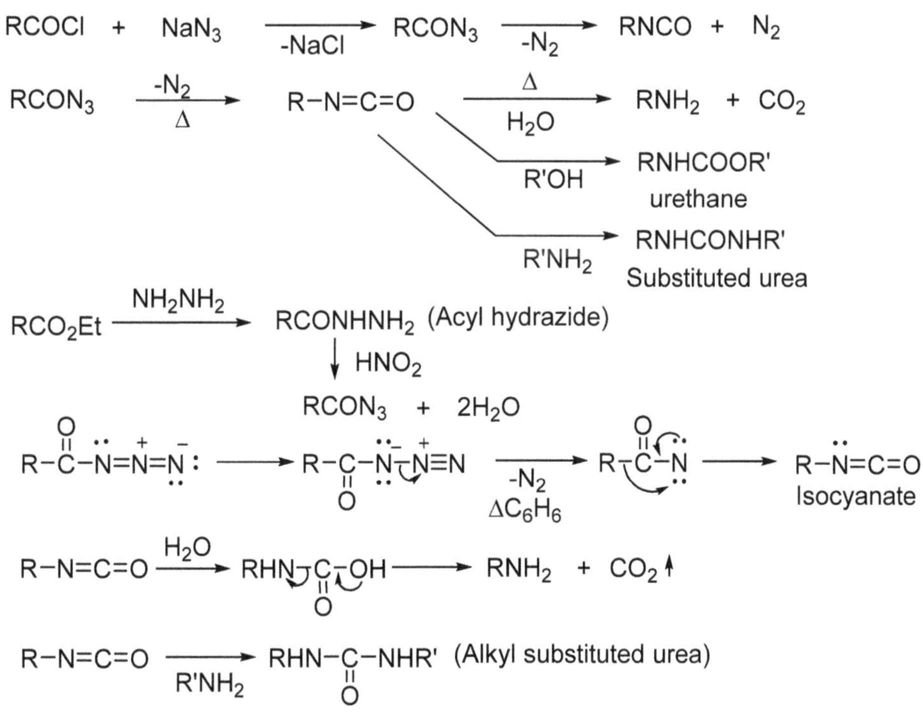

Examples and applications:

(i) Preparation of primary amines

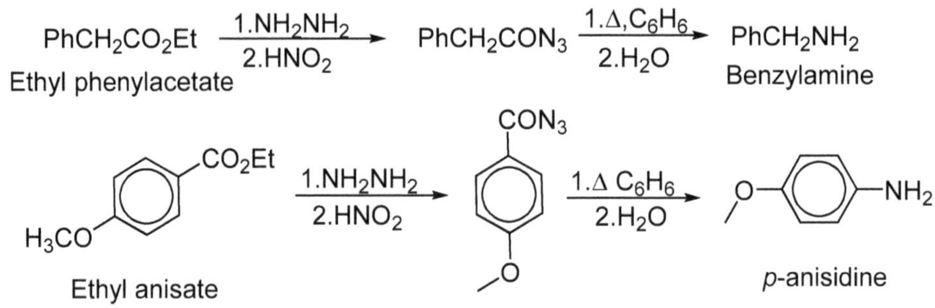

(ii) Preparation of aldehydes

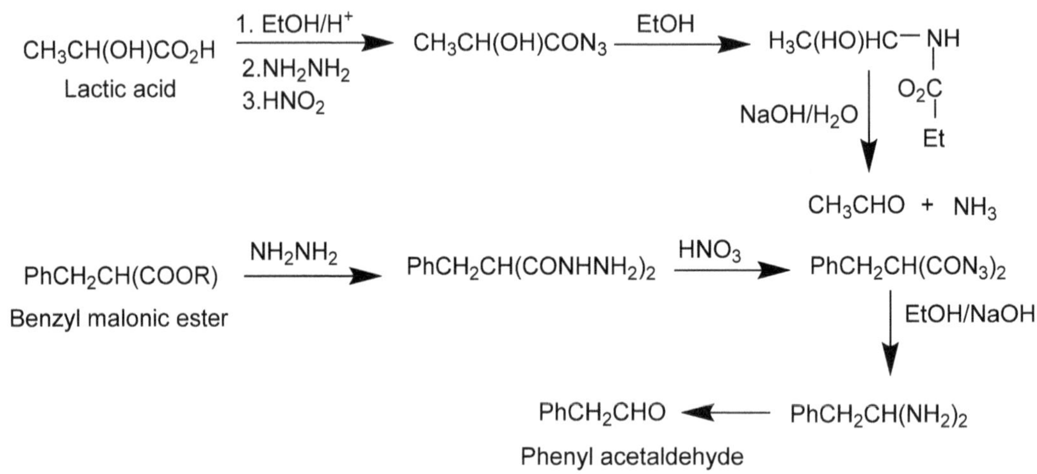

(iii) Preparation of α-amino acids

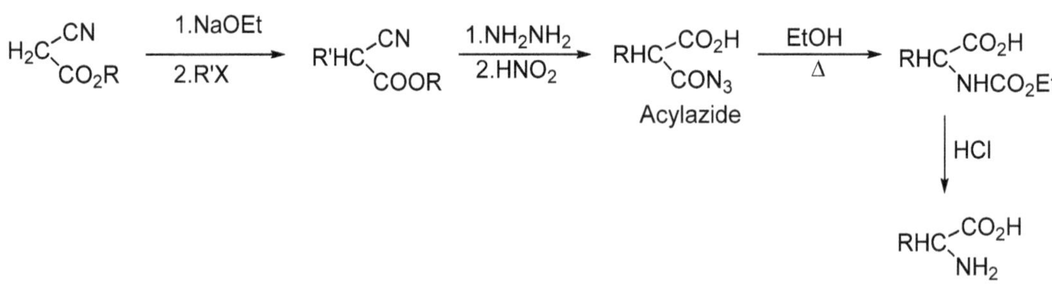

c) Lossen reaction

It is an intramolecular rearrangement, where o-acyl derivatives of free hydroxamine acids yield electron deficient nitrogen species which finally get converted to amines. O-Acyl, sulfonyl, or phosphonyl derivatives can be used in this reaction as substrates. The isocyanate obtained can be further converted to urea in the presence of amines or produce amines in the presence of water. It is named after Wilhelm Lossen.

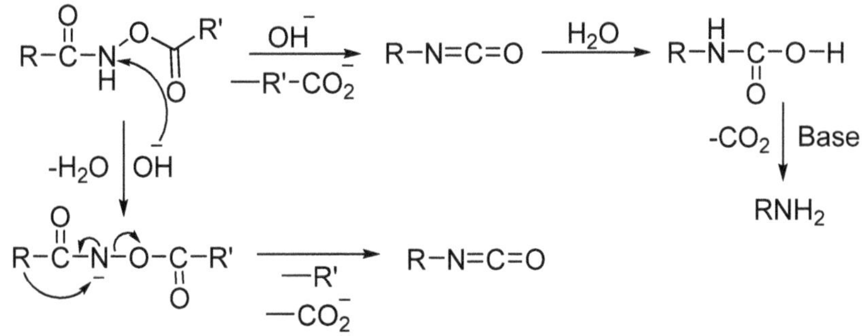

O-Acylated hydroxamic acid derivative on treatment with base produces isocyanate, which when treated with water loses CO2 to generate an amine. The reaction is initiated by the abstraction of a proton by a base. Spontaneous cycle of events releases carboxylate anion, forming an isocyanate intermediate. The rate of Lossen rearrangement is directly proportional to the acidity of the leaving groups or their conjugate acids.

i)

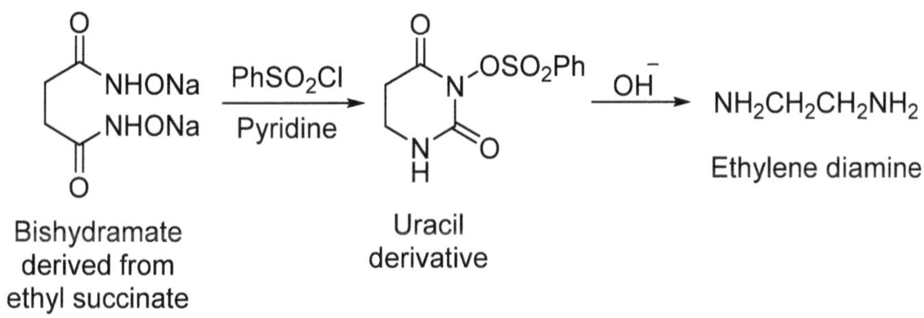

ii)

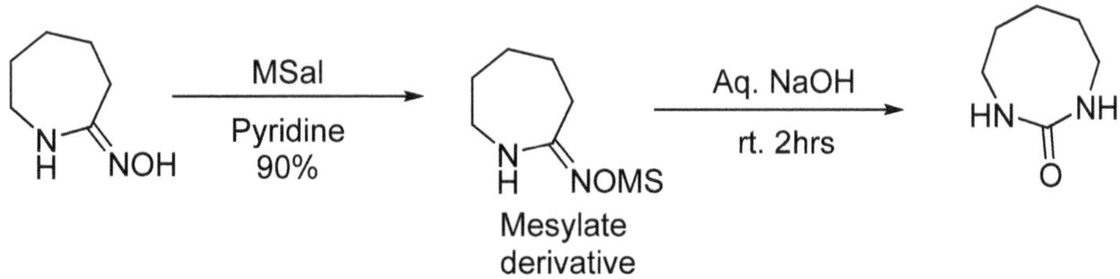

iii) 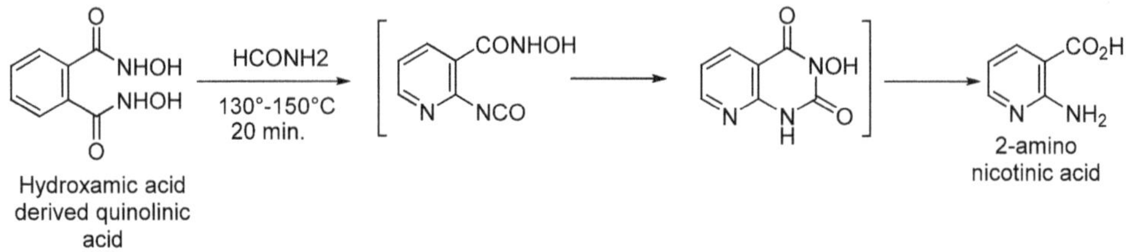

iv) $$CH_3(CH_2)_4CO_2H \xrightarrow[\substack{170°\text{-}80°C \\ 2\text{-}5\ min.}]{\substack{NH_2OSO_3H \\ \text{(Hydroxylamine } o\text{-} \\ \text{sulfonic acid)} \\ \text{mineral oil}}} H_3C{-}(CH_2)_4{-}NH_2$$

v) 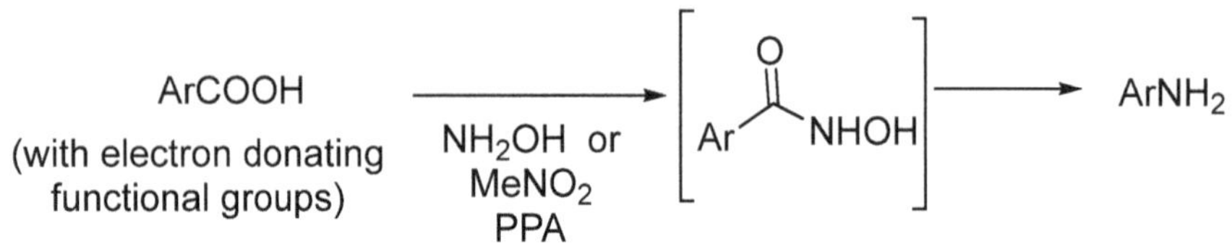

Types of reactions

Types of chemical reactions

1. Addition reaction
2. Elimination reaction
3. Substitution reaction
4. Rearrangement reaction

1. Addition reaction

An addition reaction can be defined as the reaction in which two molecules combine to form a single molecule as the product. Compounds that contain atoms sharing more than one pair of electrons or multiple bonded atoms can act as substrates in these reactions. In these types of reactions multiple bonds are converted to single bonds. The phenomenon is opposite to elimination reactions where multiple bonds are created. In addition, reactions a reagent is added to the substrate. The multiple bonds act as a source of electrons as well as base in these reactions. The electron-deficient or acidic reagents act as reagents. Therefore, these are called electrophilic reagents and the reaction is called electrophilic addition. When a free radical is involved in the reaction the reaction is called the free radical addition.

Let us examine some important addition reactions.

1. Addition of hydrogen or catalytic hydrogenation

Two kinds of hydrogenations are known.

a) Homogeneous hydrogenation

The reaction takes place in a single phase or solution phase. In this separation of catalyst is difficult. Hydrogenation is qualitative and reveals the number of unsaturation's present in the substrate molecule. Generally, organic complexes of rhodium, iridium, or other transition metals which are soluble in organic solvents act as reagents.

b) Heterogeneous hydrogenation

It is classical and widely used method wherein the reaction is conducted in two phases. Finely divided metals like palladium, nickel, or platinum are used as reagents. Reaction occurs rapidly and easily. The product is filtered and separated easily from the catalyst.

Hydrogenation is an exothermic reaction and the quantity of heat evolved when a mole of compound is hydrogenated is known as heat of hydrogenation. Hence, the function of the catalyst is to lower the activation energy (Eact). The catalyst speeds up the reaction but does not shift the position of equilibrium. Hydrogenation gives information about the relative stability of the unsaturated compounds. The greater the number of alkyl groups attached to the alkene carbon atom the more stable is the alkene.

Stability of alkenes

$$R_2C{=}CR_2 > R_2C{=}CHR > R_2C{=}CH_2,\ RCH{=}CHR > RCH{=}CH_2 > CH_2{=}CH_2$$

Stereochemistry of homogeneous hydrogenation

The alkenes exist as geometric isomers like cis and trans isomers. For example, in butane dioic acid, cis acid is maleic acid and trans acid is fumaric acid Therefore, stereochemically different substrates react differently, producing stereochemically different products. Thus, the reaction is not only stereoselective but also stereospecific. If the added groups are attached to the same face, it is "syn-addition," and if the groups are added on opposite faces, it is called "anti-addition". Deuterium addition experiments across the double bond clearly revealed the mechanism.

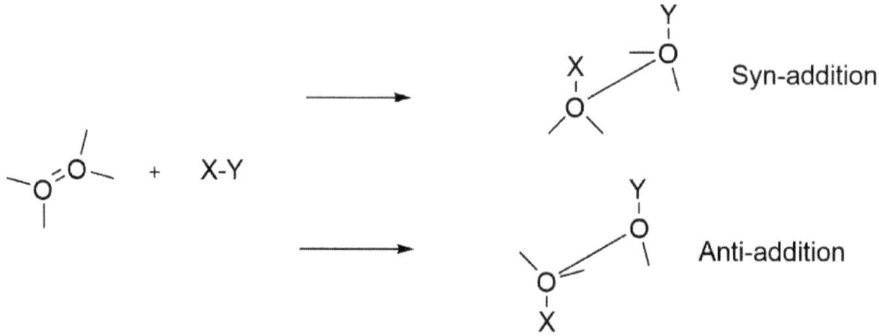

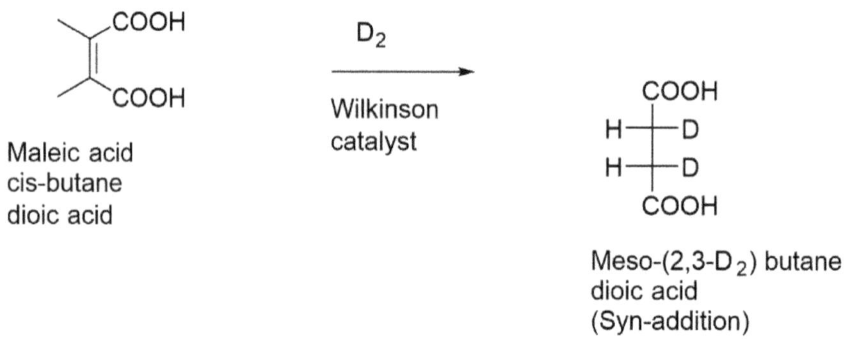

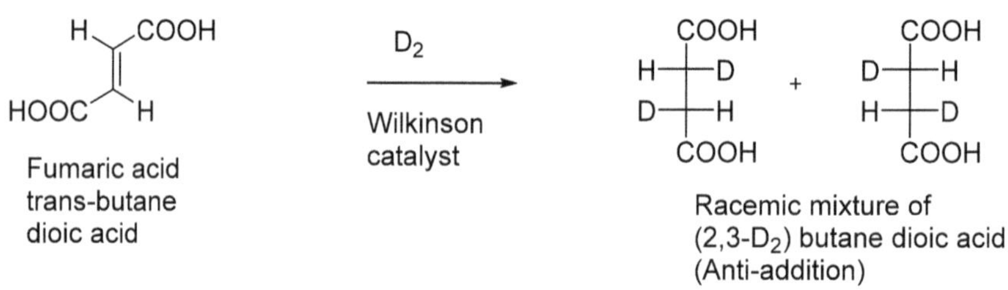

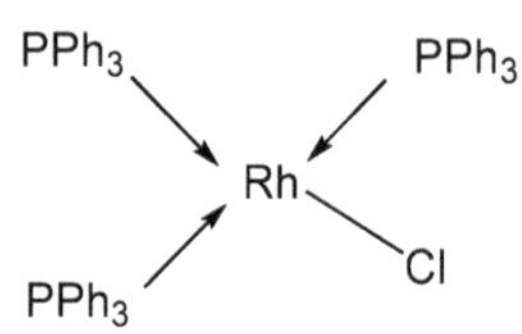

Tris (triphenyl phosphine) chloro rhodium (I)

Wilkinson catalyst

Steps of hydrogenation by Wilkinson's catalyst.

a) xchange of one PPh_3 for solvent molecule

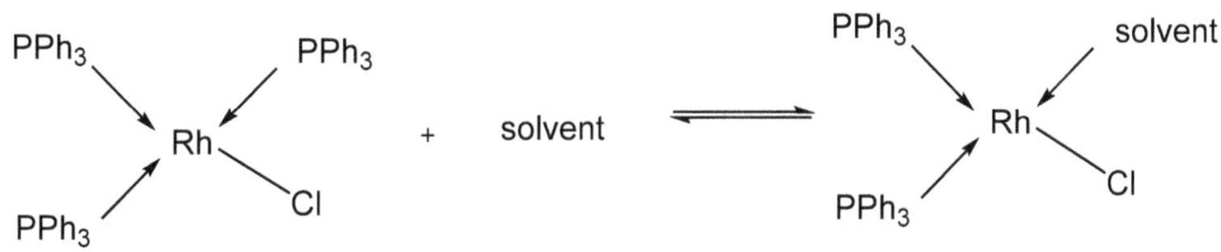

b) Reaction with H_2 molecule

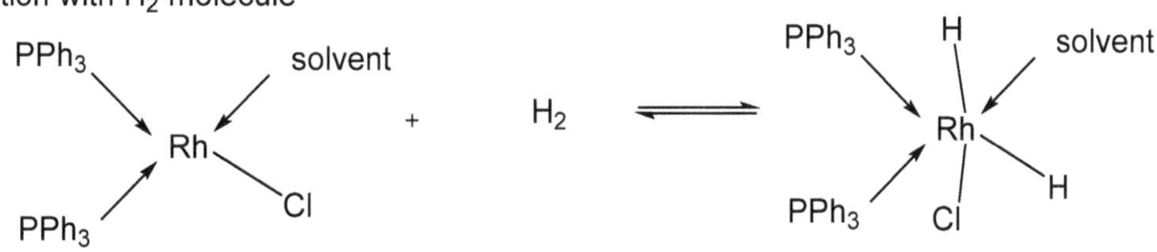

c) Reaction with alkene

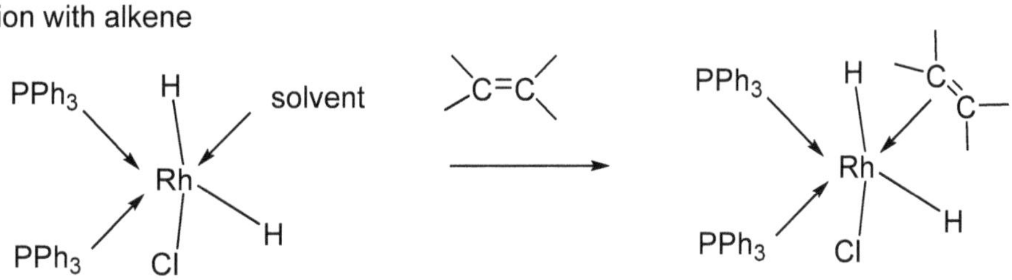

d) Migration of hydrogen from the metal to double-bond

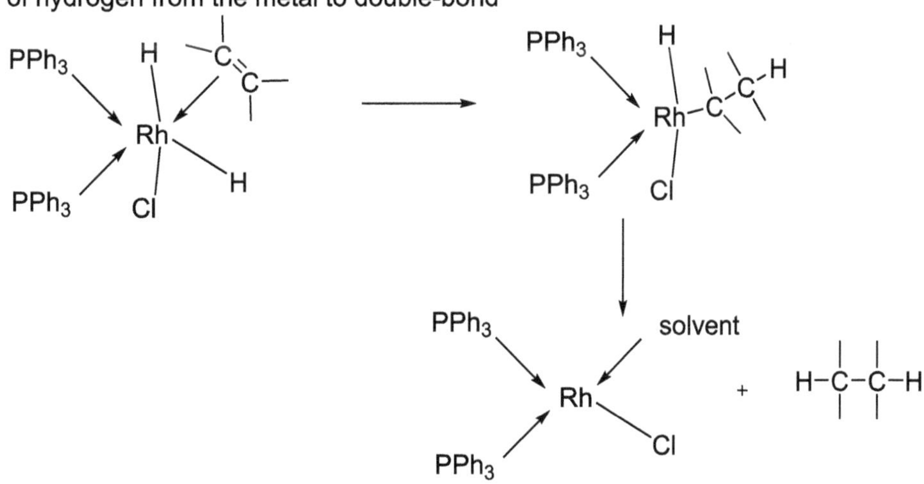

2. Addition of halogen

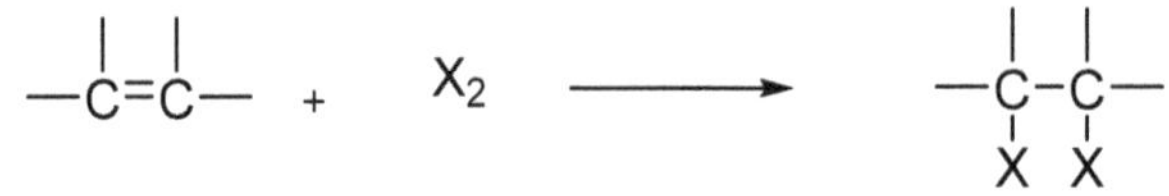

X_2= Cl_2 or Br_2

Ex a) $CH_3CH{=}CH_2 \xrightarrow{Br_2/\ CCl_4} CH_3CHBrCH_2Br$

1,2-dibromopropane
(propylene bromide)

b)

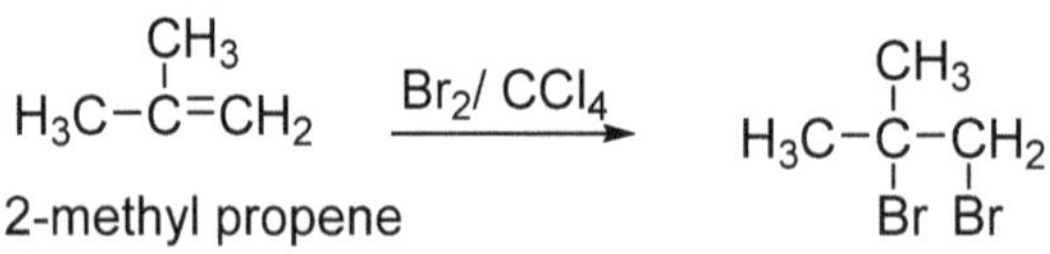

2-methyl propene
(isobutylene)

1,2-dibromo-2-methyl propane

The electrophilic addition of a halogen molecule goes by two steps.

a) Formation of halonium ion

b) Addition of second ion of halogen.

a)

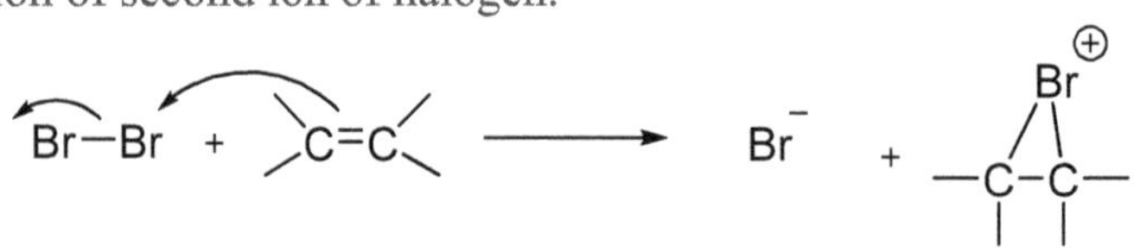

bromonium ion

b)

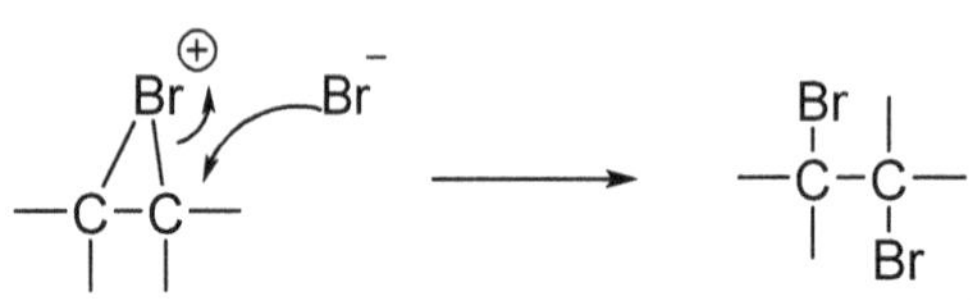

The bromonium ion formation initially is supported by the fact that when ethylene is brominated in the presence of other nucleophiles, the other nucleophile is also added onto the alkene as the other group. The bromonium or halonium ion bridge prevents free rotation of the C-C bond.

Example:

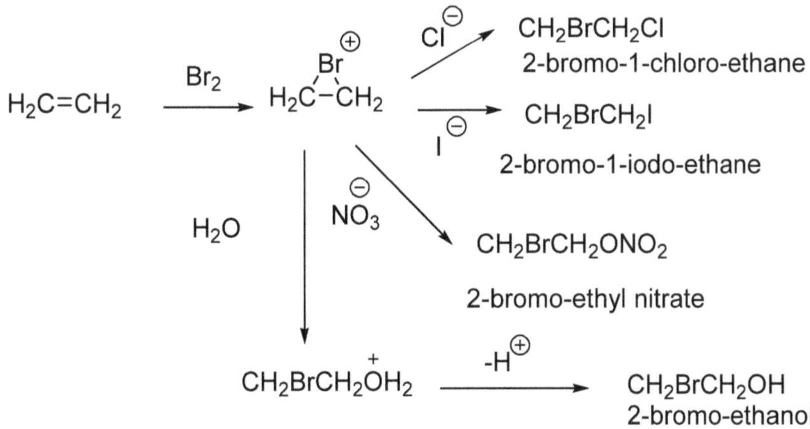

The reaction is completely stereo specific and stereo selective. Cis 2-butene on bromination yields racemic mixture of 2,3- dibromo butane whereas with trans 2- butene meso-product is obtained. The chlorination or bromination of alkene goes by anti-addition.

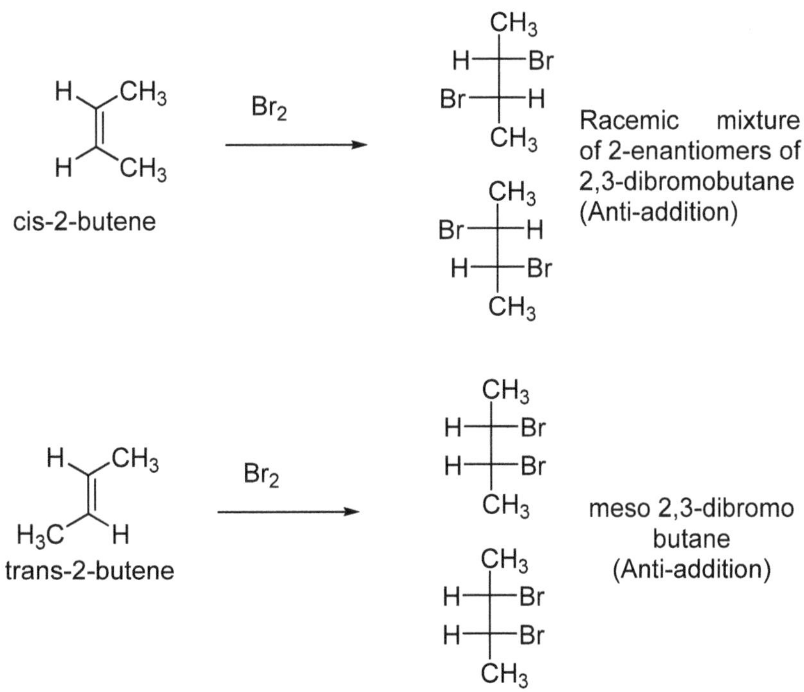

3. Addition of hydrogen halides

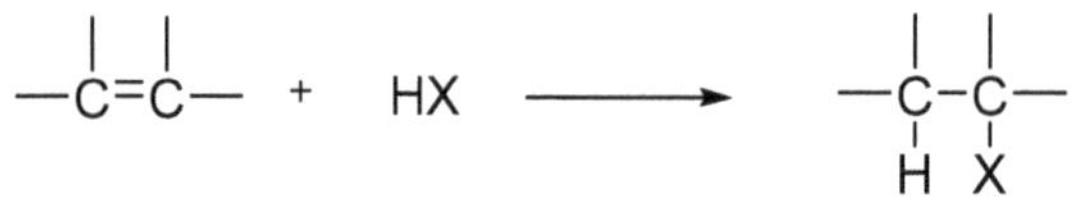

HX: HCl, HBr, HI

EX:

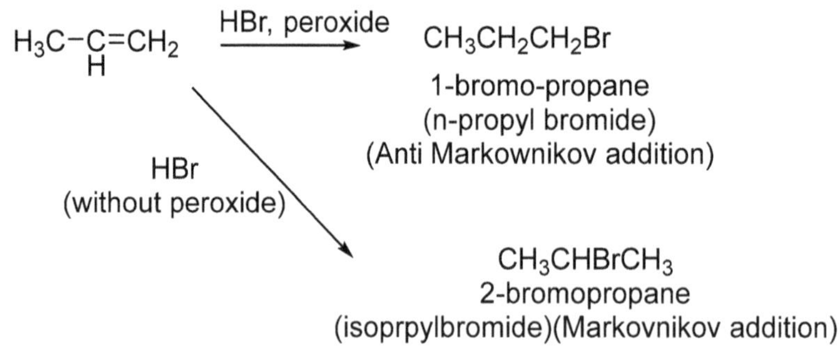

Vladimir Markovnikov observed that in the addition of an acid to the C=C double bond, the hydrogen of an acid attaches to the carbon that holds a more number of hydrogens. This is known as Markovnikov's rule.

a) $CH_3CH_2CH=CH_2 + HI \longrightarrow CH_3CH_2CHICH_3$

1-Butane → sec butyl iodide, 2-iodo butane

b)

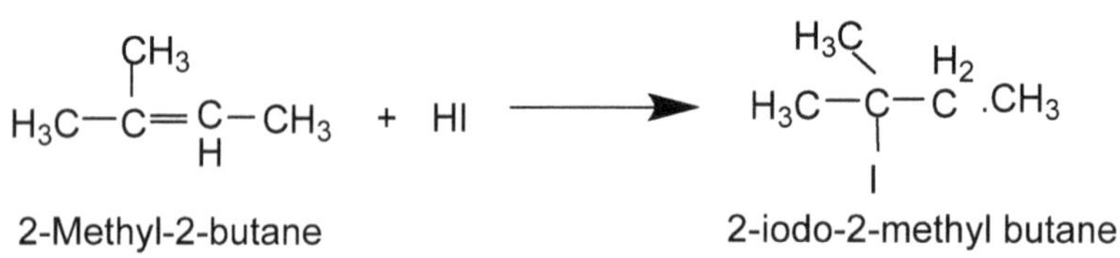

c) $CH_3CH_2CH=CHCH_3 + HI \longrightarrow CH_3CH_2CHICH_2CH_3 + CH_3CH_2CH_2CHICH_3$

2-pentene → 3-iodopentane + 2-iodo pentane

d)

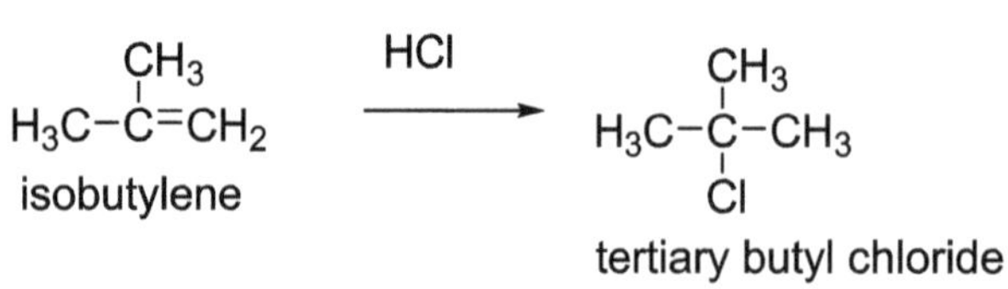

e)

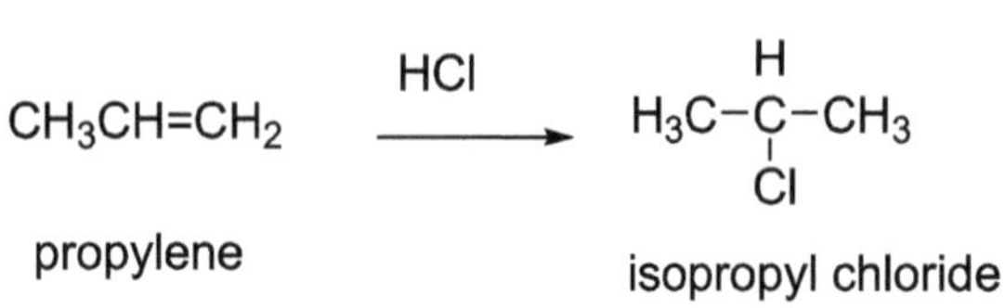

M.S. Kharash and F.R. Mayo discovered that the orientation of the addition of HBr to C=C is determined solely by the presence or absence of peroxides. Organic peroxides containing -O-O- linkage such as in tertiary butyl peroxide or benzoyl peroxide bring about the peroxide effect, generating anti-Markovnikov addition products. However, the addition of inhibitors like hydroquinone or bisphenol amine influence Markovnikov addition.

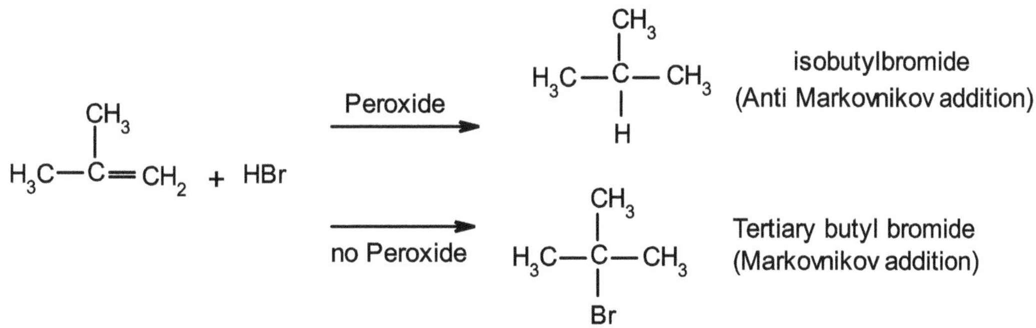

In all these reactions secondary carbonium ion is formed faster than primary and tertiary faster than secondary carbonium ion. This follows the rate of formation of carbonium ions as tertiary> secondary> primary>methyl carbonium ion. Same as that of stability of carbonium ions. Therefore, Markovnikov's rule can be interpreted as electrophilic addition to C=C involving the intermediate formation of a more stable carbocation. Therefore, the rate of addition of hydrogen ion to the double bond depends on the stability of the carbonium ion formed.

Order of reactivity of alkenes towards acids.

$$(C(CH_3)_2{=}CH_2 > CH_3CH{=}CHCH_3,\ CH_3CH_2CH{=}CH_2 > CH_3CH{=}CH_2 > CH_2{=}CH_2 > CH_2{=}CHCl$$

4. Addition of water-Hydration

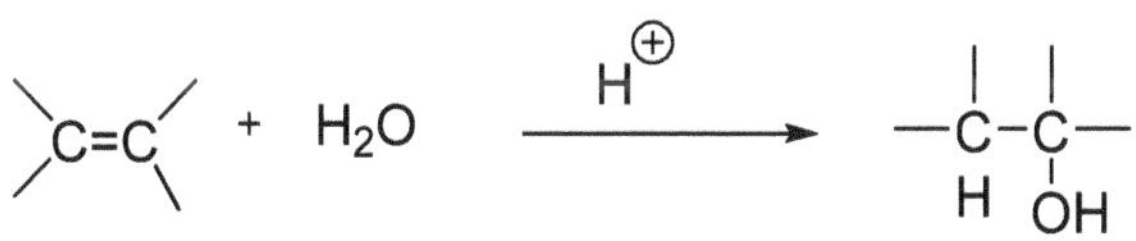

Ex a)

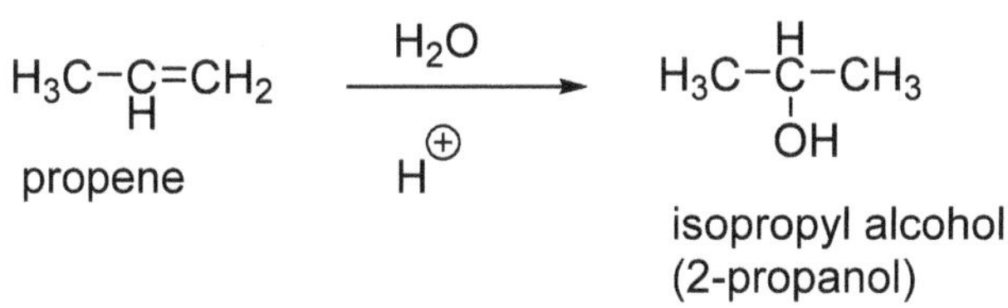

b)

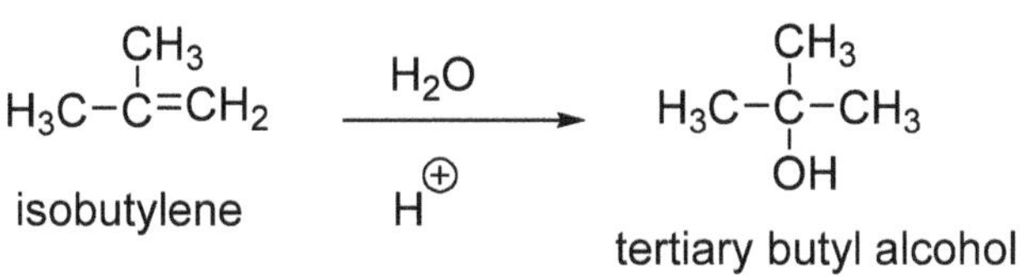

The reaction is a two-step process and consistent with Markovnikov's rule. When the hydration of alkenes via alkyl hydrogen sulphates-

a)

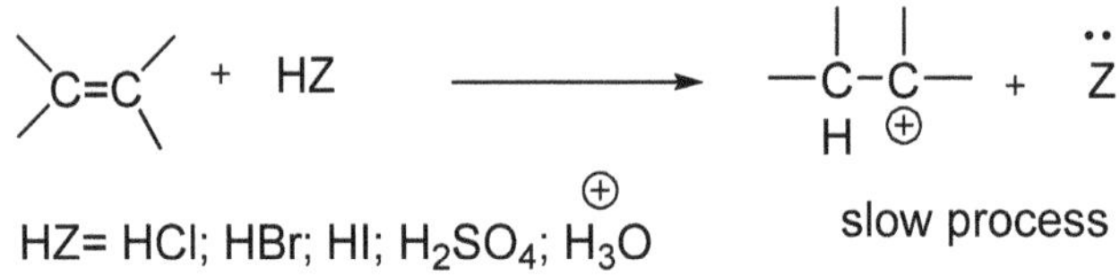

b)

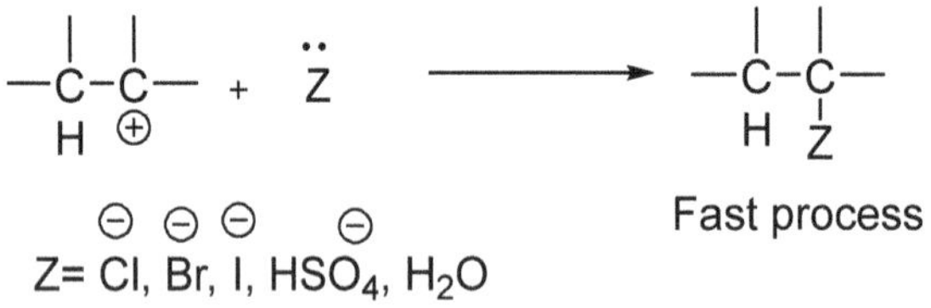

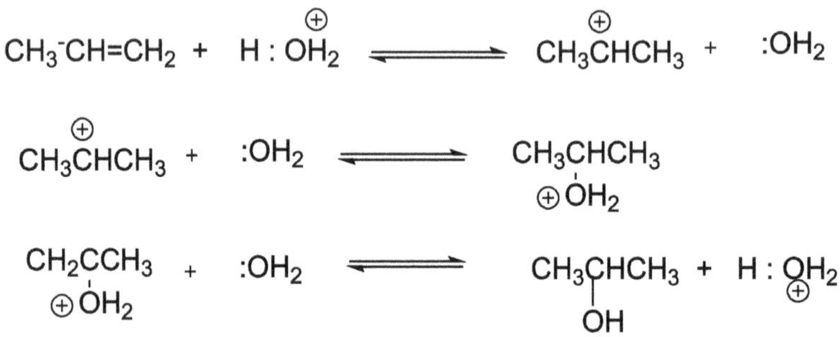

Hydrogen is transferred as a proton or electrophilic or acidic reagent.

In these reactions depending on the alkene structures, some rearrangements follow to yield more stable cations.

Examples:

a)

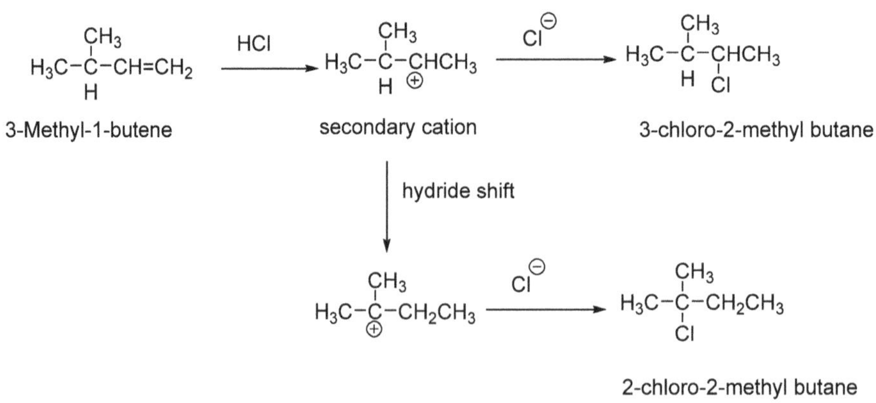

b)

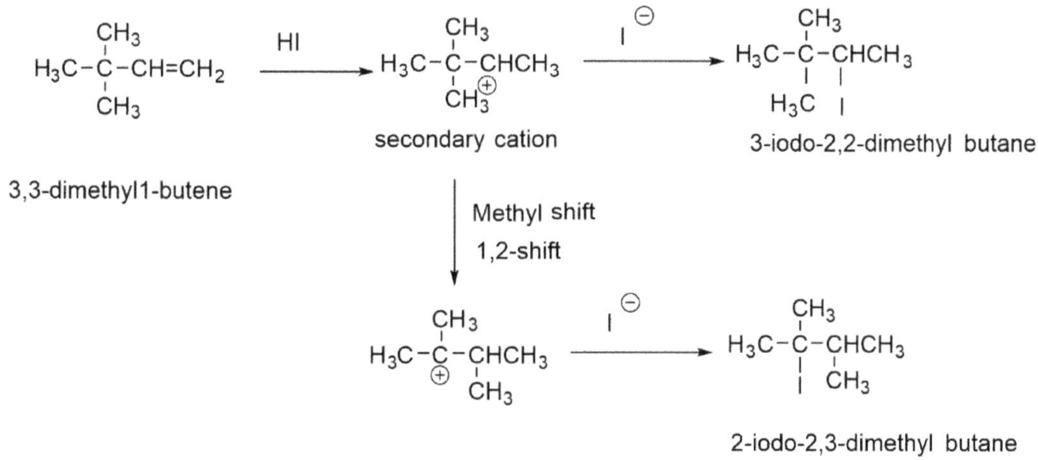

5. Addition of halogen and -OH groups-halohydrin formation

Addition of chlorine or bromine in the presence of water forms halohydrins i.e. chlorohydrins or bromohydrins.

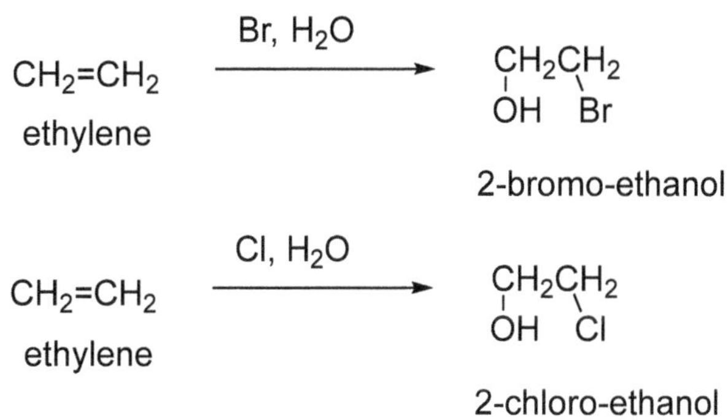

The reaction also goes by the formation of halonium ion

6. Addition of sulfuric acid

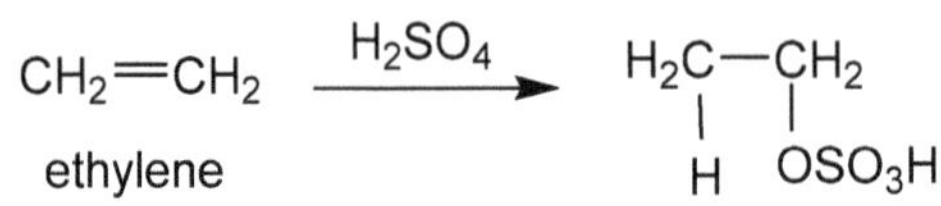

Ex : a)

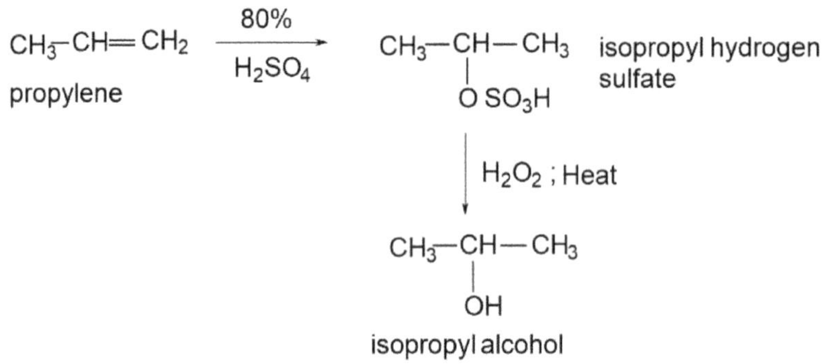

b)

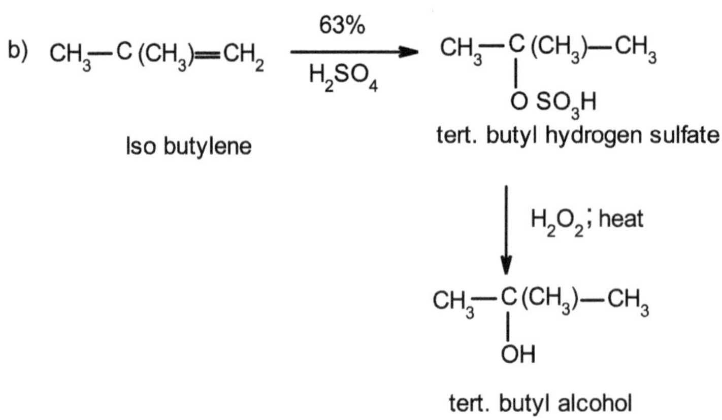

7. Alkylation

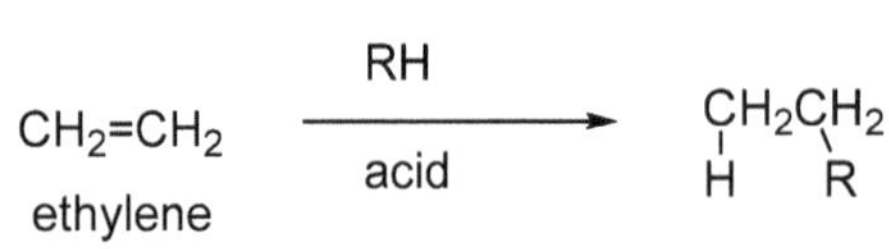

Ex:

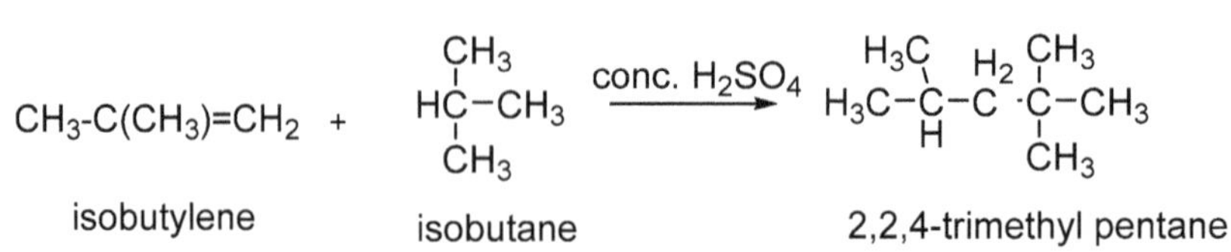

8. Dimerization

Two molecules of an alkene undergo acid catalyzed dimerization to provide a dimer of the same alkene.

Example:

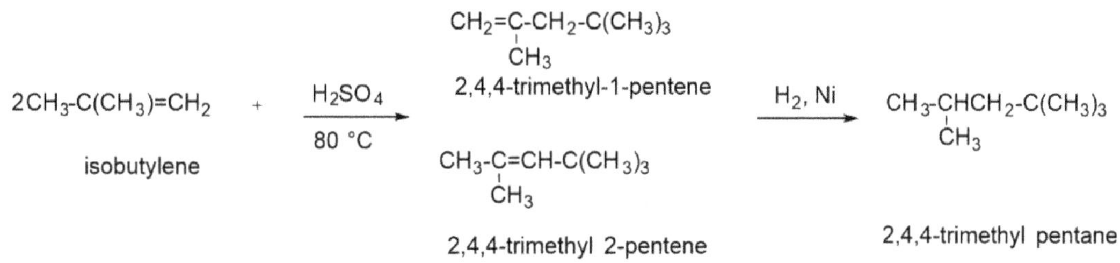

9. Hydroboration-Oxidation

Alkenes undergo hydroboration with diborane reagent $(BH_3)2$ generating alkyl boranes R_3B. These on oxidation yield alcohols. This is a simple two step high yielding reaction. The reaction was invented by Professor Herbert. C. Brown in late 1950s., for which he was awarded Nobel Prize in Chemistry in 1979.

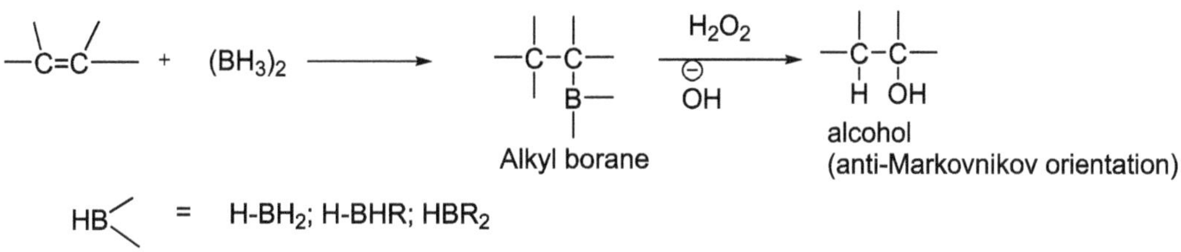

The reaction is commonly conducted in ether, tetrahydrofuran or diethylene glycol methyl ether (diglyme). Diborane is the dimer of BH3 (Borane) and is generally available in THF solution. The reagent is present in monomer form in THF as a complex.

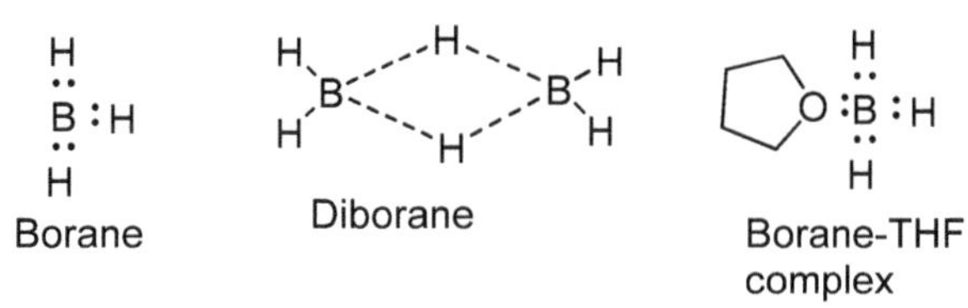

The borane group of BH3 will go on adding until all hydrogens are transferred. Generally, the reaction is initiated by the hydrogen addition to olefinic carbon followed by alkyl borane formation. The alkyl borane undergoes oxidation to give alcohol by an anti-Markovnikov orientation. The products are obtained by the anti-Markovnikov addition of water to the C=C double bond. Hydroboration does not involve any rearrangement as there is no involvement of carbonium ion.

Examples:

a)

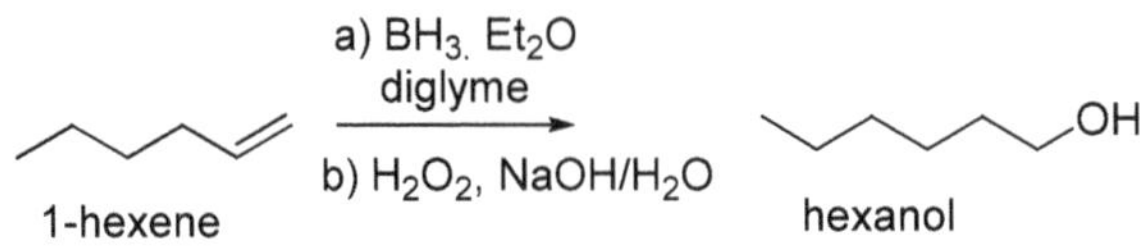

b)

$$CH_3CH{=}CH_2 \xrightarrow[\text{b) } H_2O_2,\ OH^{\ominus}]{\text{a) } (BH_3)_2} CH_3CH_2CH_2OH$$

propylene → n-propyl alcohol

c)

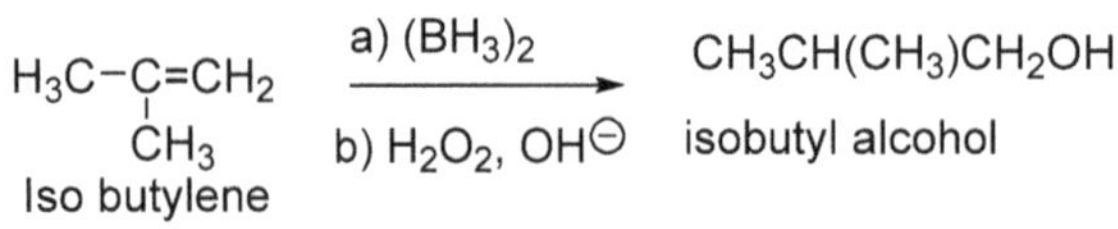

d)

$$CH_3CH_2CH{=}CH_2 \xrightarrow[\text{b) } H_2O_2,\ OH^{\ominus}]{\text{a) } (BH_3)_2} CH_3CH_2CH_2CH_2OH$$

1-butene → n-butyl alcohol

e)

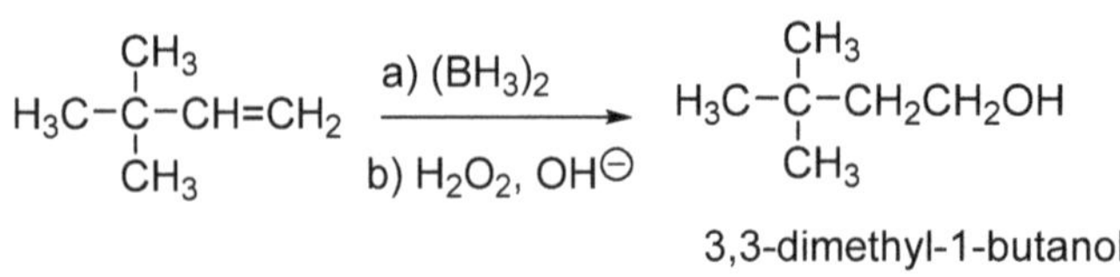

f)

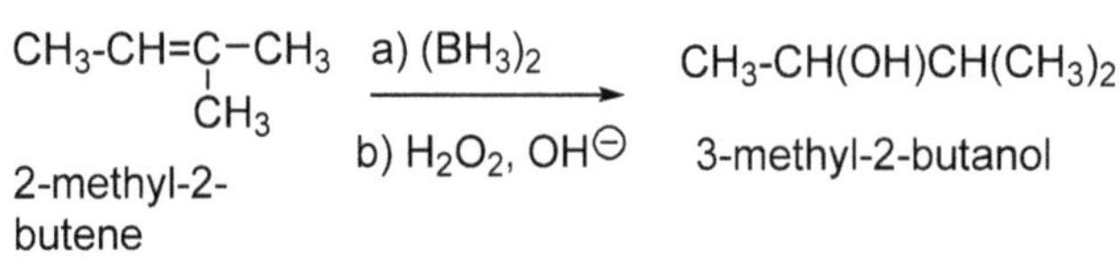

g)

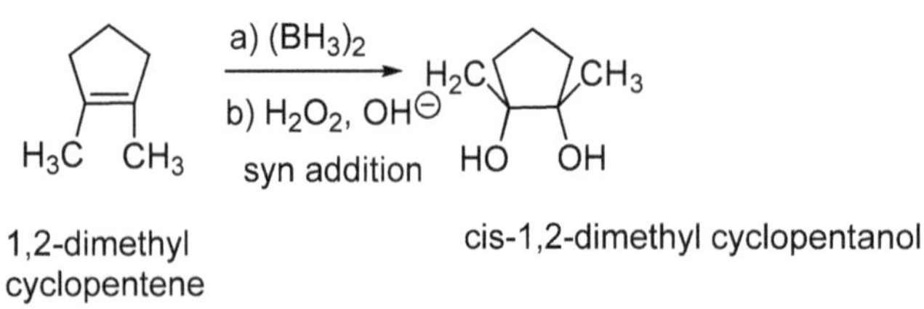

Hydroboration-Oxidation, the two-step process is a widely used reaction of importance since the Products are not obtained by other methods from alkenes. It is the most convenient approach with great synthetic utility. Many modified hydroboration agents are reported like 9-BBN Borabicyclo (3.3.1.) nonane), catecholborane or disiamylborane.

Hydroboration - Oxidation mechanism

Oxidation mechanism involves the nucleophilic hydroperoxide anion attack on Boran followed by alkyl migration to oxygen producing alkyl borane with retention of stereo chemistry.

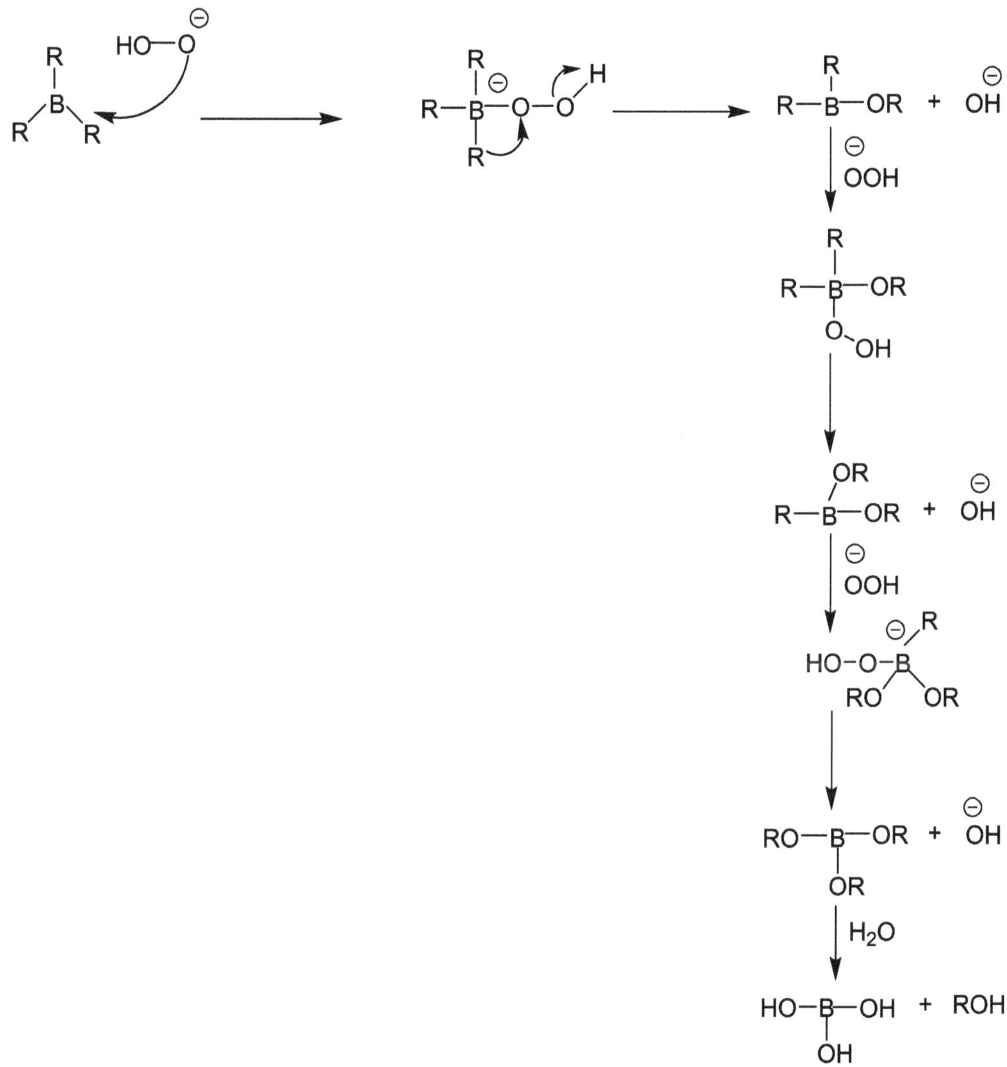

Other oxidizing agents like N- methyl morpholine N-oxide in the presence of tetra propyl ammonium perruthenate converts alkyl borane into carbonyl compound. Terminal alkenes with dichromates are reacted with chromium agents (VI) that produce carboxylic acids.

Example:

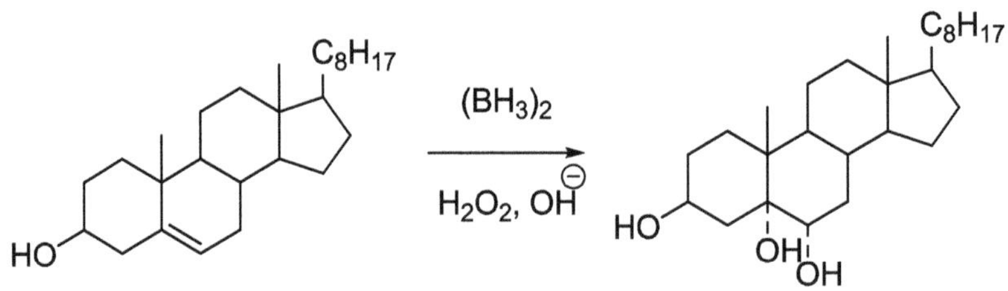

Cholesterol　　　　Cholestane-3-β,6α–diol

10. Hydroxylation

Preparation of glycols:

There are many oxidizing agents like potassium permanganate or peroxy acids like peroxy formic acid to convert alkenes into 1,2-diols.

Examples:

a)

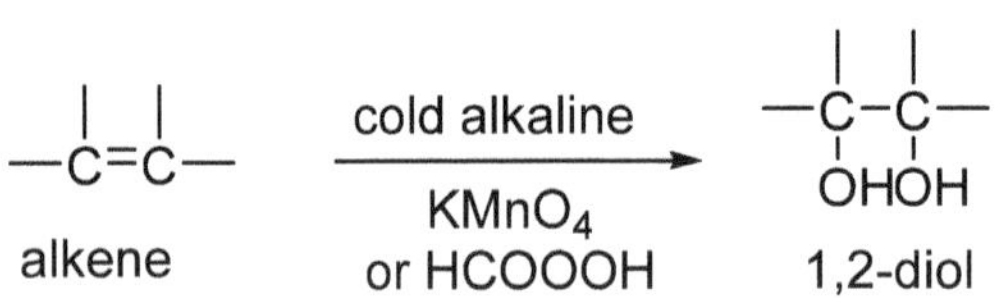

b)

$$3\ CH_2{=}CH_2 + 2KMnO_4 + 4H_2O \longrightarrow 3\ H_2C(OH){-}CH_2(OH) + 2MnO_2 + 2KOH$$

ethylene　　　　1,2-ethane diol

$$CH_3\text{-}CH{=}CH_2 \xrightarrow[H_2O]{HCOOOH} CH_3CH(OH)CH_2(OH)$$

11. Addition of carbenes

Carbene or methylene addition to C=C generating a ring is called cycloaddition. Methylene is produced by the photolysis of diazomethane (CH2N2) or ketene (CH2=C=O).

$$\overset{}{CH_2{=}\overset{+}{N}{=}\overset{-}{N}} \xrightarrow{\text{UV light}} CH_2 + N_2$$

diazomethane　　　　methylene

$$CH_2{=}C{=}O \xrightarrow{\text{UV light}} CH_2 + CO$$

ketene　　　　methylene

Methylene is a highly reactive entity and it exists in two different forms. Singlet methylene is less stable. Triplet methylene with unshared electrons not paired exist as a diradical. Singlet methylene undergoes stereo specific electrophilic addition and triplet methylene undergoes non stereo specific free radical addition. Singlet methylene is electron deficient and acts as an electrophile whereas triplet methylene being a di radical adds by a two-step free radical mechanism.

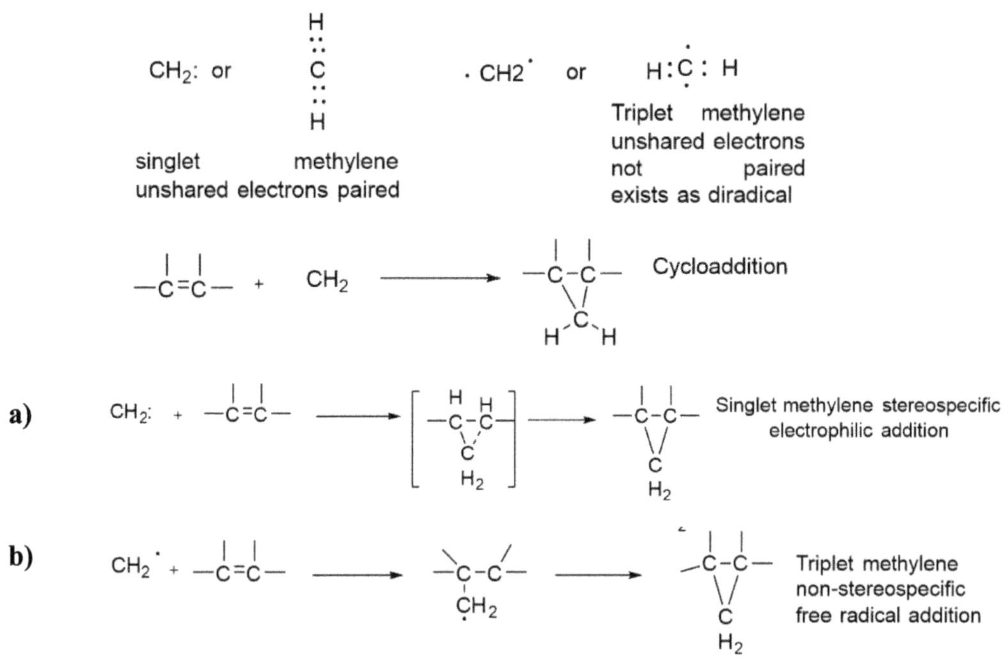

ex:

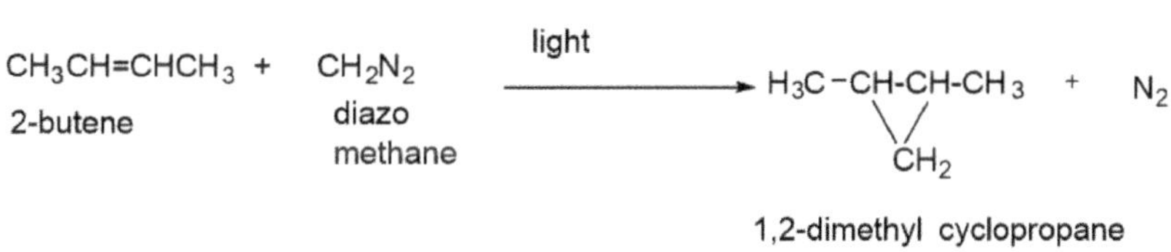

12. Addition of free radicals

To account for anti -Markovnikov addition across C=C in the presence of peroxides, Kharash and Mayo interpreted and proposed free radical mechanism for the addition reaction. The peroxides initiate the reaction by generating the radicals. Therefore, the addition does not involve carbonium ions and the reagents hydrogen and bromine in the reaction add on to the C=C homolytically and goes by the chain mechanism.

Mechanism:

a) peroxides $\longrightarrow$ radical

b) Radical$\cdot$ + H: Br $\longrightarrow$ Radical:H + Br$^\bullet$

c)

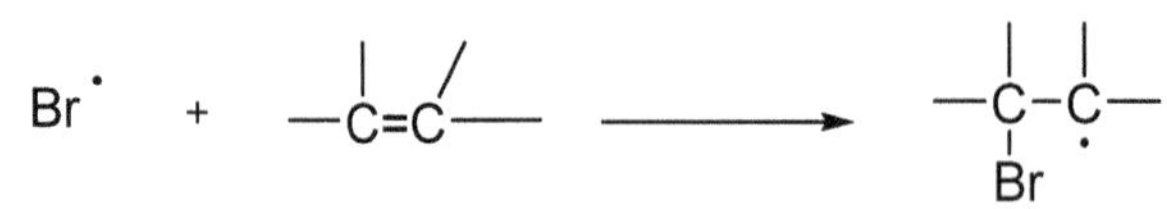

d)

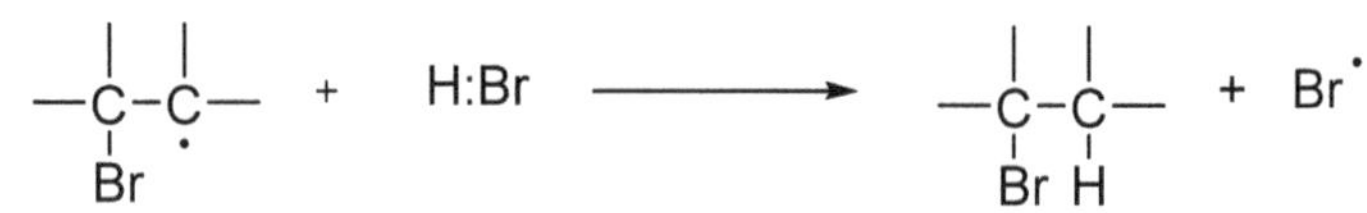

Steps a and b consist of chain initiation and c and d belong to chain propagation.

Example:

$$CH_3CH{=}CH_2 \xrightarrow{Br^\bullet} CH_3\text{-}\dot{C}H\text{-}CH_2Br \xrightarrow{HBr} CH_3CH_2CH_2Br$$

3-propylene n-propyl bromide

As secondary free radical is formed faster than primary free radical and n-propyl bromide is formed as against the electrophilic addition product of isopropyl bromide. The stability of the free radical formed, polar factors and steric factors influence the outcome of free radical addition.

Ability to accommodate partial positive charge as well as odd electron in the transition state, less hindered addition of free radical in the transaction state accounts for the stability of the transition state. As the hydrogen adds first in the electrophilic addition and bromine adds first in the free radical addition orientation of addition is reversed.

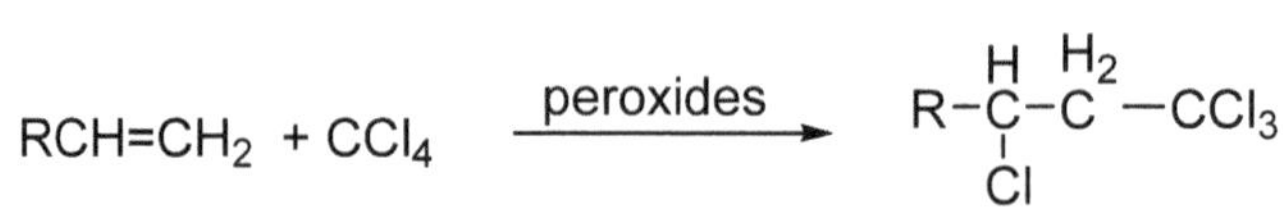

2. Elimination reactions

The elimination reaction can be defined as a reaction where in different atoms either in pairs or in groups are removed from a molecule by a one step or two step mechanism. Thus, it is a reversal of addition reaction.

a)

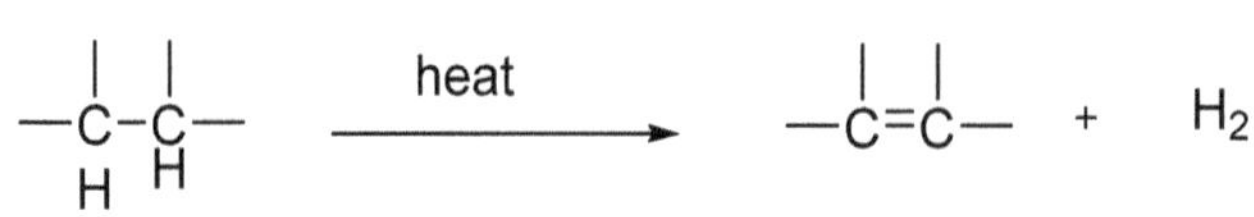

b)

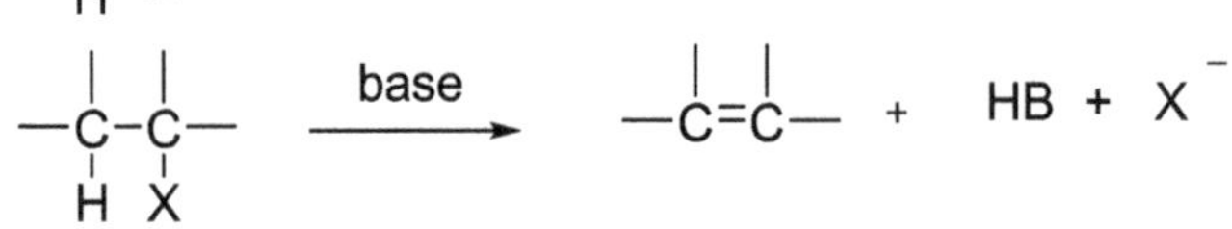

When a proton is abstracted at C and at the same time C -X is removed simultaneously in a concerted way such elimination is known as E2 elimination.

In E1 -elimination reaction which is a two-step process C-X bond is cleaved first forming a carbonium ion intermediate followed by the proton abstraction at C resulting in the formation of C=C bond.

E2 Elimination by concerted process

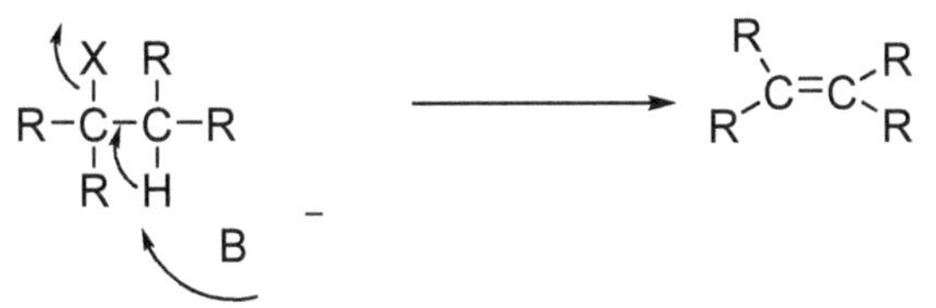

E1-Elimination by a 2 step process

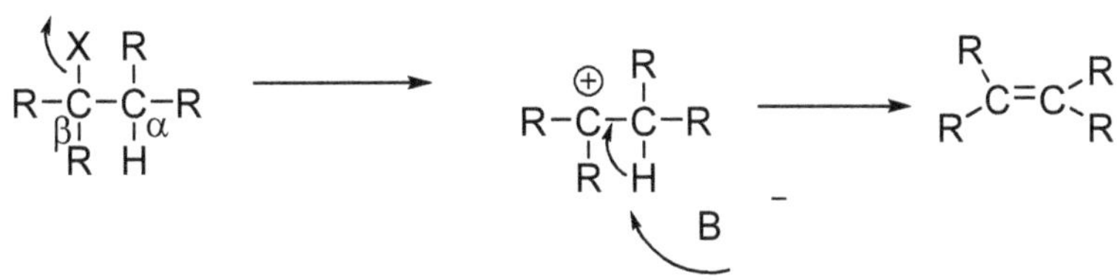

According to Hughes and Ingold, the elimination reactions like nucleophilic substitutions proceed by two different mechanisms. E1 and E2 mechanisms.

The E1 is a unimolecular elimination reaction and follows first order kinetics. It is unimolecular as the rate determining step involves only one molecule of substrate. Out of two steps, in E1, carbonium ion formation is slow and rate determining. It depends on the concentration of the substrate. Therefore, the rate of E1 reaction is independent of base concentration.

The E2 is a bimolecular elimination reaction and proceeds by second order kinetics. The rate determining step involves reaction of alkyl halide and base. Therefore, the rate of elimination reaction is proportional to the concentration of both substrate and the base.

Rate = K [RX] -E1-First order kinetics

Rate = K [RX] [B] -E2-Second order kinetics

Examples:

a)

$$H_3C-\underset{\underset{Br}{|}}{CH}-CH_3 + KOH \xrightarrow[\text{heat}]{\text{EtOH}} CH_3\,CH{=}CH_2 + KBr + H_2O$$

Isopropyl bromide $\qquad\qquad$ Propylene

b) $CH_3CH_2CH_2CH_2Br \xrightarrow{\text{KOH alc}} CH_3CH_2CH{=}CH_2$

n-butyl bromide → 1-butene

c) $CH_3CH_2CHBrCH_3 \xrightarrow{\text{KOH alc.}} CH_3CH{=}CHCH_3 + CH_3CH_2CH{=}CH_2$

sec butyl bromide → 2-butene (major) + 1-butene (minor)

d)

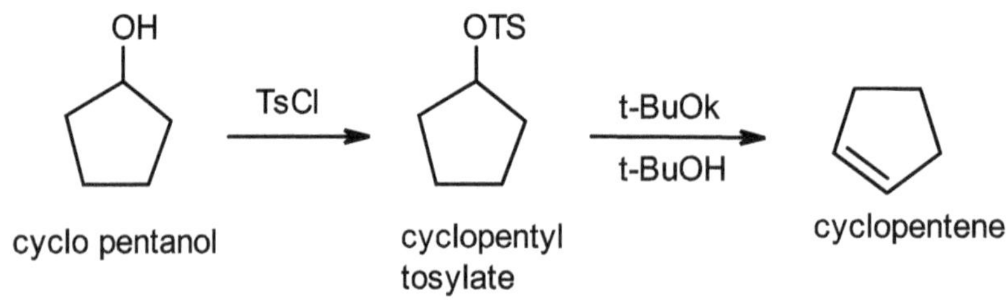

e) $CH_3CH_2OH \xrightarrow{\text{acid}} CH_2{=}CH_2 + H_2O$

Dehydrohalogenation is a typical 1,2- elimination and is brought about by strong basic anions like hydroxide or alkoxide from alcohol (EtO,t.BuO). In these reactions the leaving group is a weekly basic halide ion or tosylates, brosylates, mesylates or triflates.

Evidences for the E2 mechanism

a) Second order kinetics

b) Absence of any rearrangement

c) Exhibition of large hydrogen isotope effects i.e. during isotope experiments bond to hydrogen atom is broken more rapidly than the bond to deuterium.

d) These reactions are not followed by any hydrogen atom exchange.

e) Exhibit element effect

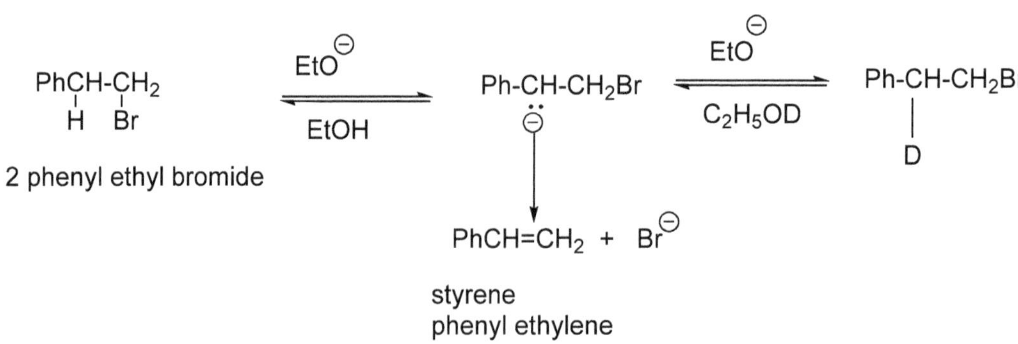

Heterolytic bond dissociation energy in these reactions follows the sequence

$$R\text{-}F > R\text{-}Cl > R\text{-}Br > R\text{-}I$$

Alkyl bromides react 25 -50 times rapidly than alkyl chlorides. These element effects are greater than isotope effects. Rate of breaking a carbon -halogen bond effect the rate of elimination reaction. The rate of reactivity of alkyl halides follows the sequence-

$$R\text{-}I > R\text{-}Br > R\text{-}Cl > R\text{-}F$$

Overall, alkyl iodides undergo elimination reaction 25000 times faster than alkyl fluorides. The stability of alkenes controls the ease of formation of alkenes. Russian scientist Alexander Saytzeff, in 1875 proposed that "in dehydrohalogenation, the preferred product is the alkene that has the greater number of alkyl groups attached to the double bonded carbon atoms." This is well known as Saytzeff's rule. Therefore, the orientation is determined by the more stable alkene, the faster it is formed. It also decides a more stable isomer. The transition state in the E2- reaction contains partly broken bonds to hydrogen and the leaving groups rendering alkene character to it.

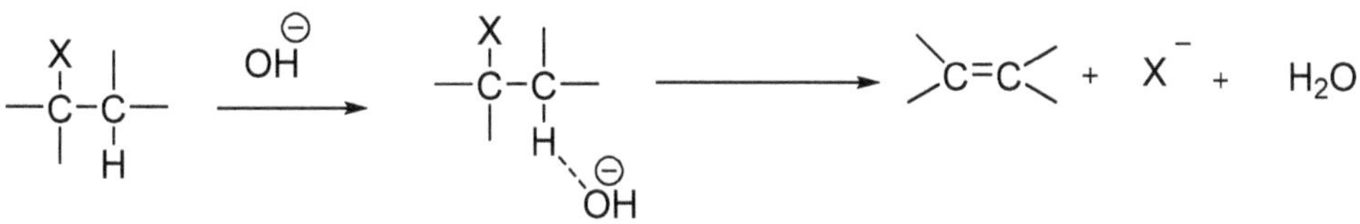

Ease of formation of alkenes

$$R_2C{=}CR_2 > R_2C{=}CHR > R_2C{=}CH_2 > RCH{=}CHR > RCH{=}CH_2 > CH_2{=}CH_2$$

Stability of alkenes

$$R_2C{=}CR_2 > R_2C{=}CHR > R_2C{=}CH_2 > RCH{=}CHR > RCH{=}CH_2 > CH_2{=}CH_2$$

Examples:

a)

$$CH_3CH_2CHBrCH_3 \xrightarrow[\text{alc}]{\text{KOH}} \underset{\text{major}}{CH_3CH{=}CHCH_3} + \underset{\text{minor}}{CH_3CH_2CH{=}CH_2}$$

b)

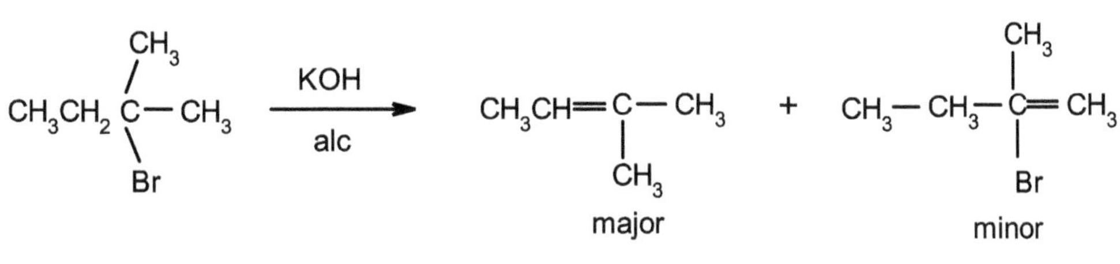

The order of the reactivity of alkyl halides in E2 dehydrohalogenation is tertiary > secondary > primary.

When elimination takes place via carbanion formation it is called E1cB elimination, the more stable the carbanion the faster will be the reaction. Electron withdrawing groups attached to the carbon disperses the negative charge and carbanion will be stabilized. Energy of the activation is lowered and the reaction becomes faster. Electron withdrawing tendency follows the order- F > Cl > Br > I.

a)

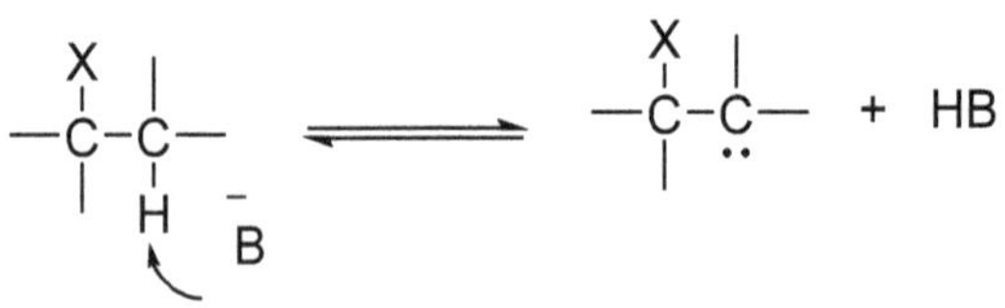

b)

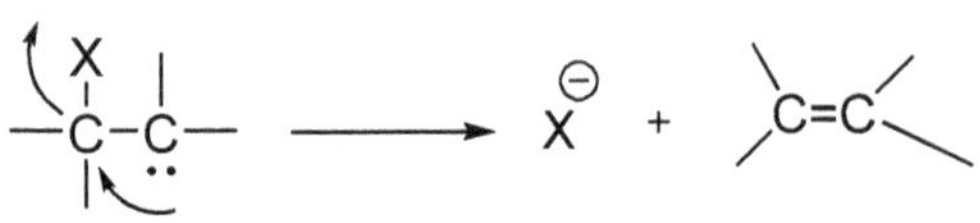

Stereochemistry of -E2 reaction

Examine the case of 1-bromo1,2-diphenyl propane, which exists as two pairs of enantiomers. Both pairs are diastereomers. On dehydrohalogenation

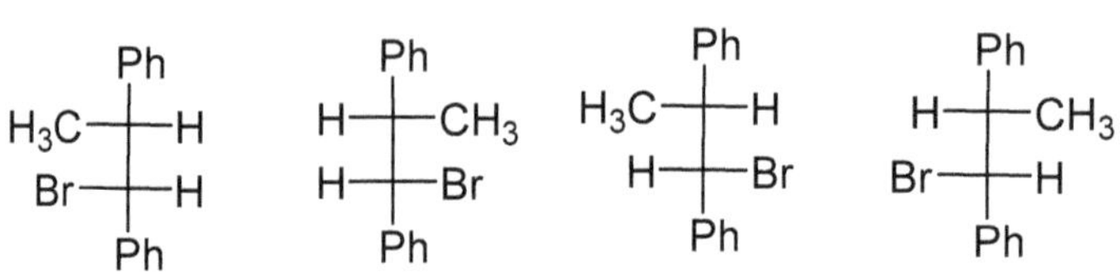

I II I II

Erythro Threo

Erythro compound gives Z-alkene and threo compound forms E-alkene. Hence it is a stereo selective and the stereo specific reaction.

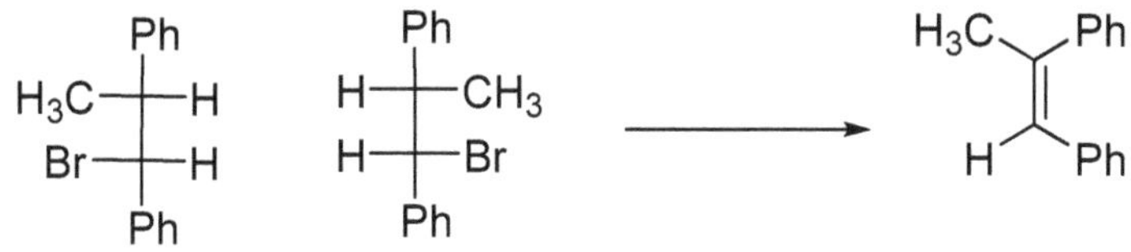

I II

Erythro
1-Bromo-1,2-diphenyl propane

(Z)-1,2-diphenyl propene

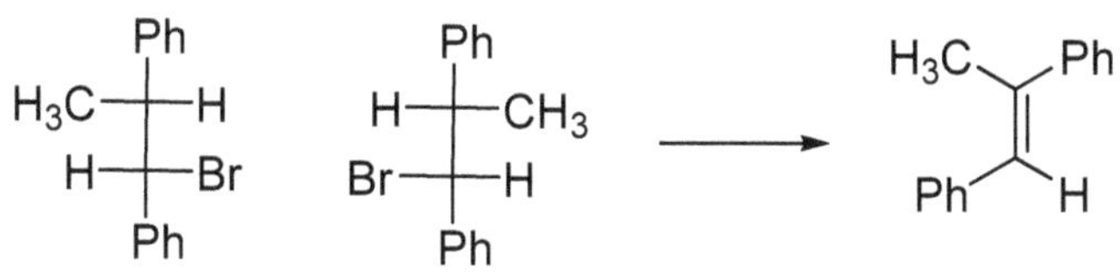

I II

Threo
1-Bromo-1,2-diphenyl propane

(E)-1,2-diphenyl propene

When eliminated groups are from the same face it is called “syn elimination” and when eliminated groups are from opposite faces it is known as “anti-elimination.” E2 elimination involves anti-elimination. Conformationally, more trans isomer is formed than cis product in these E2 reactions. Trans isomer is more stable than cis isomer due to less Vander Waals strain encountered and trans product is formed faster than cis isomer.

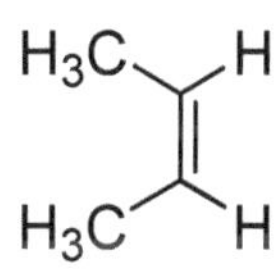

cis-2-butene

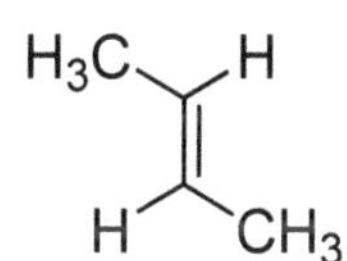

Trans-2-butene
more stable due to
less Vander Waals
strain

In the case of E1- the mechanism follows first order kinetics and involves two step unimolecular elimination as well as carbonium ion formation.

E1-Unimolecular elimination

a)

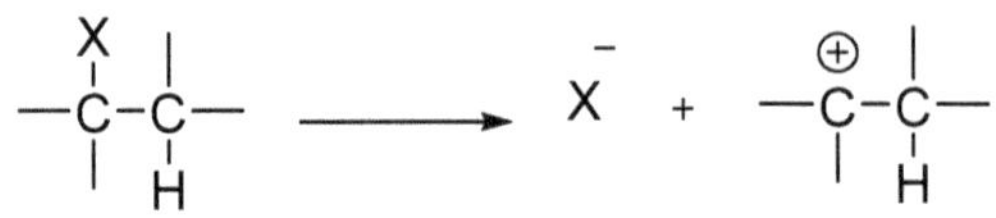

slow heterolysis
Rate determining step

b)

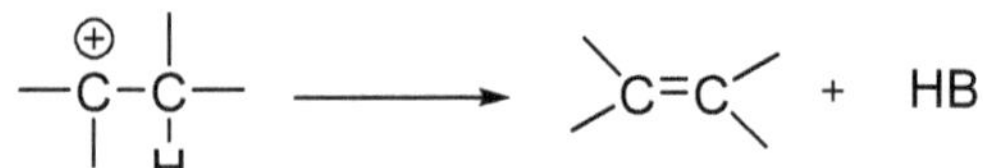

fast

alkene formation
First order kinetics

$$\text{Rate} = K[RX]$$

Evidences for E1- mechanism are as follows:

a) First order kinetics,

b) Do not show hydrogen isotope effect,

c) Accompanied by rearrangements,

d) Effect of the structure on the reactivity same as in SN1 reactions.

Order of reactivity of alkyl halides follows-

Tertiary > Secondary > Primary

E1 process follows Saytzeff's rule. In the case of highly branched substrates the more stable compound is formed.

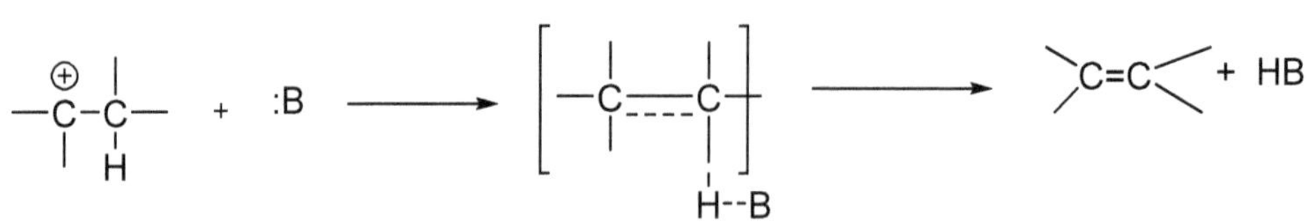

In both E1, and E2 it can be observed reactivity increases along - primary secondary tertiary. In E1, due to the greater stability of the carbonium ion formed in the rate determining step, the reactivity increases along the above lines. In E2 the reactivity increases because of the higher stability of the highly branched alkene formed.

Example:

a)

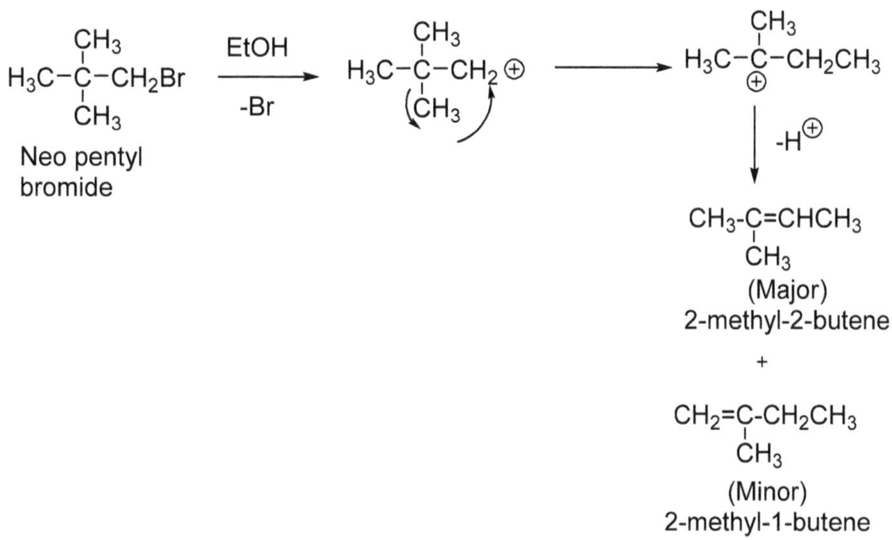
EtOH
-Br
Neo pentyl bromide
-H⊕
(Major)
2-methyl-2-butene
(Minor)
2-methyl-1-butene

b)

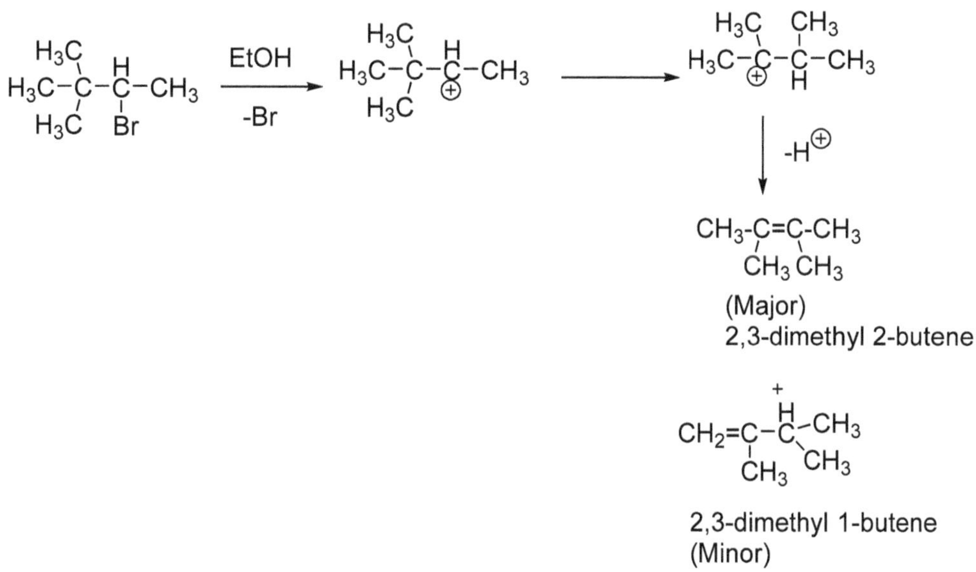
EtOH
-Br
-H⊕
(Major)
2,3-dimethyl 2-butene
2,3-dimethyl 1-butene
(Minor)

During dehydration of alcohols an elimination of water molecule takes place as 1,2- elimination.

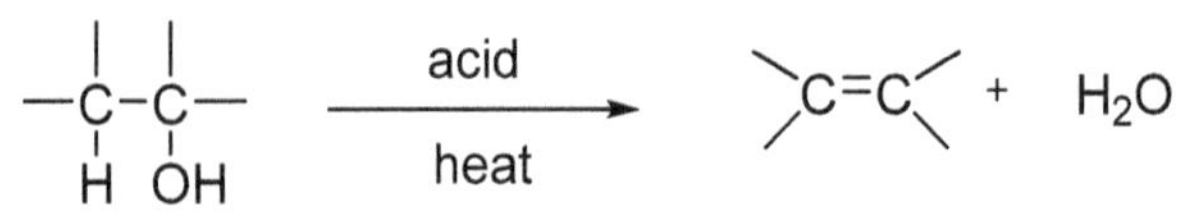

The reaction can be conducted in the presence of an acid and under heating conditions. Acid can be H_2SO_4, H_3PO_4 etc., The reaction can be performed by passing alcohol vapour over Alumina catalyst at higher temperatures. Here alumina acts as Lewis acid and Lowry Bronsted acid. The rate of reaction follows the order- tertiary secondary primary.

a)

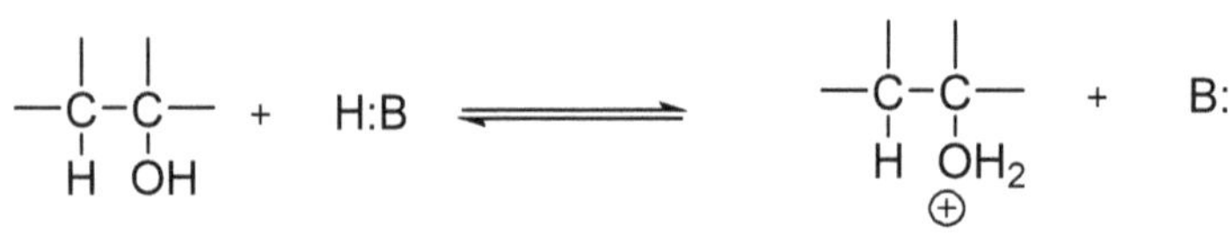

b)

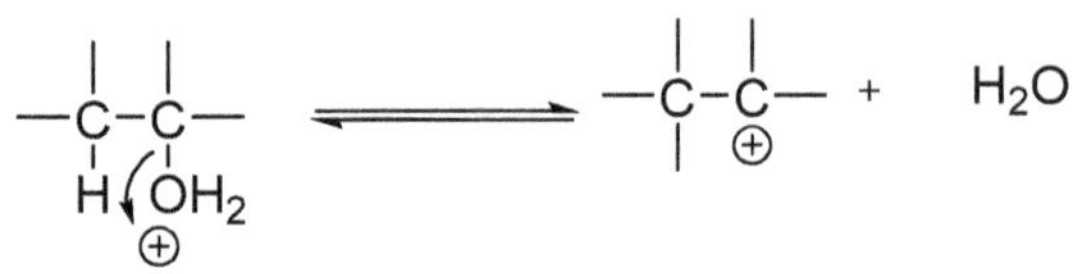

c)

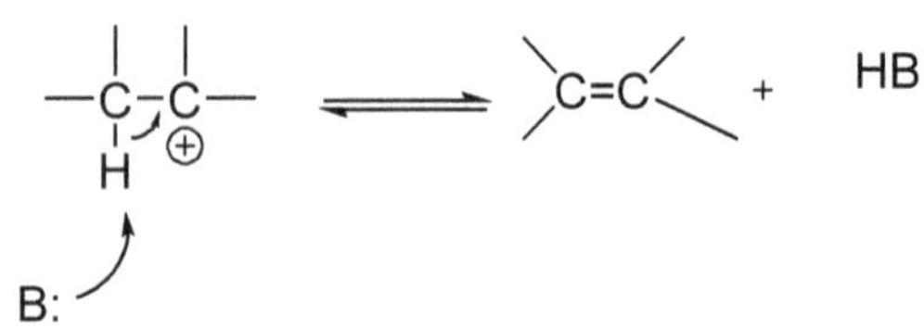

The reaction strongly follows Saytzeff's rule and a more stable carbonium ion is formed, while producing alkene molecule.

a)

$$CH_3CH_2OH \xrightarrow[170\ ^{\circ}C]{95\ \%\ H_2SO_4} CH_2{=}CH_2$$

ethyl alcohol → ethylene

b)

$$CH_3CH_2CH_2OH \xrightarrow[140\ ^{\circ}C]{75\%\ H_2SO_4} H_3CCH{=}CH{-}CH_3$$

n-butyl alcohol → 2-butene (major)

c)

$$\underset{\text{sec. butyl alcohol}}{CH_3CH_2CHOHCH_3} \xrightarrow[100\ ^\circ C]{60\ \%\ H_2SO_4} \underset{\text{2-butene (major)}}{CH_2CH{=}CHCH_3}$$

d)

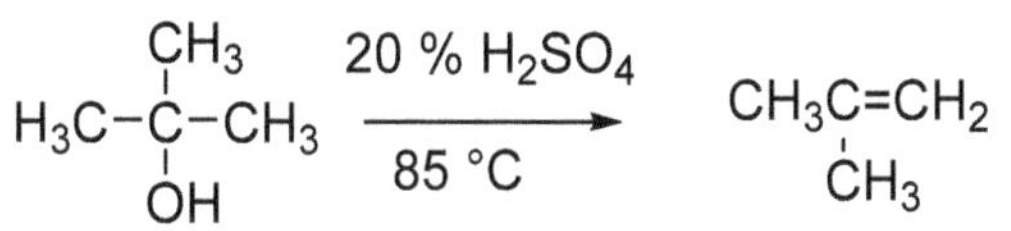

tert.butyl alcohol → isobutylene

e)

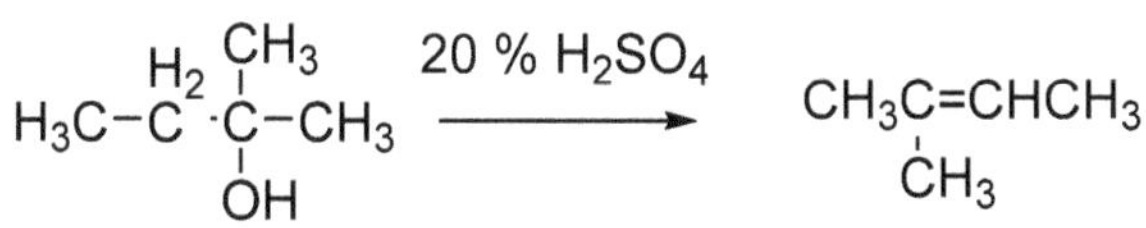

tert.pentyl alcohol → 2-methyl-2-butene (major)

3. Substitution reactions

When an electron rich reagent or nucleophile attacks the carbon nucleus resulting in the change of functional group, it is called substitution reaction or nucleophilic substitution reaction. Ex: Conversion of alcohols to alkyl halides.

$$R\text{-}OH \xrightarrow{HX \text{ or } PX_3} RX$$

Nucleophilic Substitution

$$\underset{\text{Substrate}}{R{:}X} + \underset{\text{nucleophile}}{:Z} \longrightarrow R{:}Z + \bar{X}{:}$$

In the case of aliphatic compounds generally alcohols are good substrates for conversion.

Nucleophilic substitution is the most widely practised and popular method in organic synthesis. Generally, the components of the reaction are substrates, containing good leaving groups, nucleophile and solvent. The nucleophile should be more powerful so that it can attack carbon faster. A large number of substitution reactions are known. In the above general equation, Z can be OH (alcohols), OR (ethers), CN (nitriles), NH_3 (primary amines), RNH_2 (secondary amines), R2 NH (tertiary amines), SH (thiols or mercaptans), SR (thioethers), ArH (in the presence of $AlCl_3$), I (alkyl iodides), C=C (forms alkynes), etc., Alkyl halides can also be converted to organometallic compounds with the help of lithium, magnesium, or copper metals. Apart from alkyl halides alkyl esters of sulfonic acids ($ArSO_2OR$) are commonly used in the synthesis. The following sulfonate esters are good leaving groups.

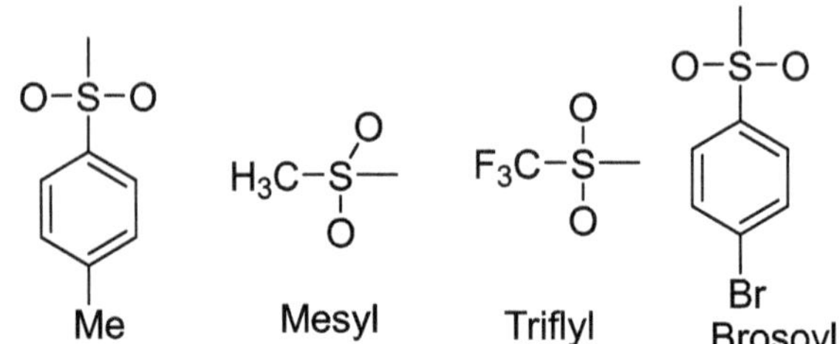

Tosyl (TS) Mesyl (Ms) Triflyl (Tf) Brosoyl (Bs)

According to E.D. Hughes and Sir Christopher Ingold, the nucleophilic aliphatic substitution proceeds by two different mechanisms.

SN1-substitution nucleophilic, unimolecular,

SN2- substitution nucleophilic bimolecular

While proposing the theory in 1935, these scientists considered kinetic order and relative reactivities.

SN1-mechanism increases from primary alkyl halides to secondary to tertiary halides.

SN2- mechanism increases from tertiary, to secondary, to primary alkyl halides.

SN 1 increases →

RX= CH_3X, primary alkyl halides, secondary alkyl halides, tertiary alkyl halides

← SN 2 increases

In the case of methyl bromide hydrolysis, the rate of reaction depends both on the concentrations of methyl bromide and hydroxide ion and the reaction goes with complete inversion of configuration or opposite configuration.

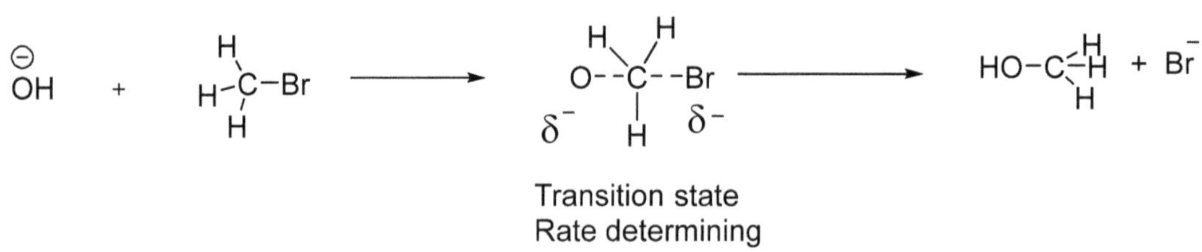

Rate= $K[CH_3Br][OH^-]$

Better leaving group speeds up both SN1, and SN2 mechanisms. In the case of SN2 reaction, it occurs in a single step. Bond breaking and bond forming occur simultaneously in a concerted fashion. Bulky electron releasing functional groups facilitate back side attack, accommodating positive charge, increases hydrolysis, making reaction faster.

In the case of SN1-reaction unimolecular, the rate of reaction is independent of OH ion concentration and depends only on concentration of RBr.

Hydrolysis of methyl bromide follows second order kinetics whereas hydrolysis of tertiary butyl bromide follows first order kinetics.

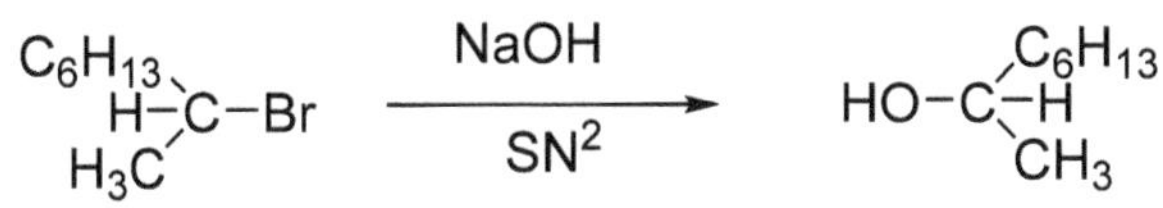

(-) 2-bromo octane (+) 2-octanol

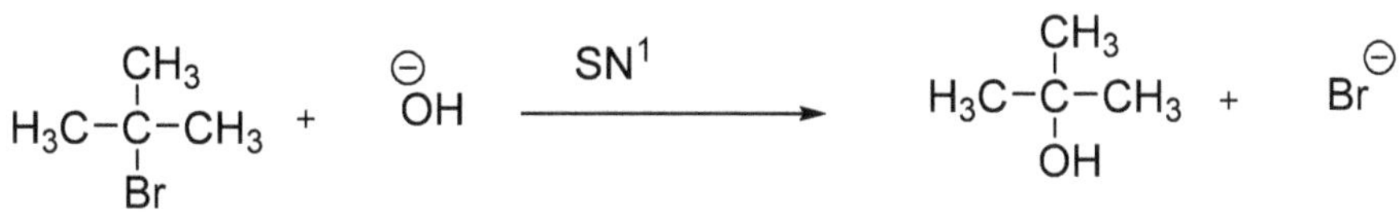

Rate= K[RBr]

$$RBr + Cl^{\ominus} \xrightarrow{DMF} R\text{-}Cl + Br^{\ominus}$$

Overall, we can observe that as the number of substituents attached to carbon with halogen group increases the reactivity towards SN2 substitution decreases. Therefore, more than polar factors steric factors are influencing the course of the reaction.

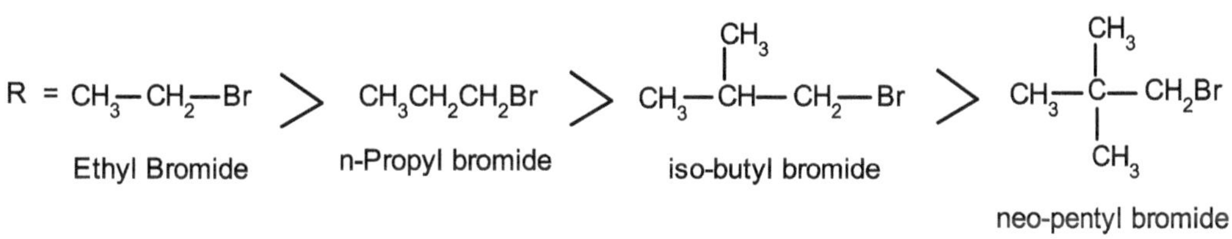

a) 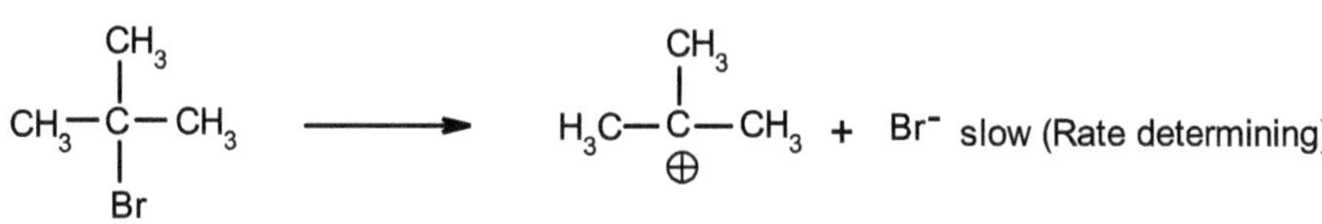

b) 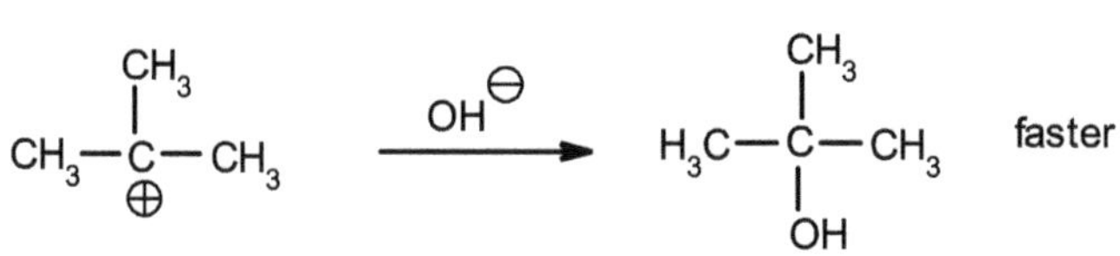

The rate determining step is the step whose rate controls overall rate of the reaction. Here in SN1 mechanism the rate of entire reaction is determined by the rapidity with which alkyl halide ionizes. It depends on the concentration of alkyl halide. When we carry out the reaction with optically pure substrates the end product will be a mixture of inverted compound and racemic compound. Thus, the reaction ends up with partial racemization plus inversion.

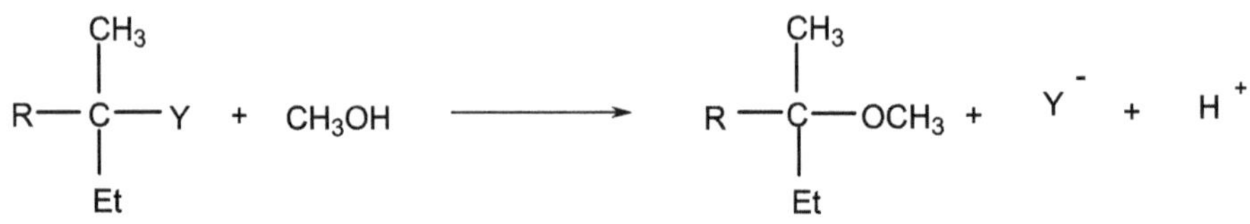

The difference between SN1 and SN2 is that an SN2 reaction proceeds with complete inversion and an SN1 reaction ends up with racemization. Complete stereo specificity in the SN2 process indicates concerted bond breaking and bond making in one step. Absence of complete stereo specificity among SN1 reactions show a stepwise completion.

Relative reactivities-SN1 VS SN2

As postulated by Hughes and Ingold reactivity towards SN2 decreases while going from CH3X, primary, secondary, and tertiary substrates.

Whereas, in the case of SN1 the reactivity order of the substrates is as follows:

Tertiary butyl > Isopropyl > Ethyl > Methyl

The stability of carbonium ion governs the reactivity and orientation in the reactions where carbonium ion is involved. The carbonium ion stability follows the order-

Tertiary > Secondary > Primary > Methyl

The stability of carbonium ion also depends on polar effects like resonance and inductive effects of the attached groups like dispersal of the charge, and ease of carbonium ion formation etc., A substrate can undergo SN1 faster when a carbonium ion can be formed faster as the rate determining step in SN1 involves the formation of carbonium ion. The more stable is a carbonium ion, the faster it can be formed.

Rearrangement of carbonium ions:

Sometimes nucleophilic substitutions accompany formation of rearranged products;

Examples:

a)

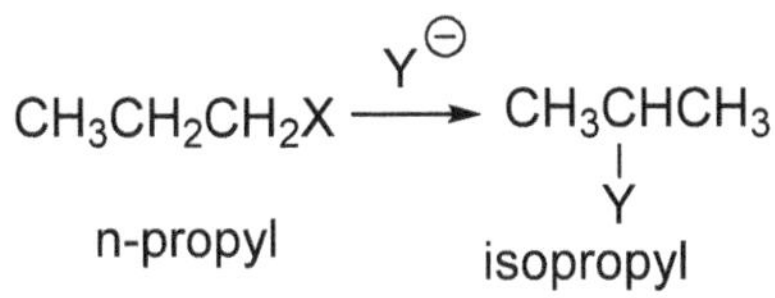

b)

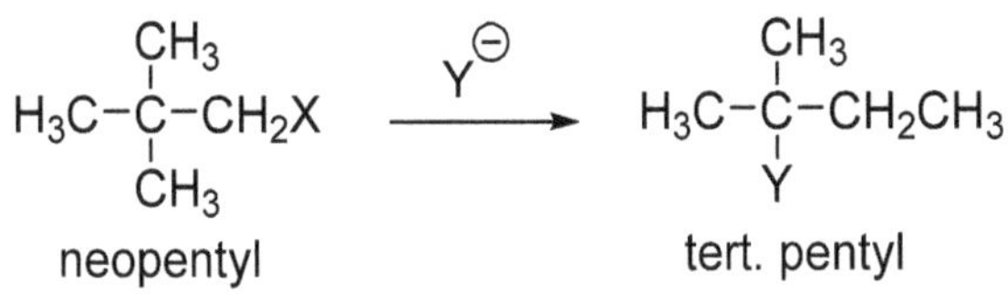

c)

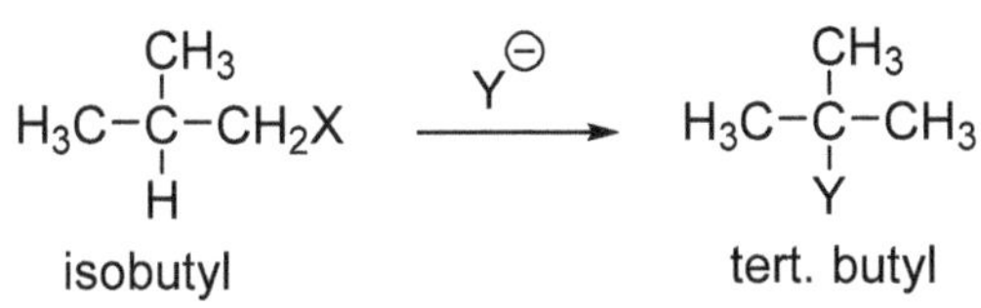

Typically, only reactions proceeding by SN1 mechanism are accompanied by rearrangements. Possibilities for such rearrangements are not there in the case of single step, concerted SN2 reactions. This is because of carbonium ion intermediate, in the slow first order reactions.

Examples:

a)

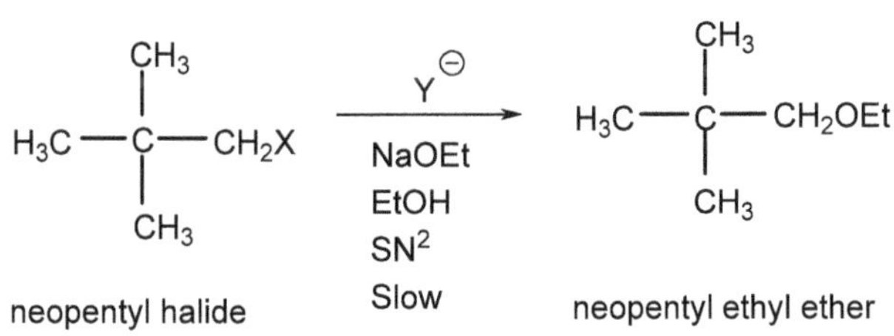

b)

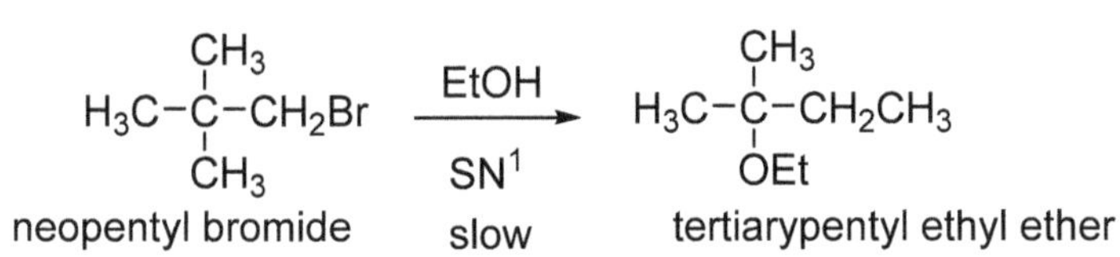

The examples illustrate that rearrangements take place to form a more stable carbonium ion. These also involve 1,2- shift of hydride or alkyl group.

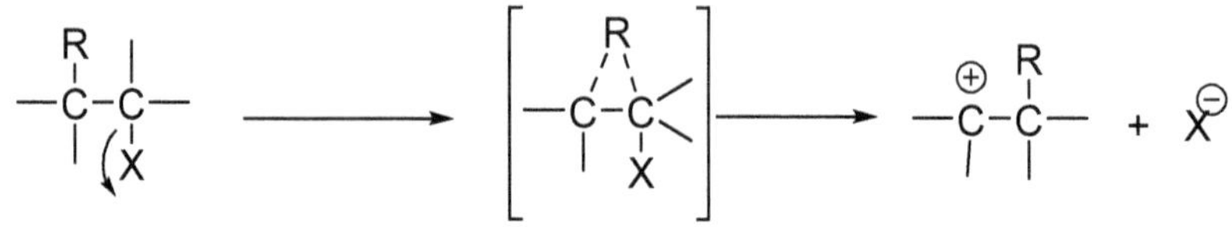

R= H, alkyl

The differences between reactivities of different substrates like primary, secondary, or tertiary compounds are also related to the lower energy of activation [Eact]. The lower the Eact the more stable will be the intermediate transition state. Moreover, the dipole-diplole interactions also play a role in the solution phase. More polar the reactant, stabilization will be more by the solvation.

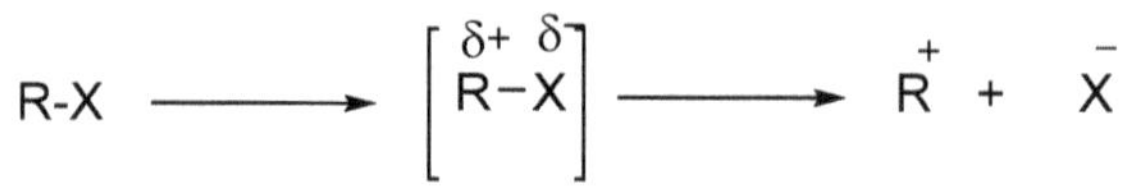

Transition state

Solvents help in lowering the Eact by stabilizing the transition state. Therefore, SN1 reactions of neutral substrates tend to complete faster in water and alcohols, than in aprotic solvents such as DMF, DMSO etc., HCO_2H, CF_3CO_2H, CF_3CH_2OHetc., act as excellent ionizing solvents, as they can stabilize the transition state, prompting heterolysis involved in the reaction. Whereas, in the case of SN2 reactions two reactants such as alkyl halides and OH are involved in the rate determining step. Both differ in forming dipole-ion bonds with the solvent. Substrates are more stabilized than transition state in the solvent.

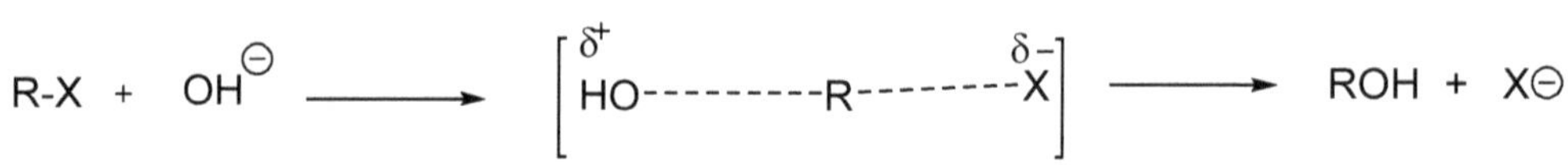

The strength of solvation and degree of deactivation of nucleophile differs from anion to anion in the case of SN2. Moreover, the effect differs from solvent to solvent. The greater the polarity of solvent, the slower will be SN2 reaction. Ideal solvent will be nonpolar solvent. Phase transfer catalysts play significant role in these reactions, minimizing two deactivating forces, solvation and ion pairing, acting on the anion.

Salient features:

S N1	SN2
1. First order kinetics	1. Second order kinetics
2. Racemization	2. Complete stereo chemical inversion
3. Rearrangement	3. Absence of rearrangement
4. Reactivity sequence Tert > Sec > Prim.> Methyl	4. Reactivity sequence Methyl> Prim>Sec>Tert
5. Step wise reaction	5.Concerted reaction

Examples:

a)

$$\underset{\text{n-butyl alcohol}}{CH_3CH_2CH_2CH_2OH} \xrightarrow[H_2SO_4]{NaBr} \underset{\text{n-butyl bromide}}{CH_3CH_2CH_2CH_2Br}$$

b)

$$\underset{\text{n-propyl alcohol}}{CH_3CH_2CH_2OH} \xrightarrow[ZnCl_2]{HCl} \underset{\text{n-propyl chloride}}{CH_3CH_2CH_2Cl}$$

c)

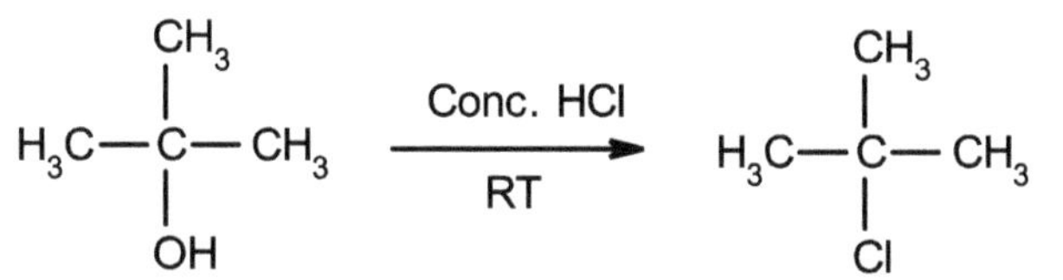

tert butyl alcohol tert butyl chloride

d)

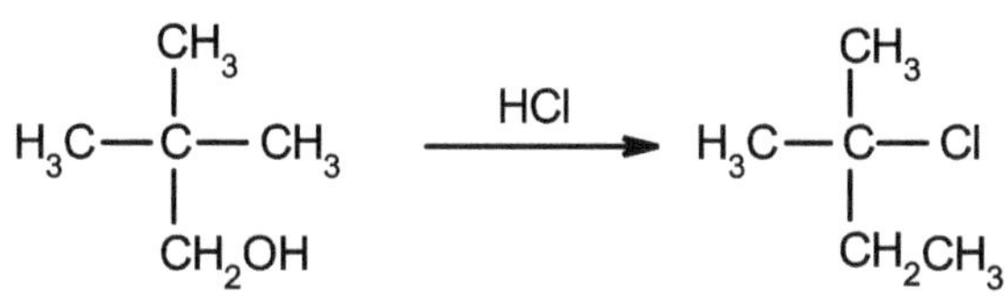

neopentyl alcohol tert. pentyl chloride

We can conclude that primary substrates undergo single step SN2 and tertiary substrates follow two step SN1 mechanism. In the case of secondary substrates, these may followSN1 like a two-step process or may involve nucleophilic assistance from the solvent (known as SN2i or SN2 intermediate). In the latter case, the intermediate is a nucleophilically solvated carbonium ion or encumbered carbo cation. This differs from SN2 kind of attack by a nucleophile. In this case, a single solvent molecule attacks the substrate from back side as a nucleophile and pushes out the leaving group from front side.

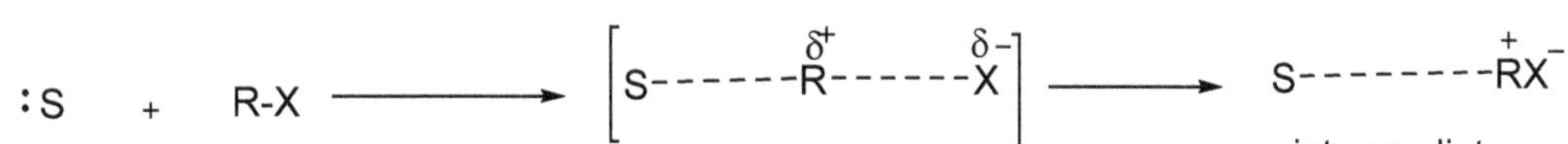

Tr. state nucleophilic assistance by solvent molecule

intermediate nucleophilically solvated carbonium ion

Alcohols also undergo SN1 or SN2 reactions just as alkyl halides, but needs strong acidic medium to protonate -OH group to make it ROH_2 as H_2O is a good leaving group than OH, which is a strong base. Protonation plays an important role in many kinds of substrates having N, O, or S, to make reaction faster.

4. Rearrangement reactions

Rearrangement reactions belong to a wide class of organic reactions in which the carbon skeleton of the substrate molecule undergoes rearrangement generating a new structural isomer of the substrate. These, which involve movement of an atom or a group of atoms, may be intramolecular or intermolecular. There are several rearrangements like 1,2- rearrangements, 1,3- rearrangements, olefin-metathesis, pericyclic reactions etc., Many name reactions come under rearrangements. These are discussed at various places in the book under the respective sections.

Examples:

a)

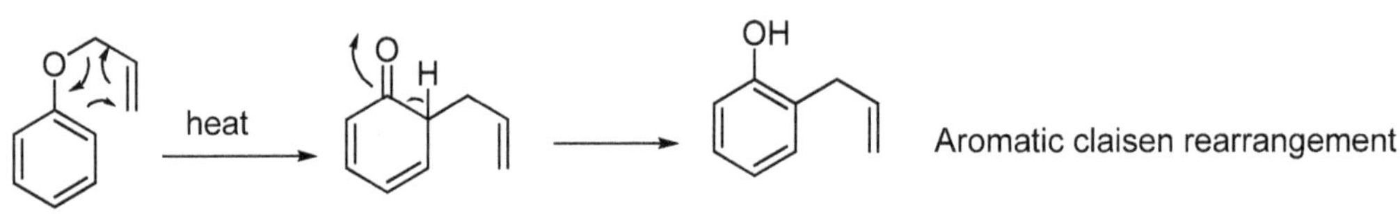

b)

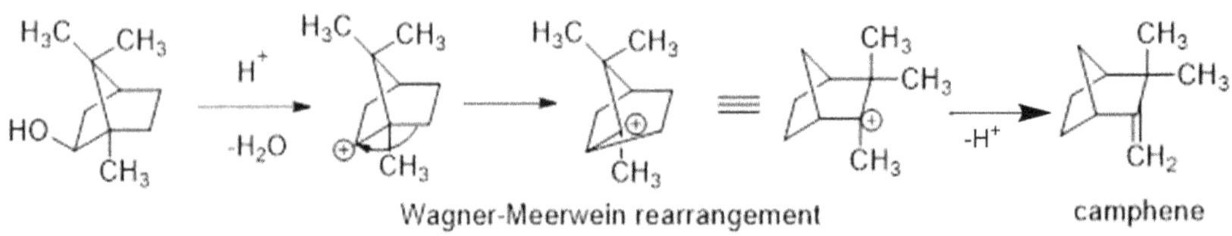

c)

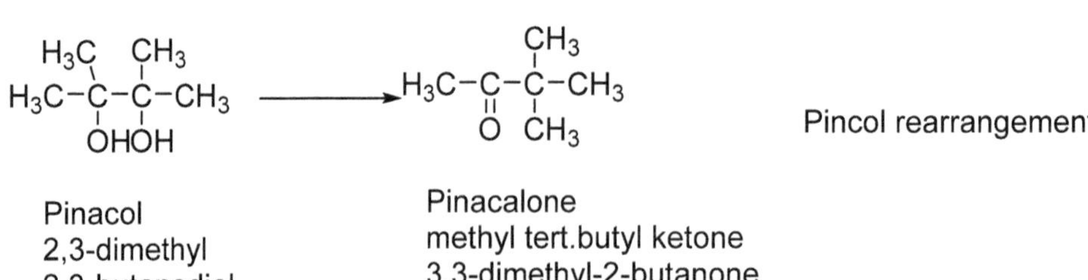

d)

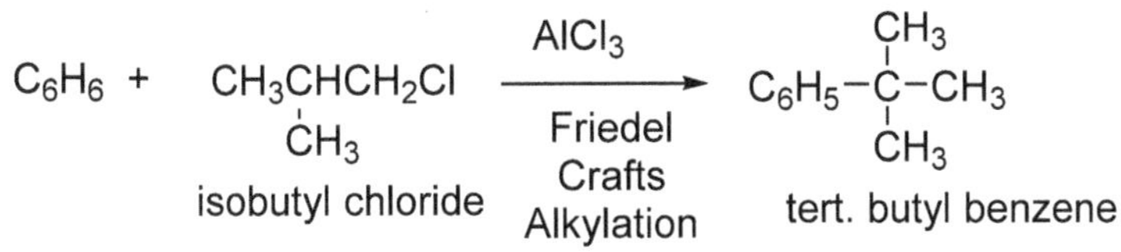

e)

$$\underset{\text{Benzil}}{C_6H_5COCOC_6H_5} \xrightarrow{OH^{\ominus}} (C_6H_5)_2C(OH)COO^- \xrightarrow[H^+]{} \underset{\text{Benzilic acid}}{(C_6H_5)_2C(OH)COOH}$$

f)

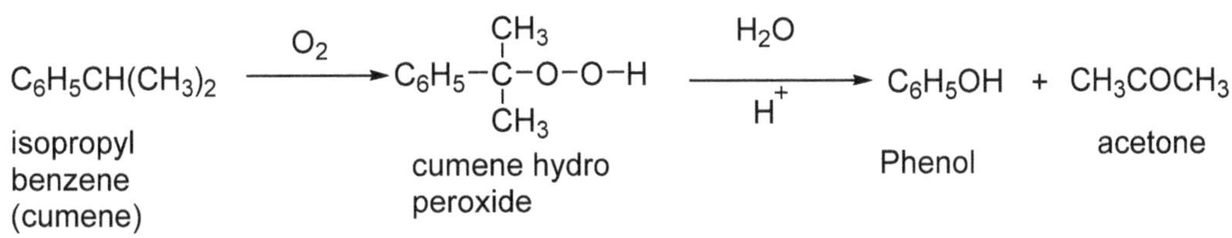

Rearrangement of hydroperoxide and migration to electron deficient oxygen species

g)

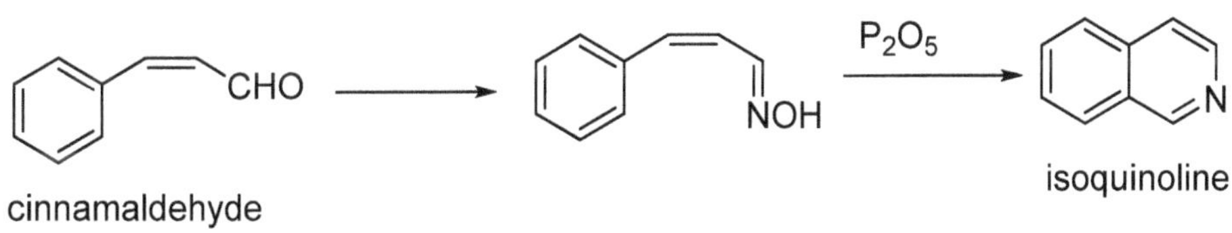

Beckmann rearrangement

h)

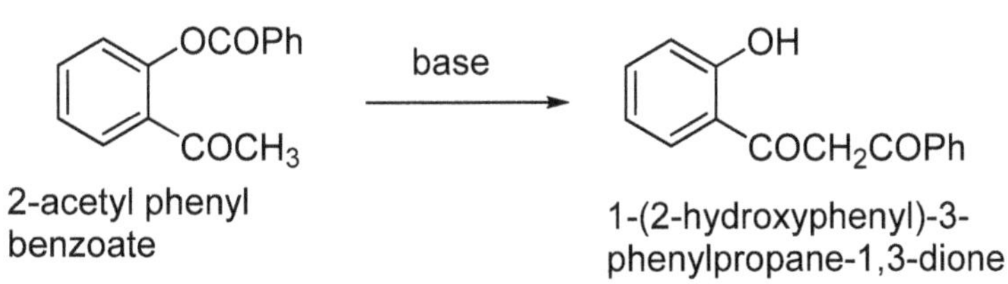

Baker-Venkataraman rearrangement

i) 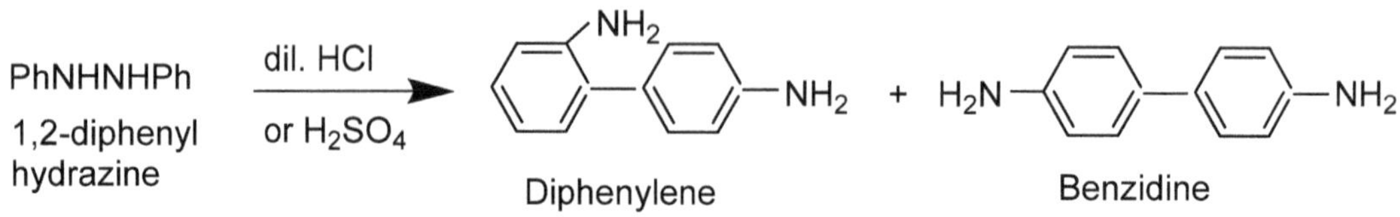

Benzidine rearrangement

j) 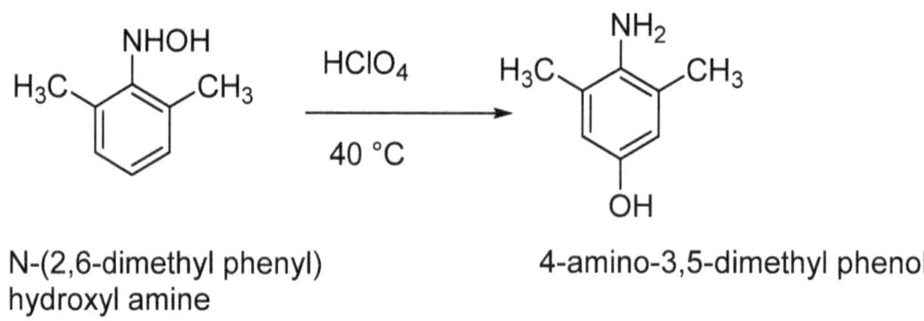

Bamberger rearrangement

CHAPTER 2

Name Reactions

2.1 Baeyer-Villiger Oxidation

It was first reported by Adolf von Baeyer, a German chemist, who synthesized indigo, and Victor Villiger, another German chemist in 1899.

In this reaction an ester or a lactone are formed from a ketone or a cyclic ketone respectively, catalyzed by oxidants like peroxyacids or peroxides like peracetic acid, perbenzoic acid, pertrifluoroacetic acid, permonosulphuric acid or BF_3-H_2O_2 etc., Cyclic ketones can be converted to lactones with ring expansion. Long chain hydroxy esters can be prepared from large ring size ketones.

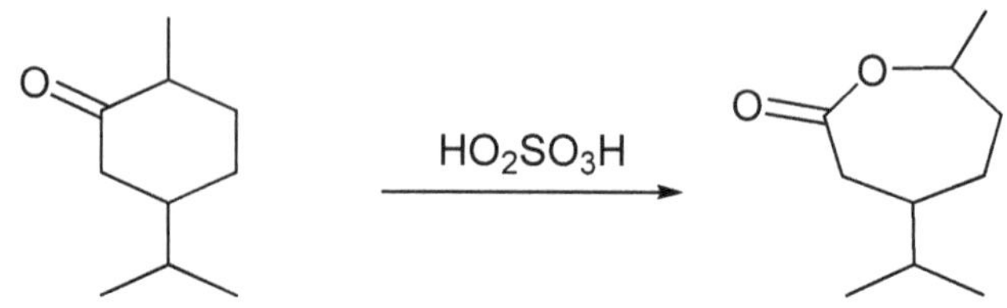

Tetrahydrocarvone

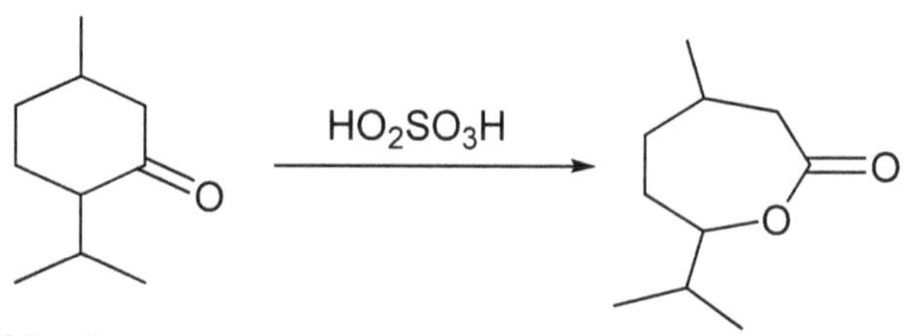

Menthone

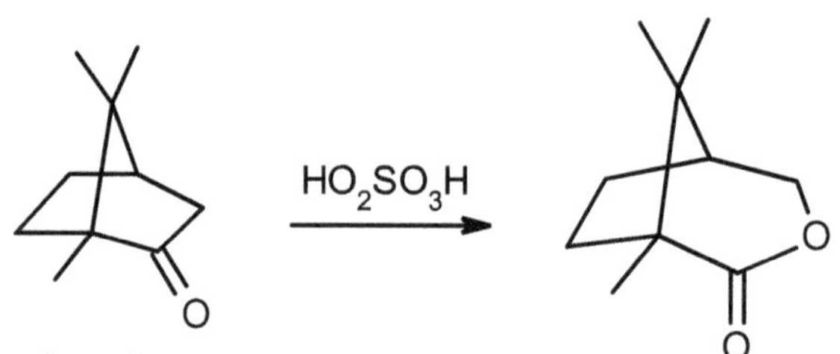

Camphor

General reaction:

Mechanism:

About three mechanisms involving the formation of three different intermediates followed by two modes of attacks of peroxyacid attack – on either the oxygen or the carbon of the carbonyl group are suggested. Attack on oxygen forms two possible intermediates, a) a dioxirane intermediate as suggested by Baeyer and Villiger, b) a peroxide as suggested by Georg Wittig and Gustav Pieper, and c) attack on carbon as suggested by Rudolf Criegee producing Criegee intermediate. However, oxygen-18 labelling concluded that the correct pathway involves the formation of the Criegee intermediate.

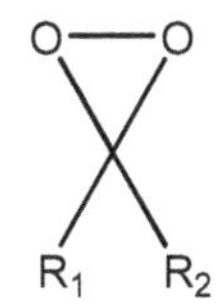

Baeyer and Villiger Intermediate

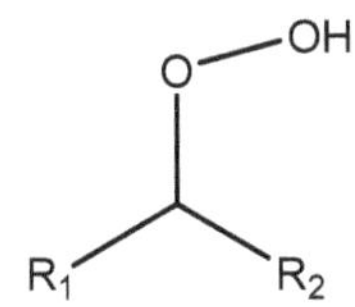

Wittig and Pieper Intermediate

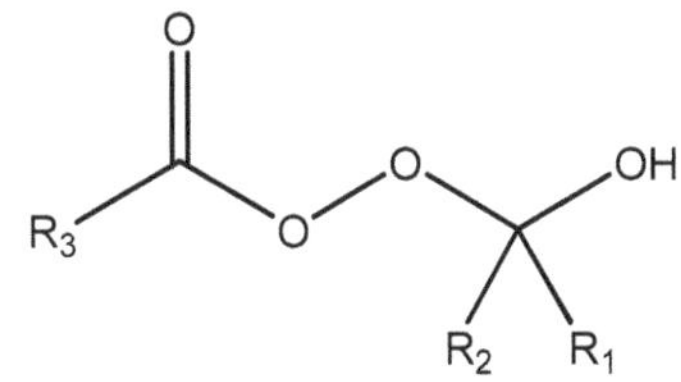

Criegee Intermediate

Now in the actual mechanism the initial protonation of the carbonyl group by peroxyacid, is followed by the attack of peroxyacid on the carbonyl carbon forming the Criegee intermediate. Next one of the substituents on the ketone group migrates to the oxygen of the peroxide group and the carboxylic acid leaves. The ester is formed by the deprotonation of the oxocarbenium ion. This migration is the rate determining step. Migratory group retains its configuration as in any other concerted mechanisms. The migratory aptitude of alkyl group follows the order tertiary>secondary>primary>methyl. Electron releasing substituents favour migration. In aryl groups the order is p-anisyl>p-tolyl>phenyl>p-chlorophenyl>p-nitrophenyl.

Both primary and secondary stereoelectronic effects control the outcome of the products.

a) The oxygen-oxygen bond in the peroxide group should be antiperiplanar to the group that migrates, making optimum overlap of the **σ** orbital of the migrating group to the σ* orbital of the peroxide group.

b) The lone pair on the oxygen of the hydroxyl group should be antiperiplanar to the migrating group, making optimum overlap of the oxygen nonbonding orbital with the σ* orbital of the migrating group.

Trifluoroperacetic acid (TFPAA), 4-nitroperbenzoic acid, *meta*-Chloroperoxybenzoic acid (mCPBA), performic acid, peracetic acid, hydrogen peroxide, tert-butyl hydroperoxide are some of the important oxidant catalysts useful in the Baeyer–Villiger oxidation reaction. In this the lower is the pK_a of the carboxylic acid or alcohol (in the case of the peroxides) the higher is the reactivity. The peroxyacids are more reactive than the peroxides. However, sometimes the Baeyer–Villiger oxidation can cause the undesirable oxidation of other functional groups.e.g., alkenes/amines. Hydrogen peroxide is known to be environmentally benign as the byproduct is only water.

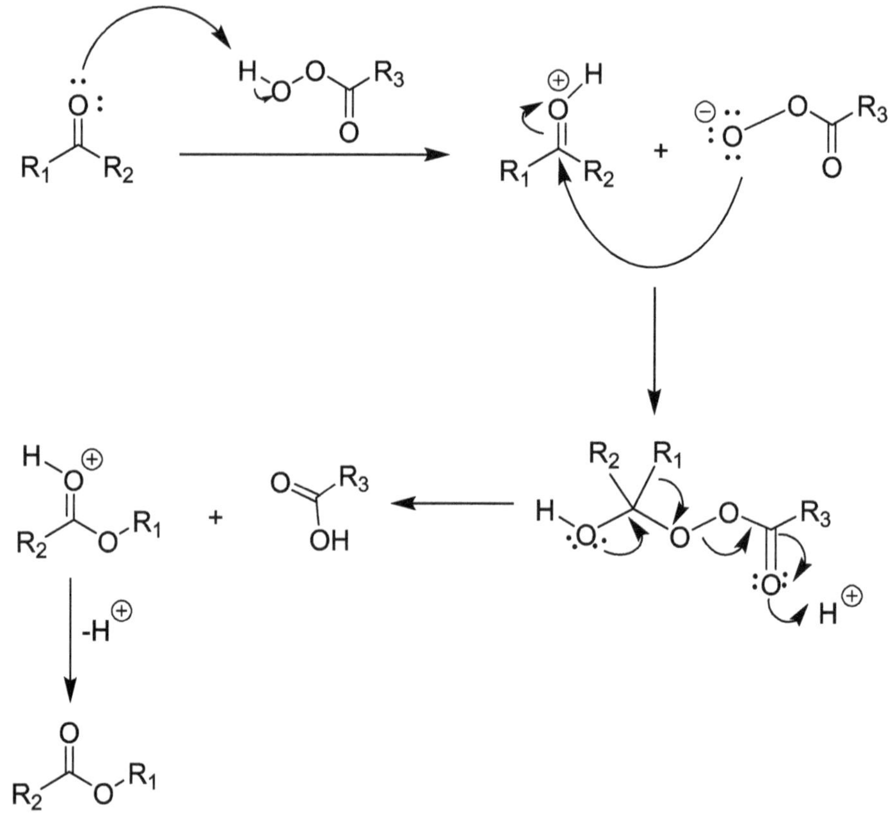

1. Preparation of esters from ketones

a) $PhCOCH_3$ (acetophenone) $\xrightarrow{CF_3CO_2H}$ CH_3COOPh (Phenylacetate)

b) $CH_3COC(CH_3)_3$ $\xrightarrow{CF_3CO_2H}$ $CH_3COOC(CH_3)_3$ (t-butylacetate)

c)

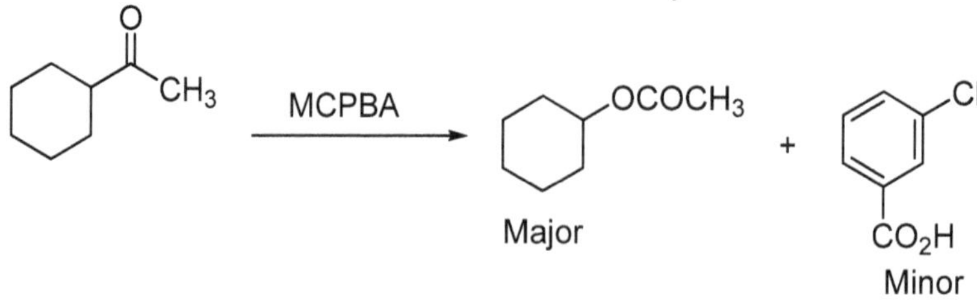

d) Sodium percarbonate in trifluoroacetic acid was employed as an effective reagent for the Baeyer-Villiger oxidation of ketones to esters[1].

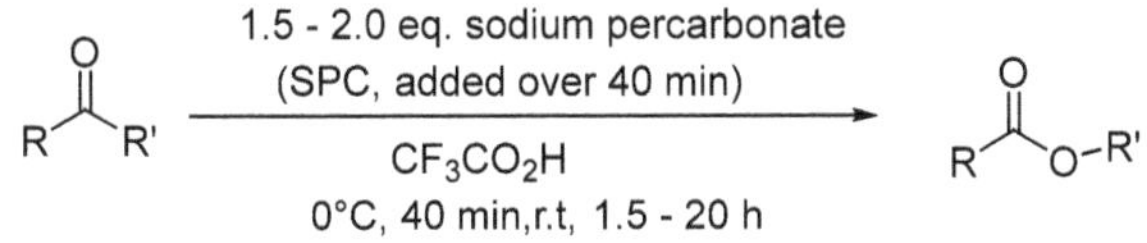

EX:

PhCOPh -------------------→ PhCOOPh (Na_2CO_4,CF_3CO_2H, 0°C,40 min, rt 1-4 hrs, 76%)

2. Preparation of anhydrides

a) $CH_3COCOCH_3 \xrightarrow{RCO_3H} CH_3COOCOCH_3$ acetic anhydride

b)

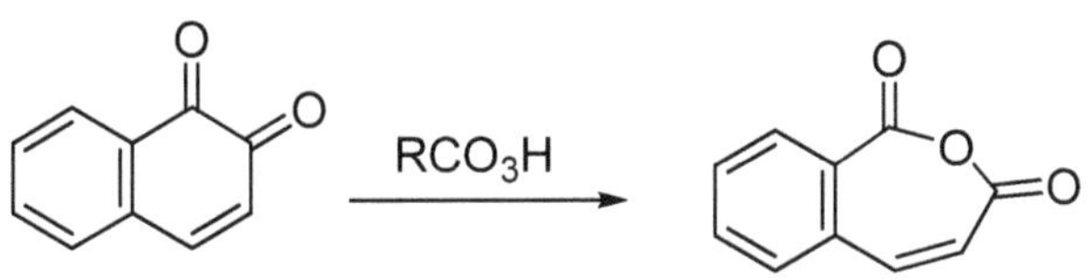

3. Preparation of epoxides

The epoxidation of various olefinic substrates and the Baeyer-Villiger oxidation of aldehydes and ketones with hydrogen peroxide was reported using aryl benzyl selenoxides[2].

4. Preparation of lactones

a)

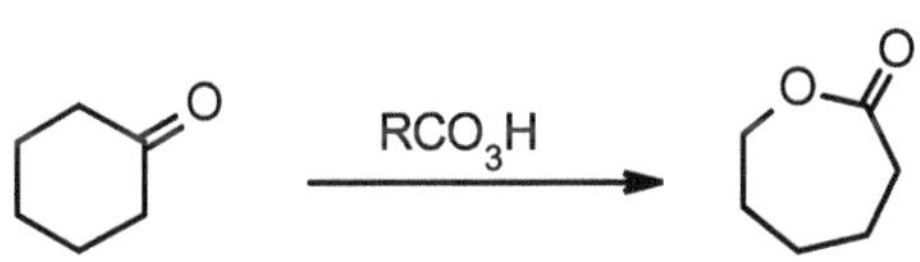

Cyclohexanone → E-caprolactone

b)

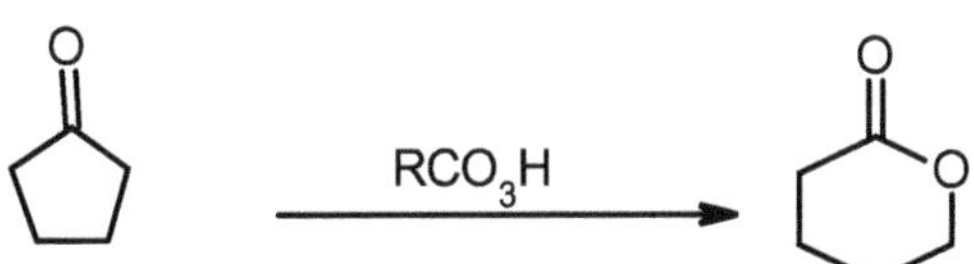

Cyclopentanone → Tetrahydro 2H- pyran-2-one

c)

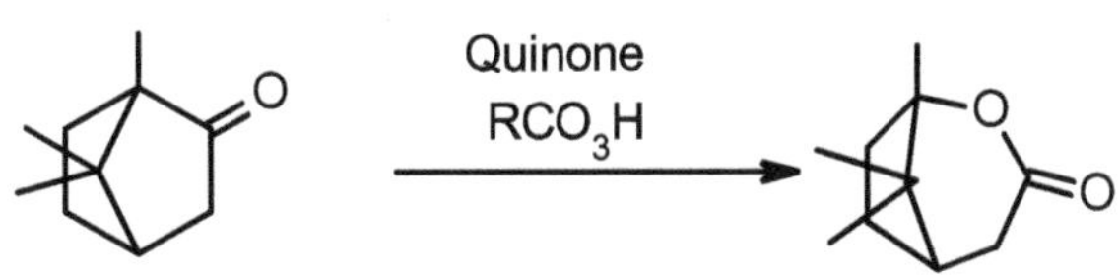

Camphor → Major

5. Preparation of hydroxy alkyl esters

Hydroxy alkyl esters are also reportedly generated by the oxidation of cyclic acetals in the presence of MCPBA.

6. Microwave-assisted Baeyer–Villiger Oxidation

Preparation of lactones by the oxidation of cyclic ketones. The Baeyer–Villiger oxidation of cyclic ketones to the corresponding lactones was improved with *m*-CPBA under microwave irradiation.

Ex: Cycloheptanone into oxocan-2-one.

7. Ultrasound-assisted Baeyer–Villiger oxidation

Ex: Preparation of ε-caprolactone.

Baeyer–Villiger oxidation of cyclohexanone to ε-caprolactone was studied in a new sonochemical reactor. Ultrasound intensified the rates of reactions and also increased the yield of product. Facile oxidative conversion of cyclohexanone to yield ε-caprolactone using molecular oxygen and benzaldehyde was developed[3].

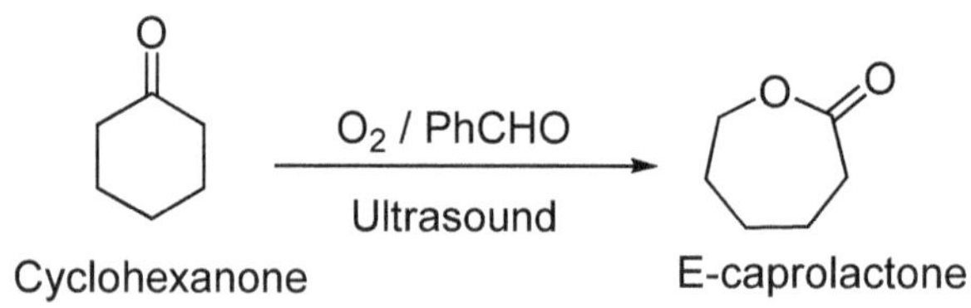

2.2 Brook rearrangement

The Brook rearrangement introduced by Adrian Gibbs Brook, involves rearrangement of any [1,*n*] carbon to oxygen silyl migration producing silyl ethers as products which is driven by the stability of the oxygen-silicon bond. They can take place under basic/acidic conditions or thermally or photolytically. Anionic rearrangements are most common. It is an intramolecular 1,2-anionic migration of a silyl group with the formation of a cyclic pentavalent silicon species in the transition state. The rearrangement is known to occur with retention of configuration at the silicon.

The silyl substituents can be aliphatic or aromatic. An electron-withdrawing R group facilitates the reaction. Analogous Brook rearrangements are known including nitrogen, phosphorus, and sulfur as the nucleophilic components. When an intramolecular migration of a silyl group from oxygen to carbon take place, it is known as retro-Brook rearrangement.

General Reaction:

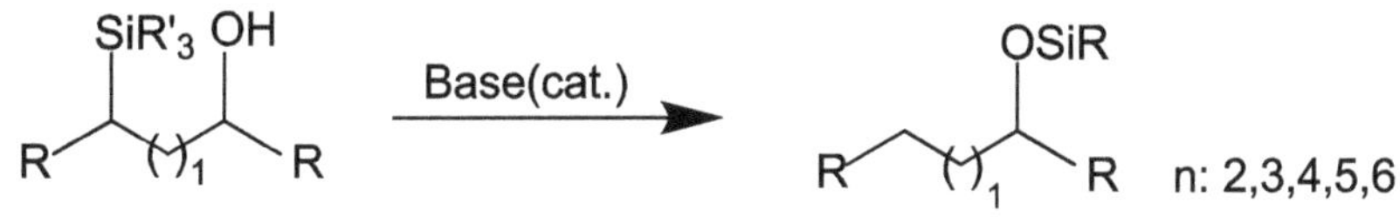

Mechanism:

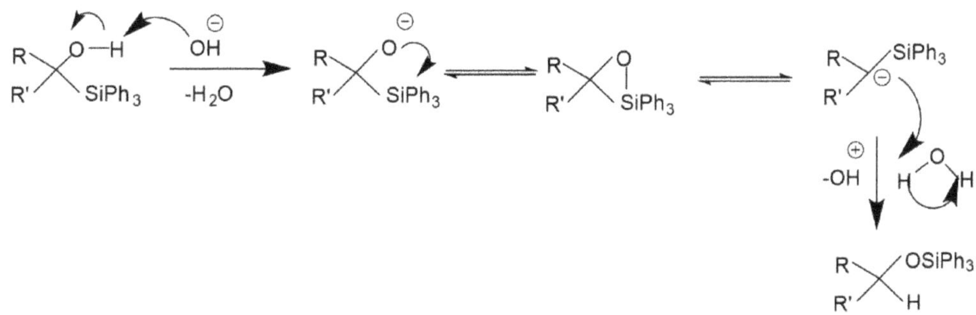

Applications and examples:

1. **Preparation of silyl ether**

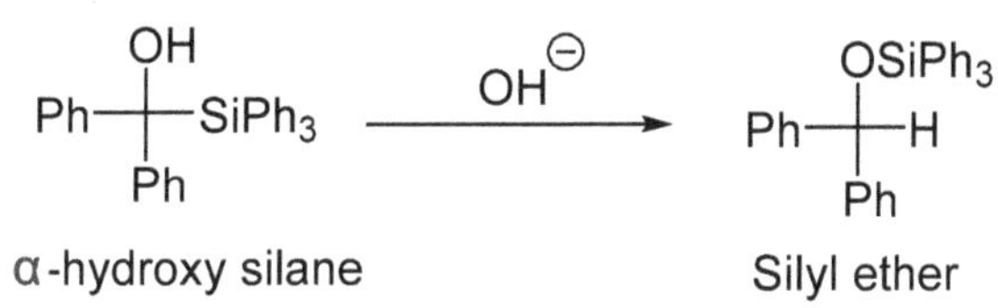

2. **Allylation of β-Triphenyl silyl Allylic Alcohols**

Copper(I) *tert*-butoxide and allylic halides are efficiently used in the preparation of β-triphenylsilyl allylic alcohols[4].

3. **Preparation of α-Hydroxy Acid Derivatives**

A wide range of α-substituted α-siloxy silanes were carboxylated under CO_2 atmosphere *via* Brook rearrangement, in the presence of CsF[5].

4. **Synthesis of tetrasubstituted furans via [1,2]-phospha Brook rearrangement**

Tetrasubstituted furan derivatives were prepared by utilizing the [1,2]-phospha-Brook rearrangement under Brønsted base catalysis. The two step one-pot [3 + 2] cycloaddition involves the nucleophilic addition of a propargyl anion, generated through the [1,2]-Phospha-Brook rearrangement, to an aldehyde followed by an intramolecular cyclization promoted by *N*-iodosuccinimide (NIS) to afford 2,4,5-trisubstituted-3-iodofurans[6].

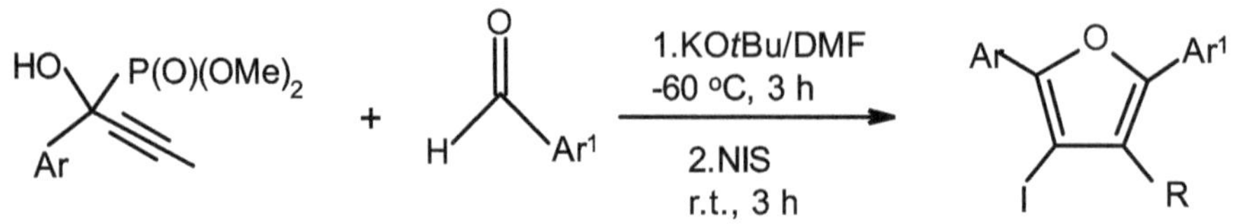

R : alkyl

5. Conversion of silyl ketones to silyl ethers

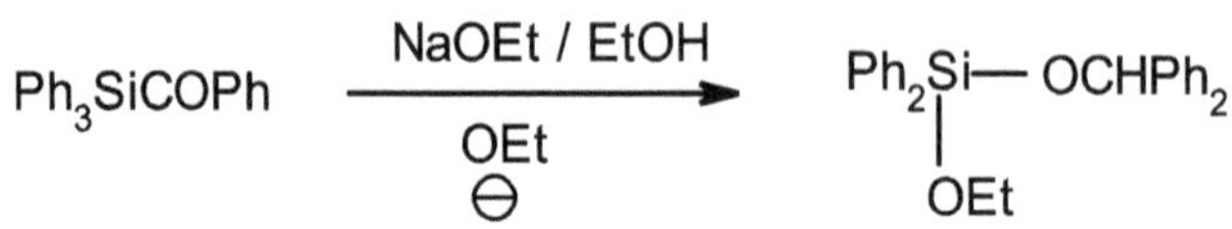

2.3 Dieckmann Reaction

It is the intramolecular conversion of diesters to β-keto esters in the presence of a base and is named after the German chemist, Walter Dieckmann. The Dieckmann condensation along with its intermolecular version are classic and interesting reactions studied because of their great importance in organic synthesis and biochemical transformations. An enolate ion is formed by the deprotonation of an ester at the α-position. It undergoes a 5-exo-trig nucleophilic attack to give a cyclic enol. A Bronsted-Lowry acid protonates (H_3O^+ for example) to form the β-keto ester. Five-membered and six-membered β-keto esters are formed from 1,6 diesters and 1,7 diesters respectively. Bases like tBuOK, tBuONa, EtOK, and EtONa etc., can be used as catalysts.

General reaction

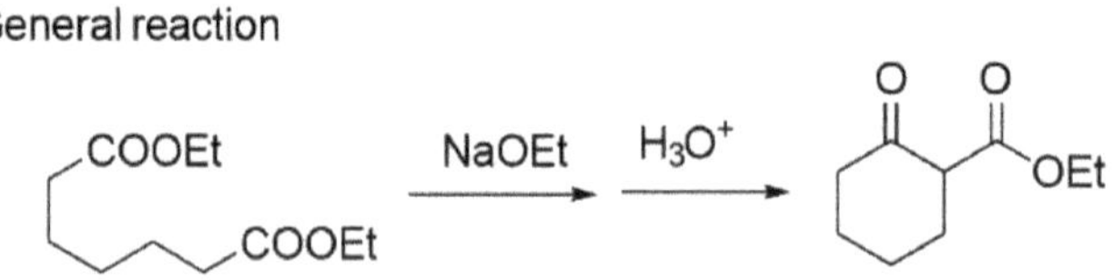

Mechanism:

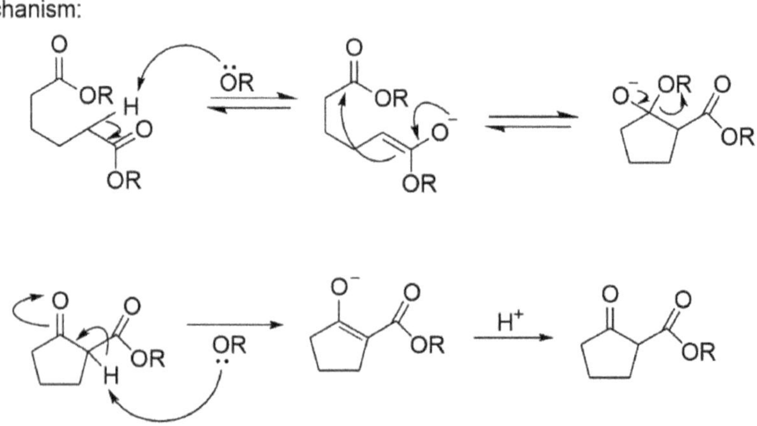

Applications and examples:

1. 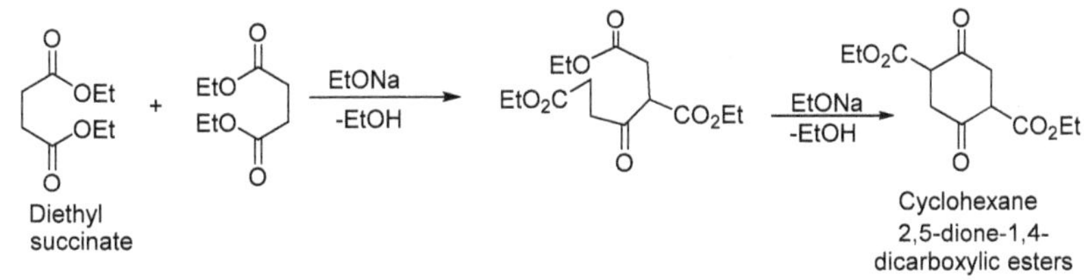

2. 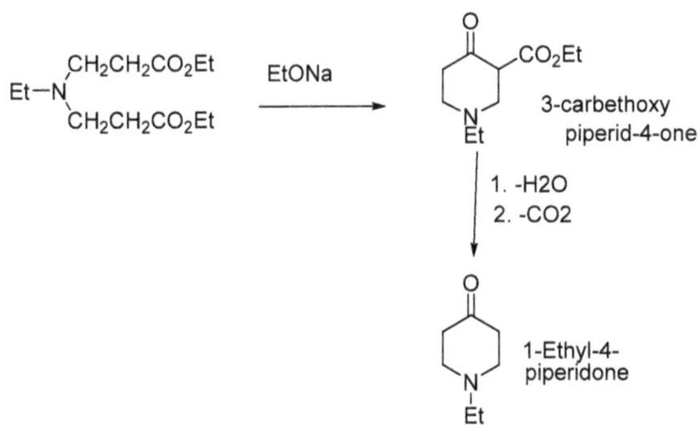

3. 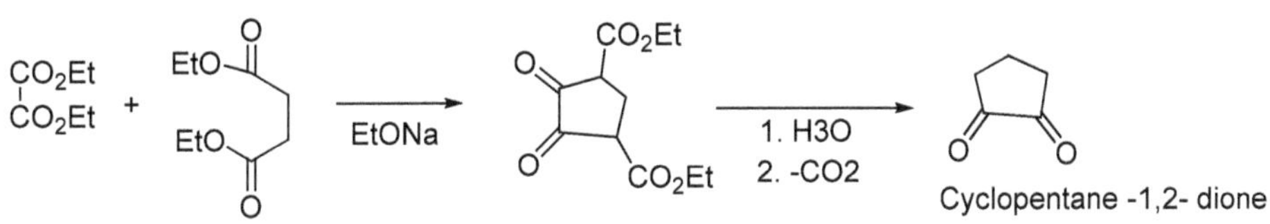

4. 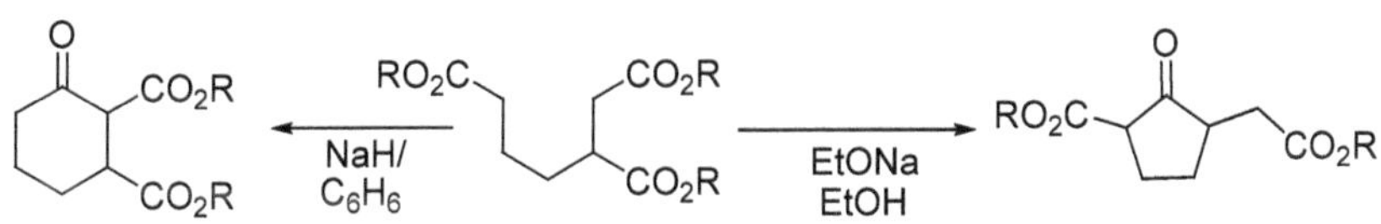

5. 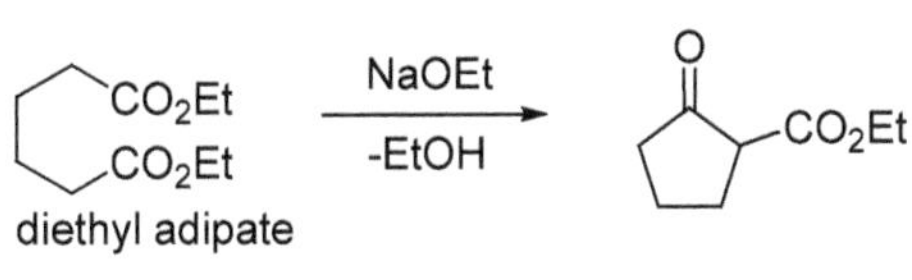

From Synthesis of Camphoric Acid

6.

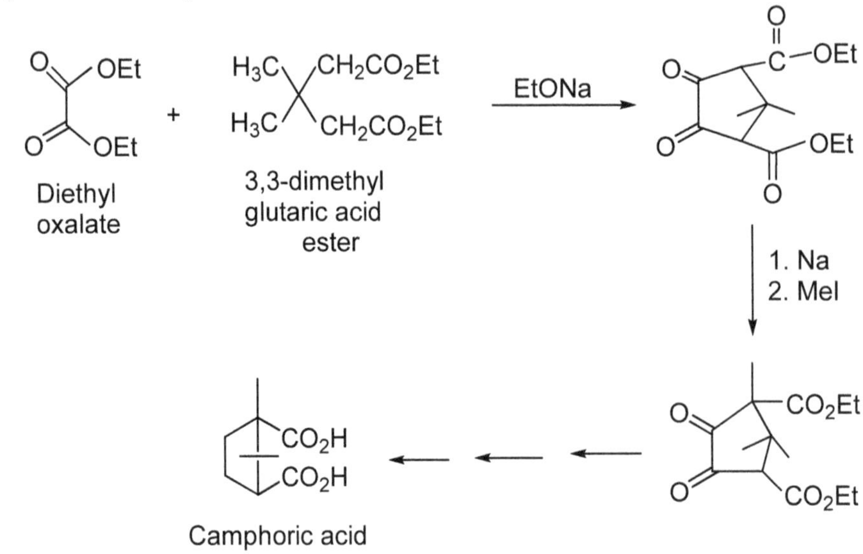

From Total Synthesis of α–pinene

7.

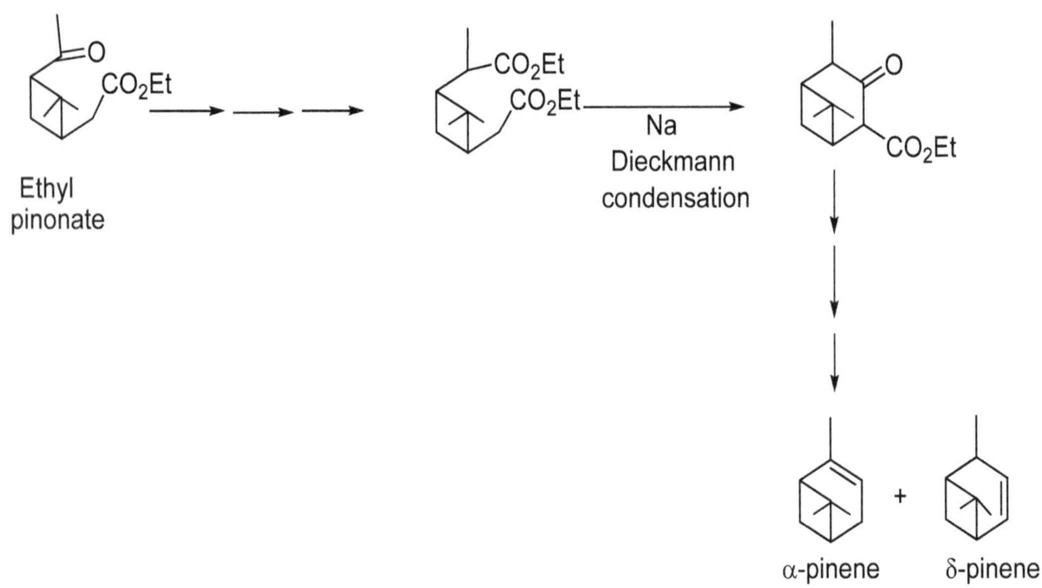

8. Conversion of diethyl succinate and diethyl adipate by microwave irradiation[7]

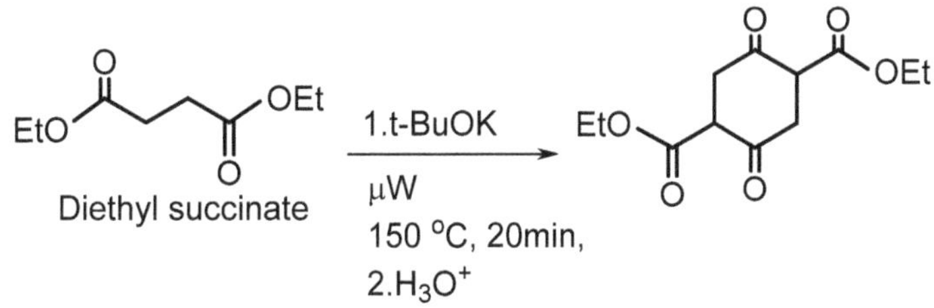

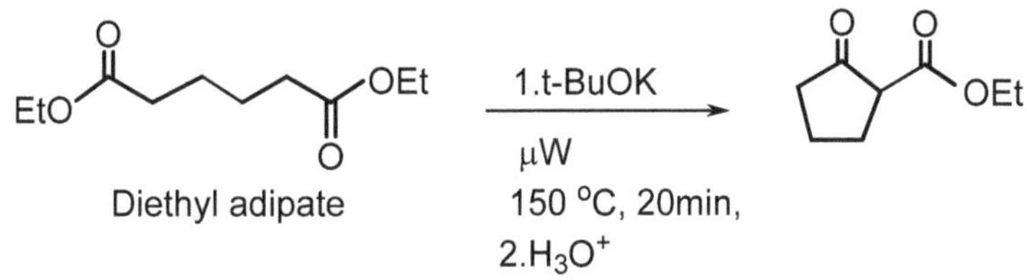

9. Preparation of thiophene derivatives promoted by base catalysis[8]

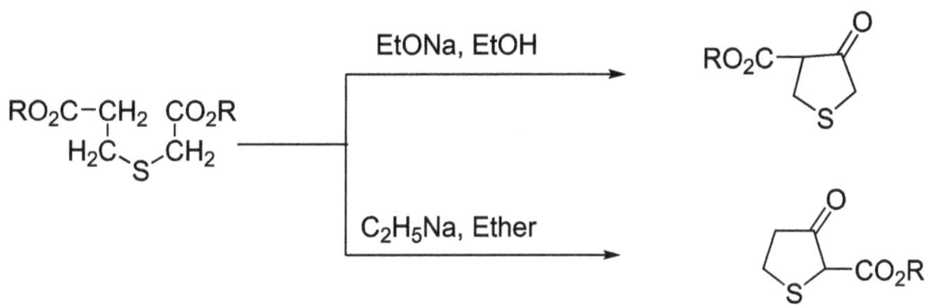

10. Solid-state Dieckmann condensation reaction[8]

Diethyl adipate and diethyl pimelates can be easily prepared by green methods like solid state reaction in the absence of any solvent in the presence of a base from powdered reaction mixture.

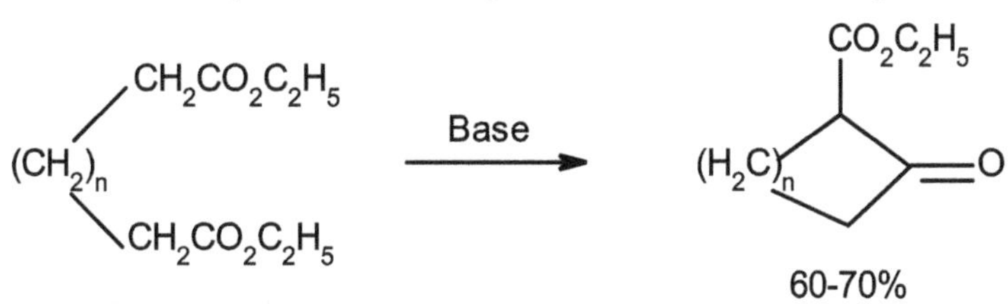

Diethyl adipate n = 2
Diethyl pimelate n = 3

11. Dieckmann condensation under sonication[8]

The reaction took place well under the influence of sonication and dispersed potassium in toluene catalyzed the reaction efficiently.

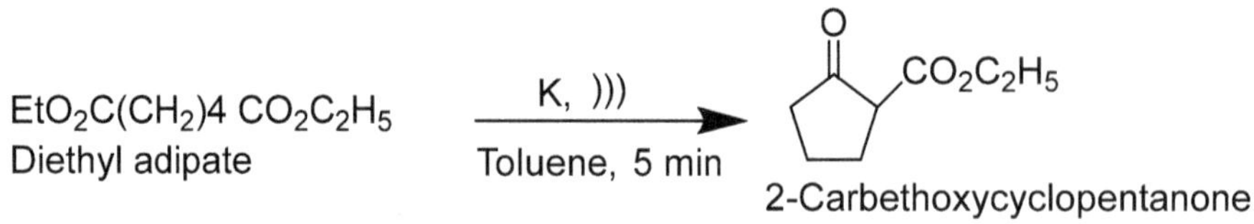

12. Microwave assisted synthesis of *N*-phenylsuccinimide[9]

By heating a mixture of aniline and succinic anhydride in a domestic microwave oven for four minutes, *N*-phenylsuccinimide is obtained in moderate yields.

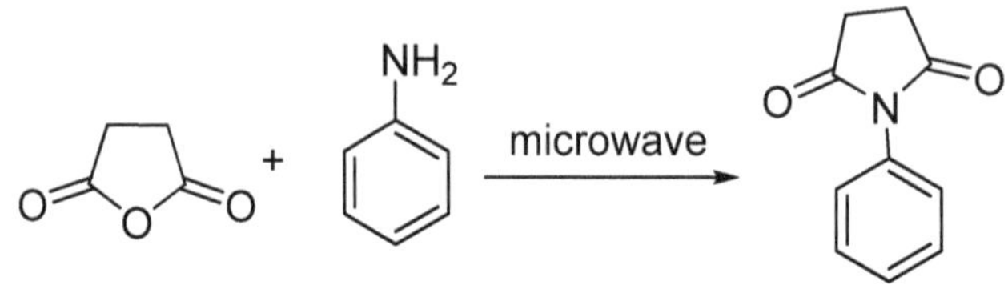

2.4 Doebner-Miller Reaction

Named after the Czech chemist Zdenko Hans Skraup and the German chemists Oscar Döbner (Doebner) and Wilhelm von Miller, this reaction is also known as Skraup-Doebner-Von Miller quinoline synthesis. This reaction is also a variant of the Skraup quinoline synthesis.

Primary aromatic amines (e.g., anilines) and α, β-unsaturated carbonyl compounds (mostly α, β-unsaturated aldehydes) undergo condensation to afford 2,3-disubstituted quinolines, catalyzed by Lewis acids or Brønsted acids. It can also be performed from primary aromatic amines, aldehydes and α-keto acids like 2-oxopropanoic acid or pyruvic acid. In such cases the reaction proceeds through three steps. **1.** Formation of β, γ-unsaturated alpha keto acid **2.** Michael addition with primary aromatic amine **3.** Air oxidation. Different catalysts like tin tetrachloride ($SnCl_4$), scandium (III) triflate $Sc(OTf)_3$, Ytterbium (III) trifluoromethanesulfonate (Yb (OTf)3), Zinc chloride ($ZnCl_2$), Indium (III) chloride ($InCl_3$), p-toluenesulfonic acid ($CH_3C_6H_4SO_3H$- PTSA or *p*-TsOH), perchloric acid ($HClO_4$), amberlite or iodine can be used. Moreover, microwave irradiation with the assistance of Lewis acid activators like montmorillonite K-10 is also reportedly employed to achieve this reaction.

General reaction:

a)

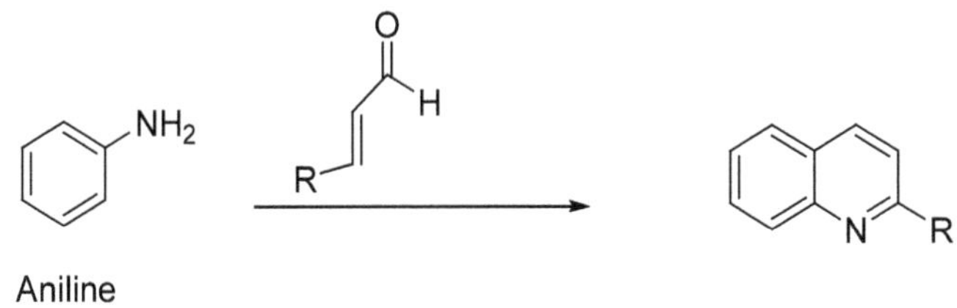

b)

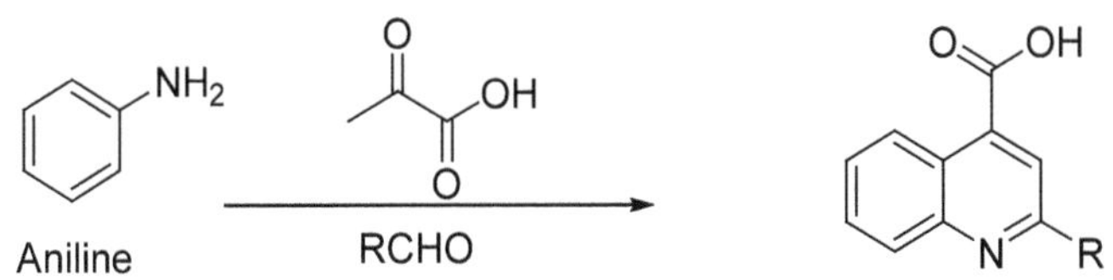

c)

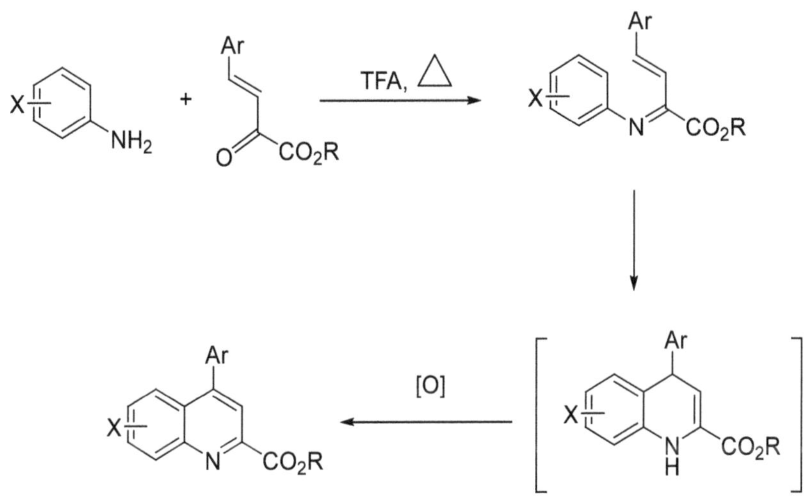

Mechanism:

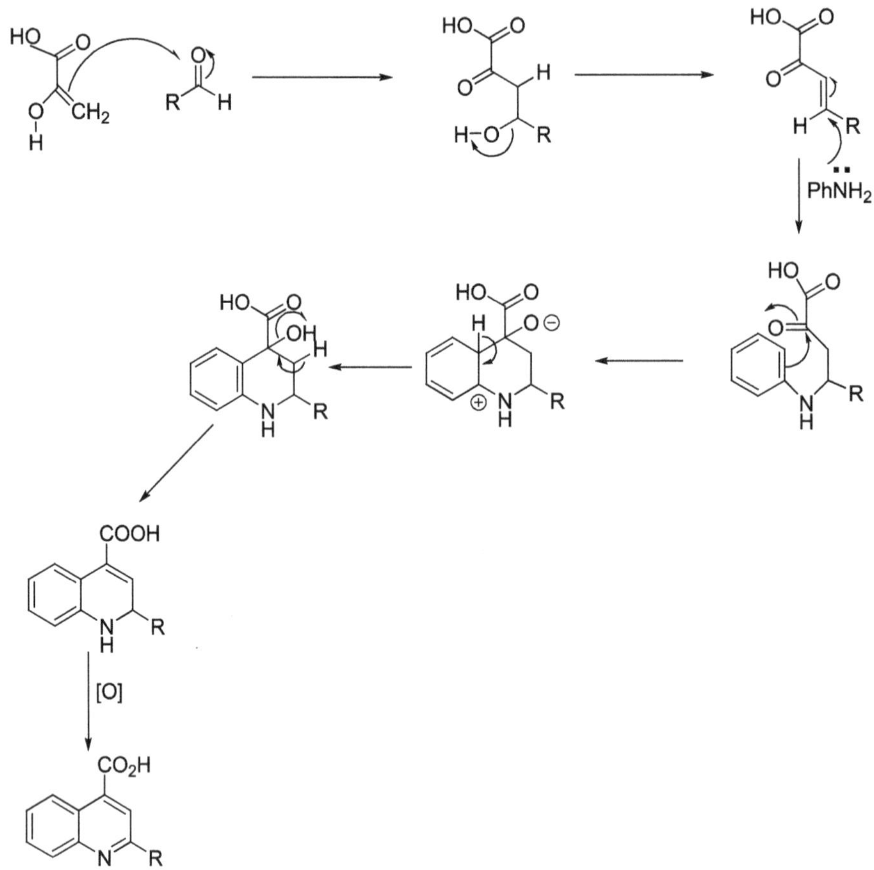

Applications and examples:

1.

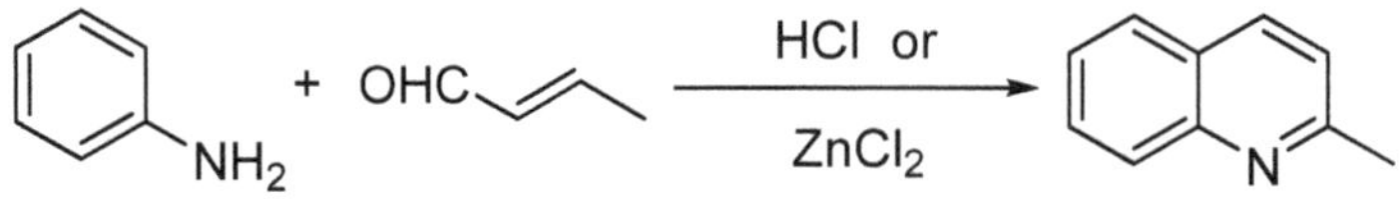

2. Synthesis of quinaldines and lepidines under thermal and microwave irradiation[10]

Quinaldines and lepidines can be produced by a one-pot reaction of anilines with crotonaldehyde or methyl vinyl ketone using phosphotungstic acid, a Keggins-type heteropoly acid, under both thermal and microwave irradiation conditions.

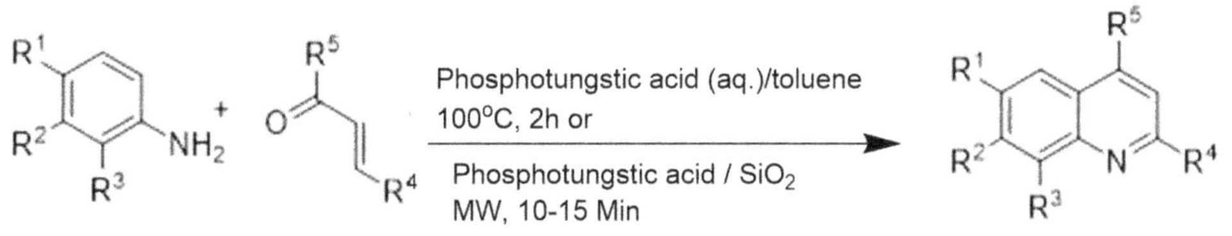

3. Preparation of Quinoline Derivatives[11]

Various substituted quinoline derivatives can be prepared from anilines and both aromatic and aliphatic α, β-unsaturated aldehydes catalyzed by recyclable Ag(I)-exchanged Montmorillonite K10.

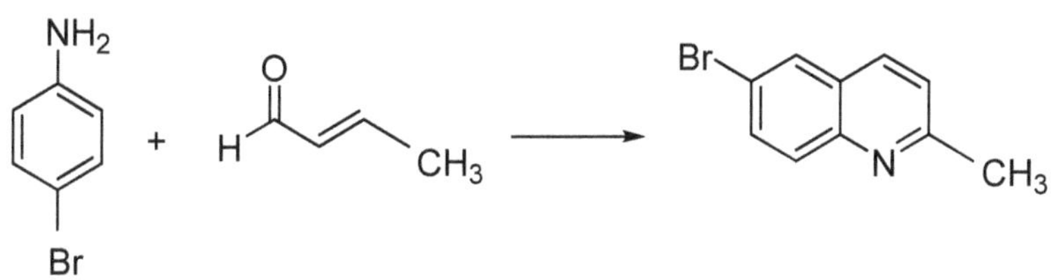

2.5 Mannich Reaction

This multicomponent condensation reaction, developed by Carl Mannich, involves the aminoalkylation of an acidic proton next to a carbonyl group by formaldehyde and a primary or secondary amine or ammonia. The product is a β-amino-carbonyl compound, known as Mannich base. Tertiary amines cannot participate in this reaction as these do not have N–H proton. Aryl amines generally do not participate in the reaction. Apart from carbonyl compounds phenols, nitriles, acetylenes, aliphatic nitro compounds, α-alkyl-or γ-alkyl pyridines or α-alkyl-or γ alkyl quinolines, imines can also react with Schiff base. Others like activated phenyl groups and electron-rich heterocycles such as furan, pyrrole, thiophene and indole derivatives also participate in this reaction. If the compound possesses more than one active hydrogen, all of them can be substituted by amino methyl groups. This reaction can be catalyzed by acid or base. It is extensively studied and applied.

The Mannich reaction is applied in many areas like agrochemicals, alkaloids, organic intermediates, catalysts, nucleotides, peptides, pharmaceuticals (in the production of fluoxetine, a powerful antidepressant, and nonsteroidal anti-inflammatory drug tolmetin), polymers, and soap and detergents etc., It is involved in many biological pathways.

General reaction

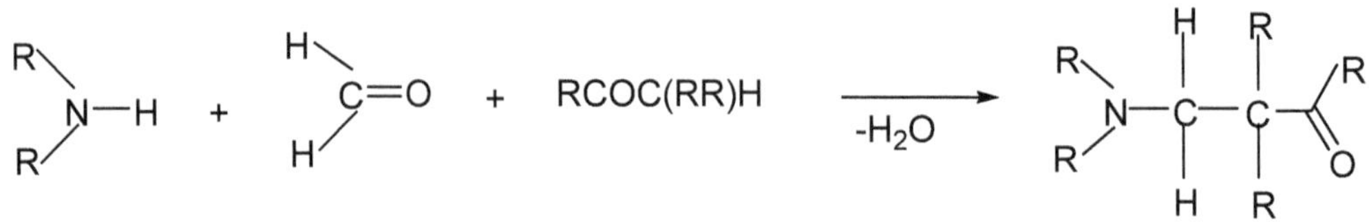

Mechanism

The reaction is initiated by the nucleophilic addition of an amine to a carbonyl group, via the formation of an iminium ion from the amine and formaldehyde, followed by dehydration to the Schiff base. The enol formed from the carbonyl compound containing an acidic α-proton undergoes electrophilic addition with the Schiff base.

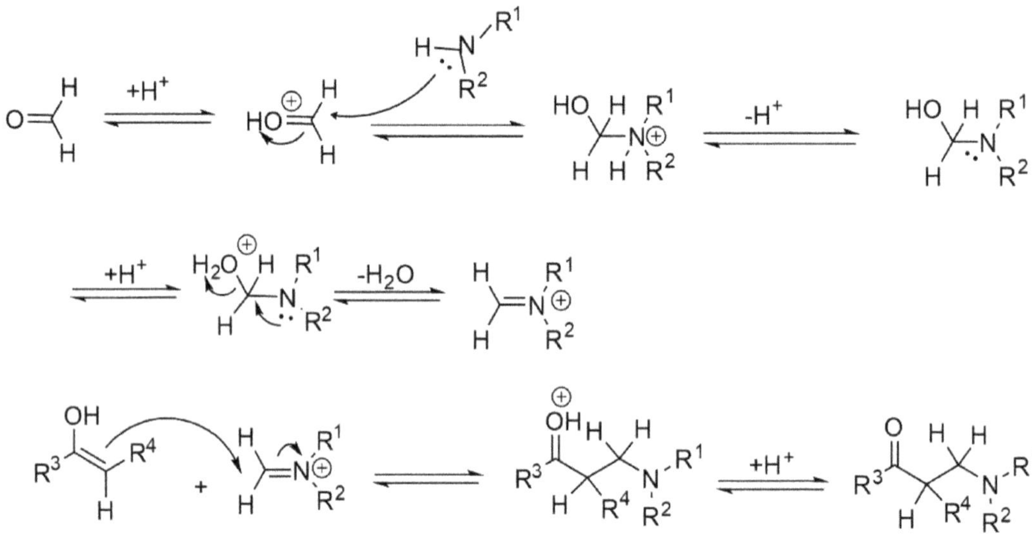

Applications and examples

1. $PhCOCH_3 + HCHO + (CH_3)_2NH.HCl \longrightarrow PhCOCH_2CH_2N(CH_3)_2.HCl + H_2O$

2.

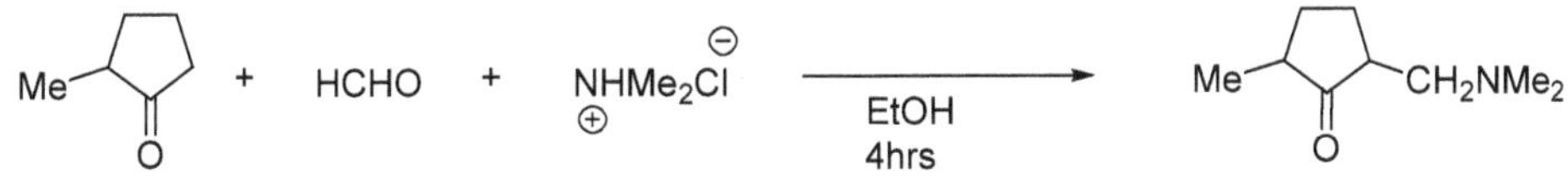

3.

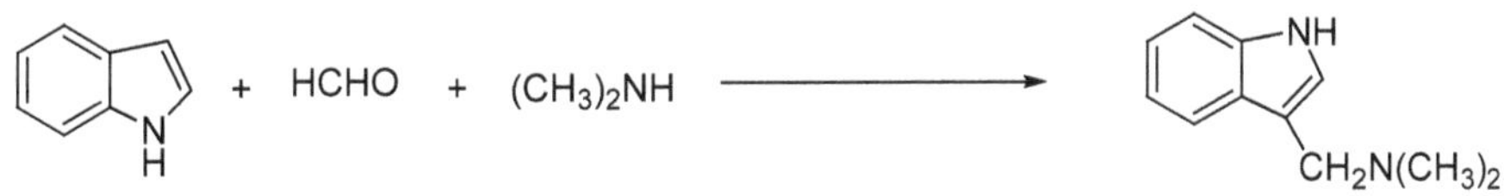

4.

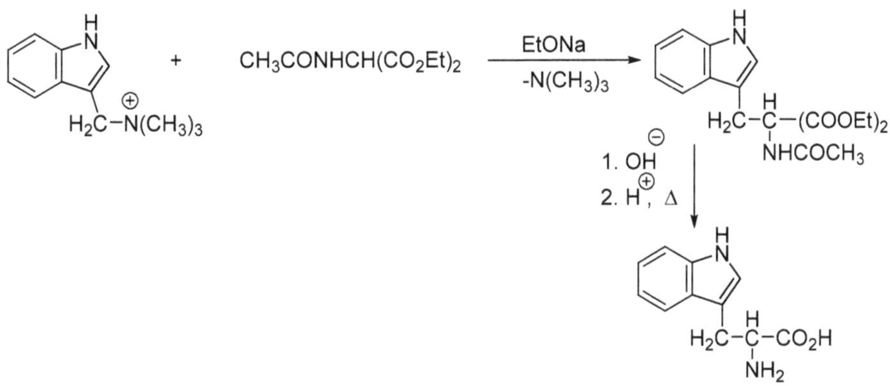

5.

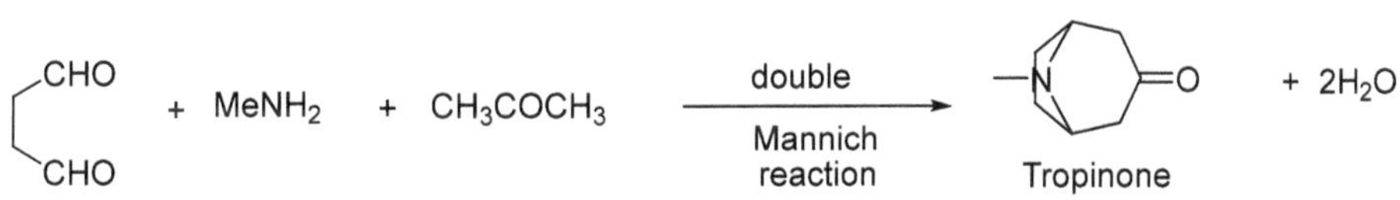

2.6 Michael Addition Reaction

The Michael reaction, invented by Arthur Michael, is the addition of an enolate of a ketone or aldehyde to an α,β-unsaturated carbonyl compound at the β carbon., or the 1,4-addition of a doubly stabilized carbon nucleophile to an α,β-unsaturated carbonyl compound. It can also be viewed as an addition reaction between α,α-disubstituted carbonyls, nitriles, sulfones, etc., called Michael donors and α,β-unsaturated carbonyls, nitriles, nitro, etc., called Michael acceptors. It is an important, widely applicable and atom-economical conjugate addition reaction, leading to the formation of C-C bonds (Michael adducts). These reactions can be enantioselective or/and diastereoselective. Tandem sequence of Michael and aldol additions is called the Robinson annulation.

General reaction:

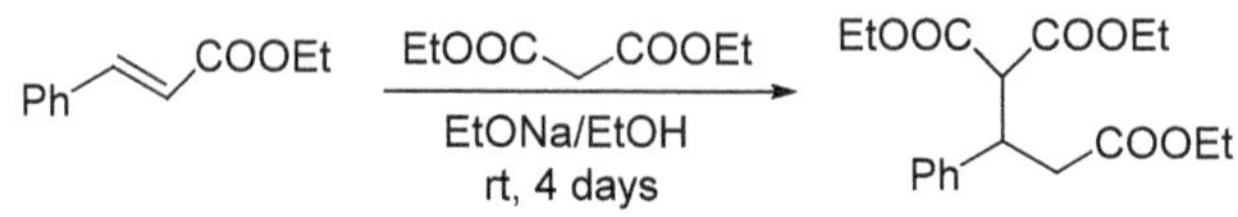

Mechanism

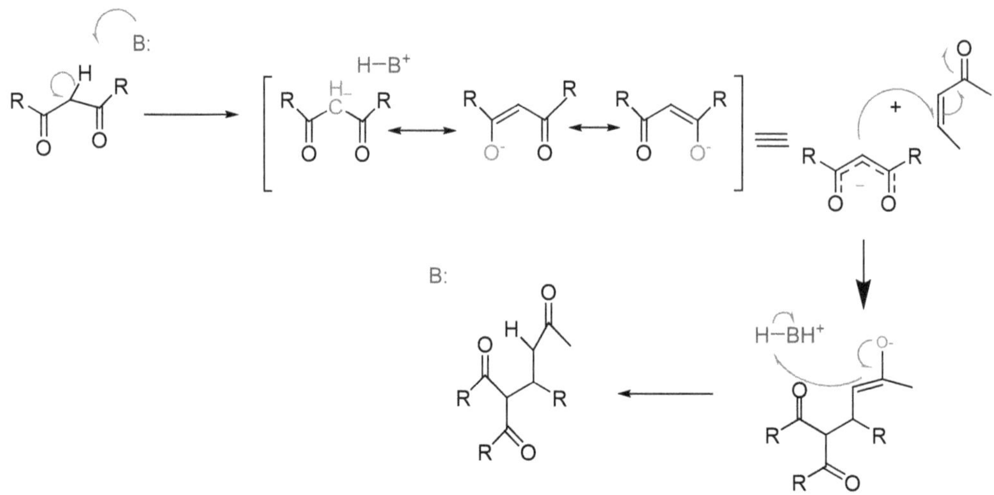

Applications and examples:

1. Preparation of ethyl propane-1,1,2,3-tetracarboxylate[12]

The addition reaction between diethyl malonate (Michael donor) and diethyl fumarate (Michael acceptor) in the presence of Na/EtOH under reflux generates the title compound.

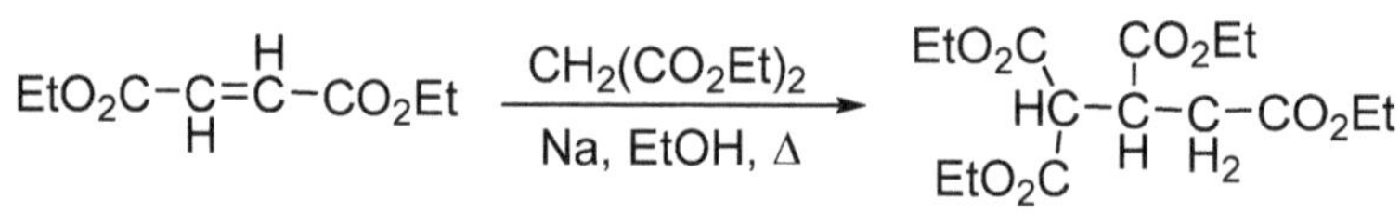

2. Preparation of methyl γ-methyl-γ-nitro valerate[13]

The reaction between and 2-nitropropane and methyl acrylate in the presence of 40% aqueous solution of benzyl trimethylammonium hydroxide (Triton B) in dioxane under reflux conditions forms the product.

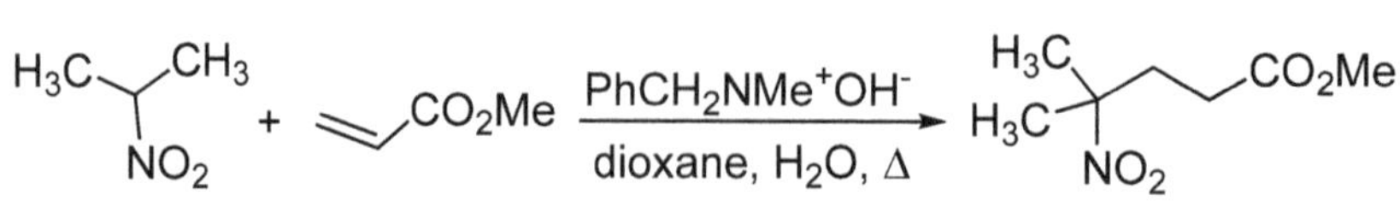

3. Preparation of 5-nitroheptan-2-one[14]

Methyl vinyl ketone reacts with 1-nitropropane catalyzed by diisopropylamine in CHC13 under reflux to generate the product.

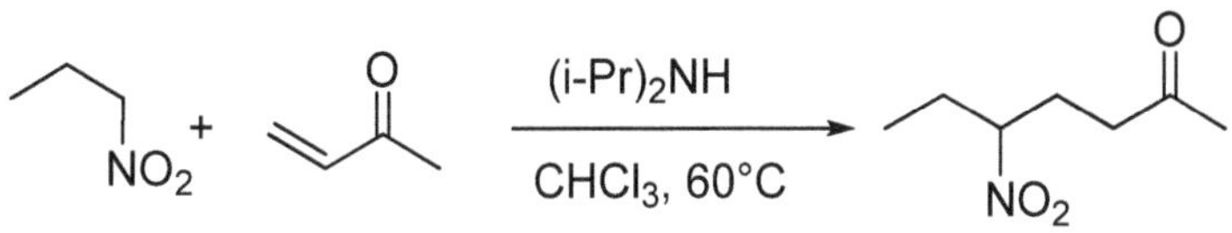

4. Preparation of warfarin[15]

The addition reaction between 4-hydroxycoumarin and benzylideneacetone produces Warfarin by Michael reaction.

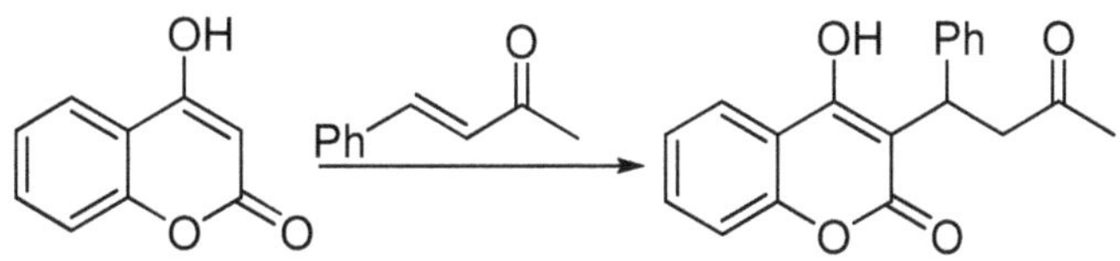

5. A step from the synthesis of cincholoiponic acid

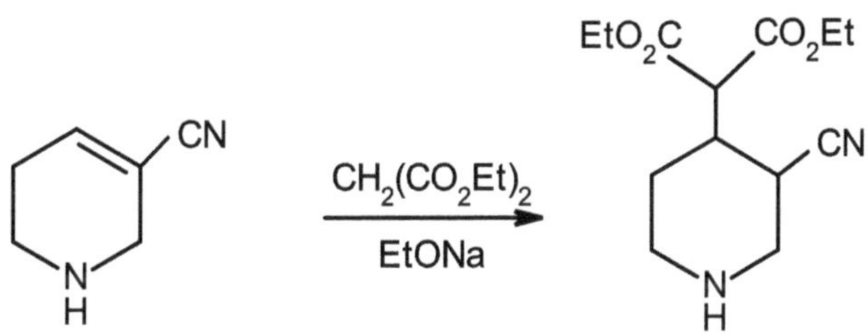

6. An example from the total synthesis of Cholesterol by Woodward.

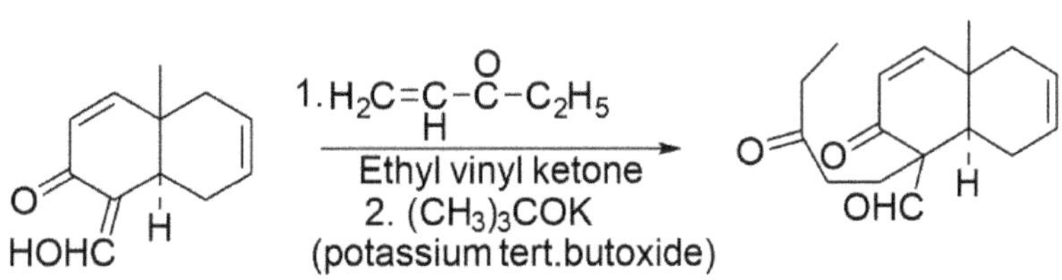

7. Perkin and Thorpe employed Michael condensation as a step in the synthesis of caronic acid from ethyl cyanoacetate and ethyl β, β dimethyl acrylate.

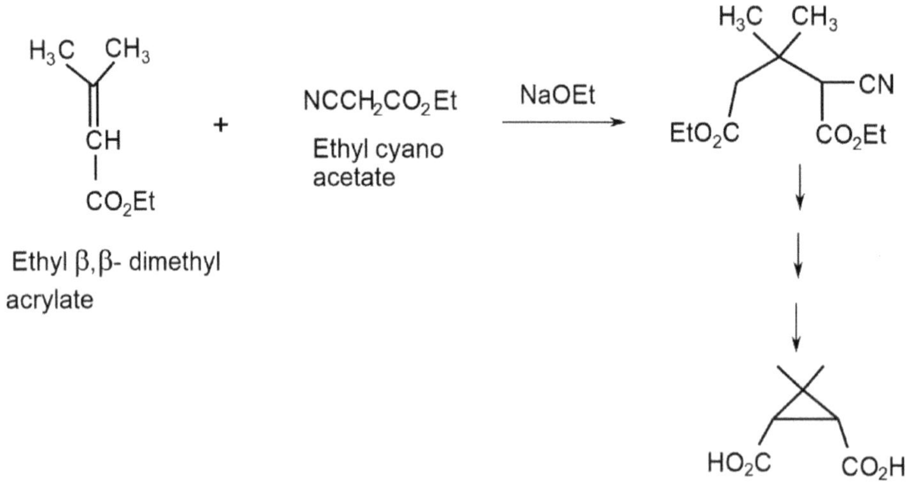

Caronic acid

8. Michael addition reaction mediated by microwave irradiation[16]

Michael addition of active methylene compounds to, α,β -unsaturated carbonyl compounds take place on the surface of potassium carbonate under solvent-free microwave irradiation conditions.

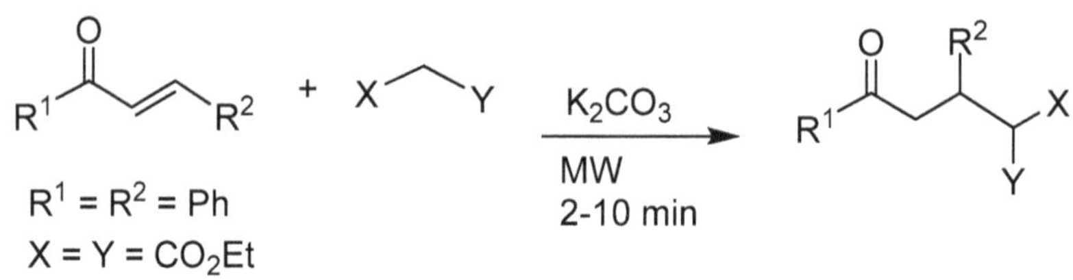

2.7 Mitsunobu reaction

Discovered by Oyo Mitsunobu, the reaction deals with the conversion of primary and secondary alcohols into a variety of functional groups, such as an ester, phenyl ethers, thioethers, etc., using triphenyl phosphine and an azodicarboxylate like diethyl azodicarboxylate (DEAD) or diisopropyl azodicarboxylate (DIAD). Apart from DEAD, DIAD some other azodicarboxylates also facilitate the reaction. Apart from carboxylic acids, imides, phenols, hydrazoic acid, arylsulfonylhydrazine and sulfonamides can also act as nucleophiles. Many variations and modifications as well as applications of this reaction are in practice. When a nitrogen nucleophile is involved, it is known as a Fukuyama–Mitsunobu reaction.

General reaction:

a)

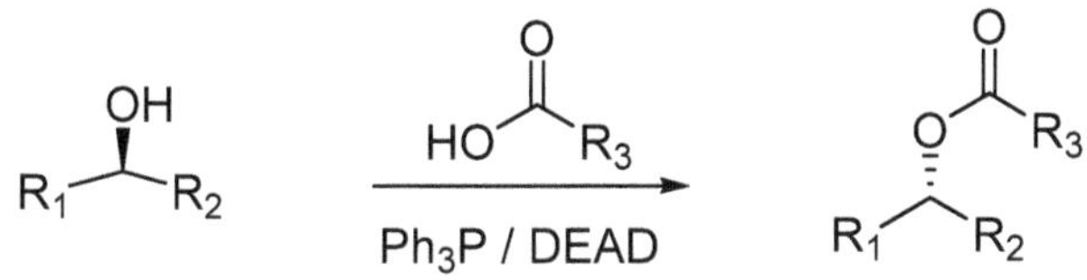

b)

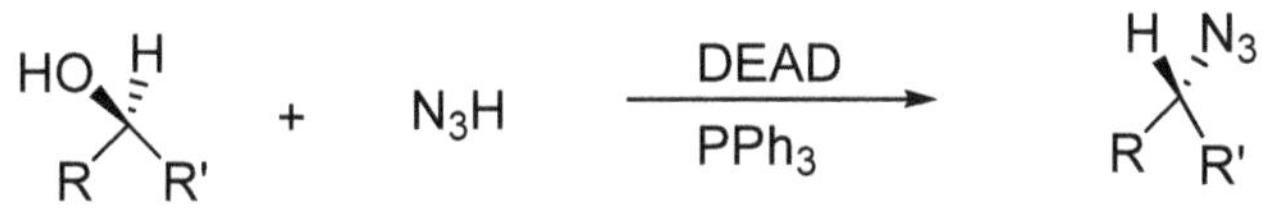

Mechanism:

Initially, a betaine intermediate is formed by the nucleophilic attack of triphenyl phosphine upon diethyl azodicarboxylate. This deprotonates the carboxylic acid to form the ion pair. The key oxophosphonium ion is formed by the alkoxide, which is produced by the deprotonation. The desired product is generated by the attack of the carboxylate anion on key oxophosphonium ion. The alcohol reacts with the phosphine and undergoes an inversion of stereochemistry in classic S_N2 mode.

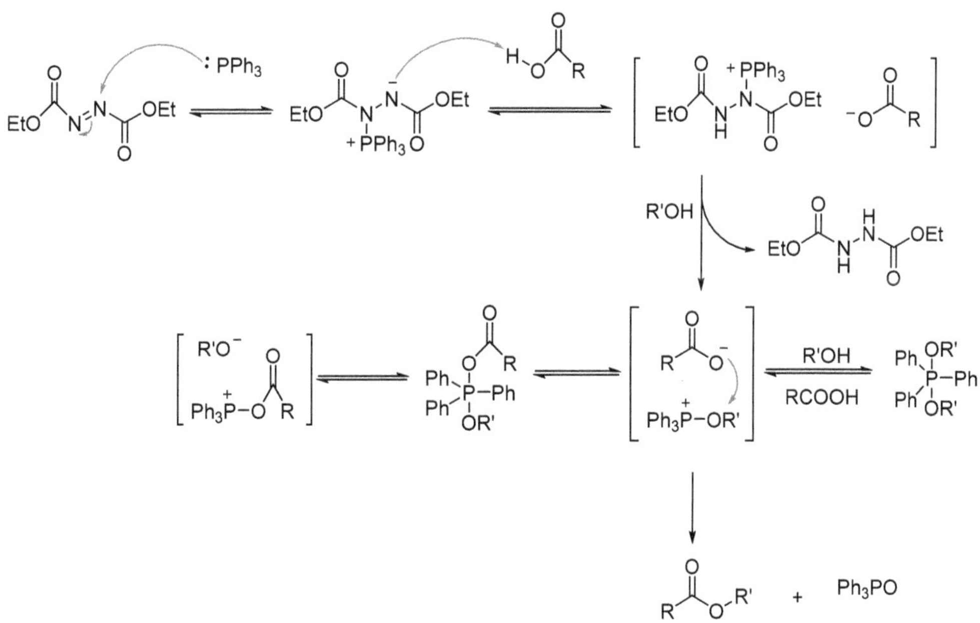

Applications and examples:

1. The Synthesis of Substituted Allylic Amines from Allylic Alcohols

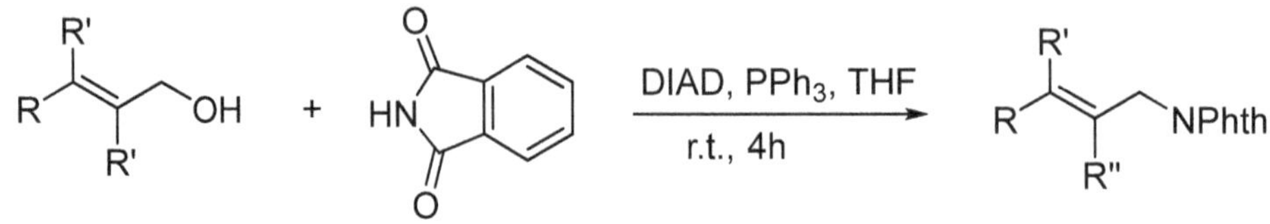

2. Mitsunobu Reaction under sonication[17]

The research scientists observed that the coupling reaction of sterically hindered phenols and alcohols is greatly accelerated by the use of high reaction concentrations under sonication. The mono- and di-o-substituted phenols were reacted with cyclohexanol and neopentyl alcohol successfully.

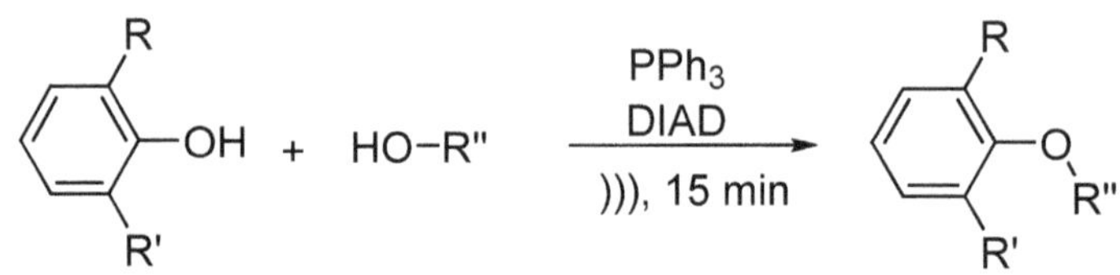

2.8 Ozonolysis Reaction

Ozonolysis is a chemical reaction where ozone is used to cleave the unsaturated bonds like alkene (C=C), alkyne, and azo compounds to determine the position of unsaturation. Ozone is a very reactive allotrope of oxygen and reacts readily with unsaturated compounds. It is discovered in 1845 by Christian Friedrich Schönbein, who discovered ozone in 1840. It is used extensively in the determination of the structure of natural products and aromatic compounds. It leads to the formation of ozonides. On hydrogenation or treatment with acid, ozonide forms a mixture containing aldehydes, ketones, or carboxylic acids. The azo compounds on ozonation give nitrosamines (N–N=O). Alkynes generally give an acid anhydride or diketone product and the anhydride hydrolyzes to give two carboxylic acids in the presence of water. The products depend on the type of multiple bonds being oxidized and the workup conditions. Ozonolysis is considered an organic redox reaction. It is conducted by bubbling ozone through the reaction medium generally in methanol at −78 °C until the solution turns to blue due to unreacted ozone. The completion of the reaction can be ascertained by the use of indicators. The ozonide is further worked up by reduction or oxidation. Reaction with NaBH4 produces alcohols. Aldehydes or ketones are produced on treating with of triphenylphosphine, thiourea, zinc dust, or dimethyl sulfide. Treatment with hydrogen peroxide generates carboxylic acid.

General reaction:

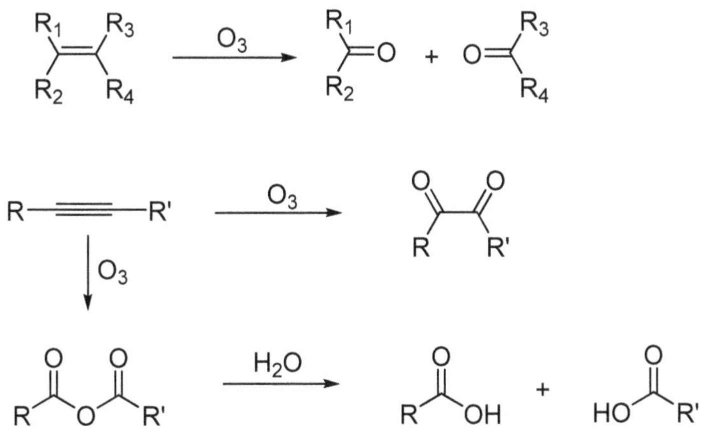

Mechanism:

Rudolf Criegee in 1953 proposed reaction mechanism. The reaction follows 1,3-dipolar cycloadditions. Initially an intermediate molozonide is formed in a 1,3-dipolar cycloaddition, followed by reversion to the Criegee intermediate or Criegee zwitterion. Stable ozonide intermediate called trioxolane is formed by further 1,3-dipolar cycloaddition.

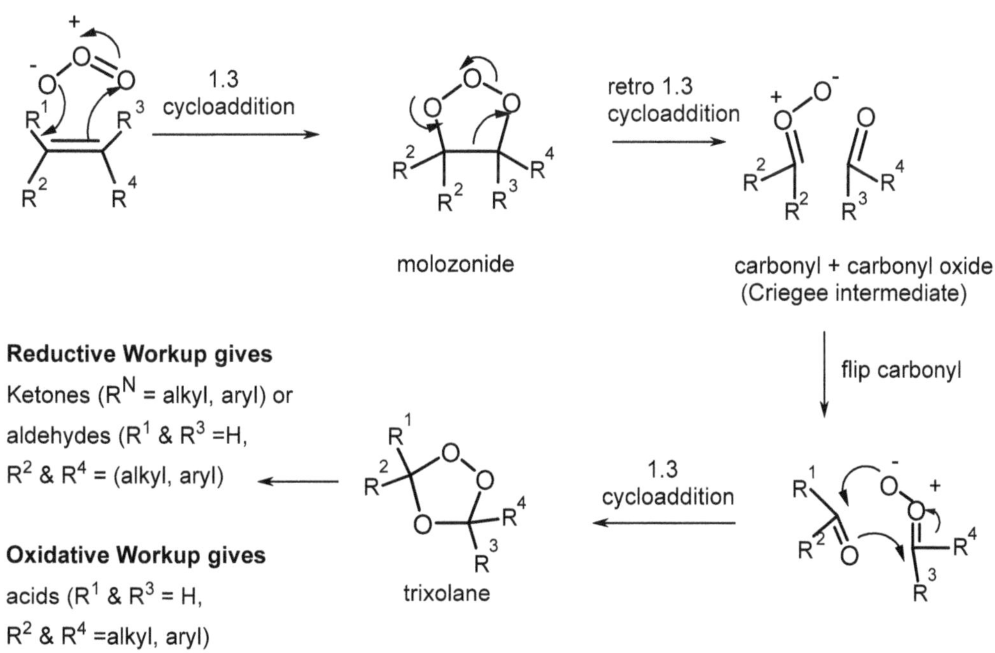

Applications and examples:

Reductive Workup

1.

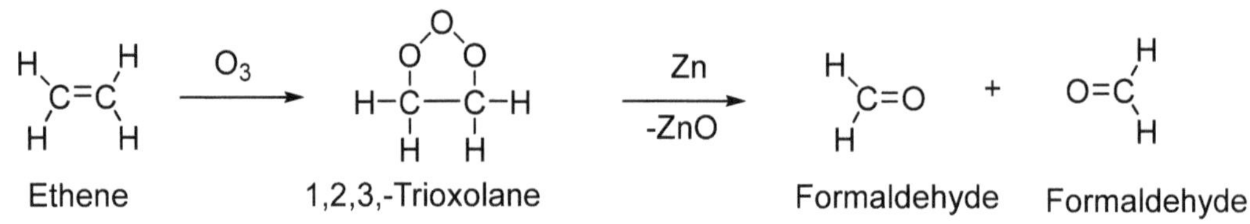

2.

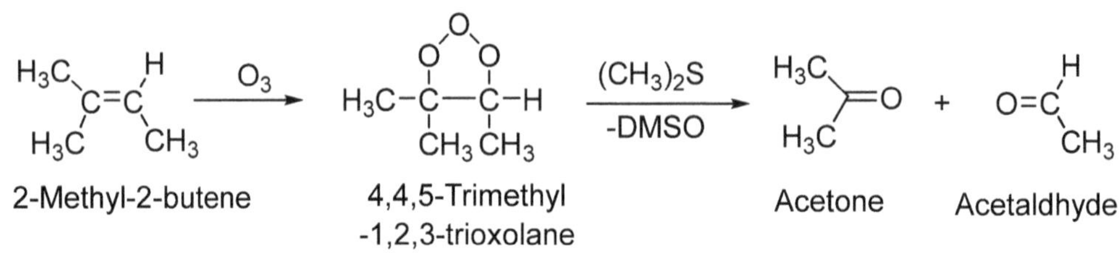

3.

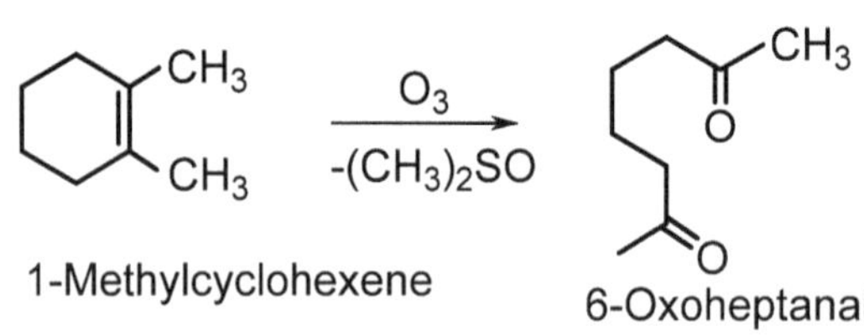

Oxidative workup (Aldehyde get oxidized to carboxylic acid)

4.

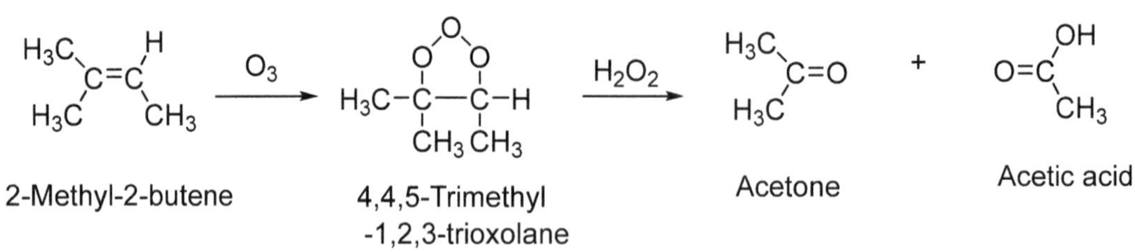

5. Ozonolysis of oleic acid

$$C_8H_{17}CH{=}CHC_7H_{14}CO_2H + 4\,O_3 \longrightarrow \underset{\text{Azelaic acid}}{HO_2C{-}C_7H_{14}{-}CO_2H} + \underset{\text{Nonanoic acid}}{C_8H_{17}{-}CO_2H}$$

6.

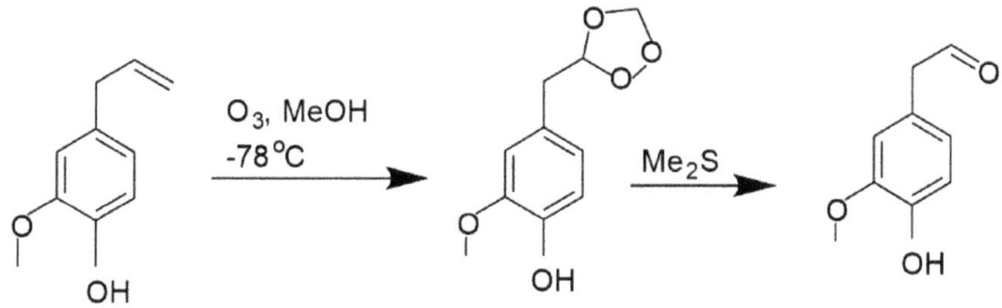

Eugenol

7.

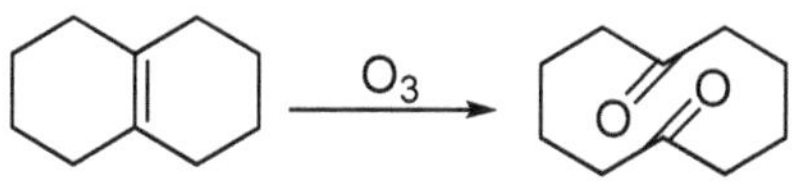

Cyclodecane 1,6-dione

8.

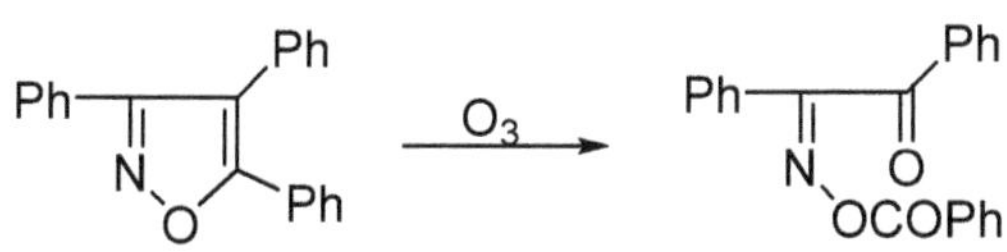

Triphenyl isoxazole

Benzyl derivative of anti-phenyl benzil monooxime

9.

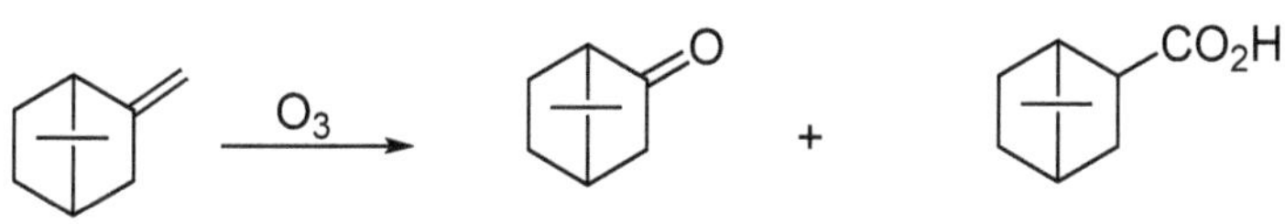

α–Fenchene

α–Fencho camphorone (Major)

(Minor)

10.

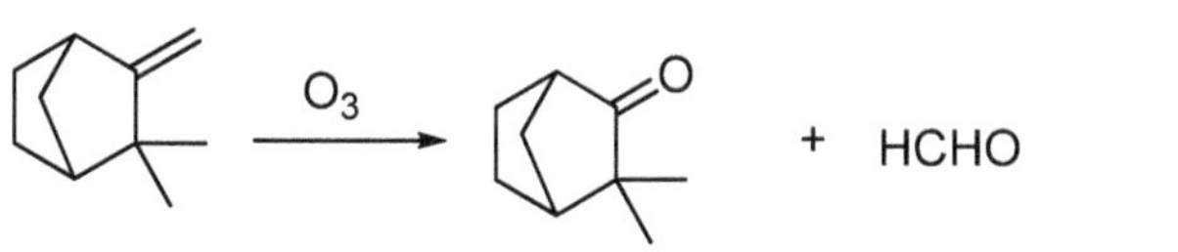

Camphene

Camphenilone

Formaldehyde

11

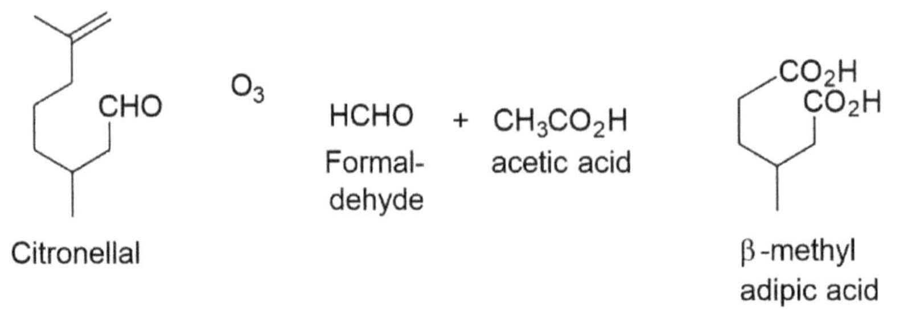

12

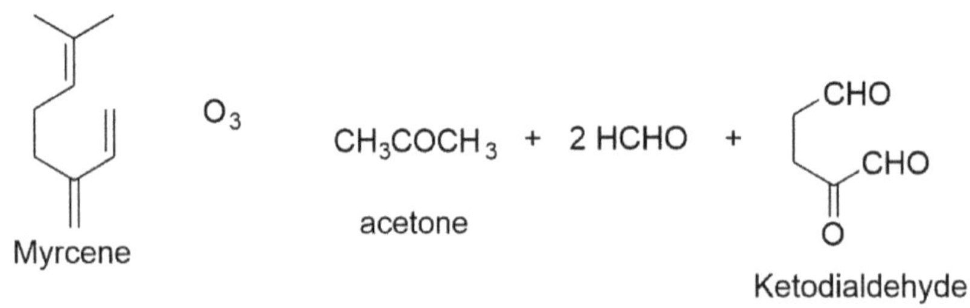

13

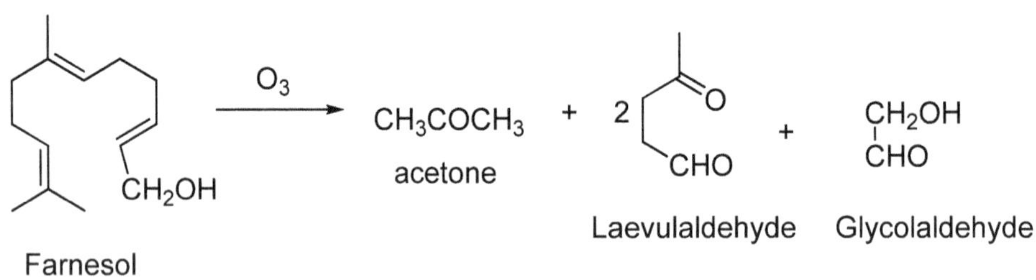

14

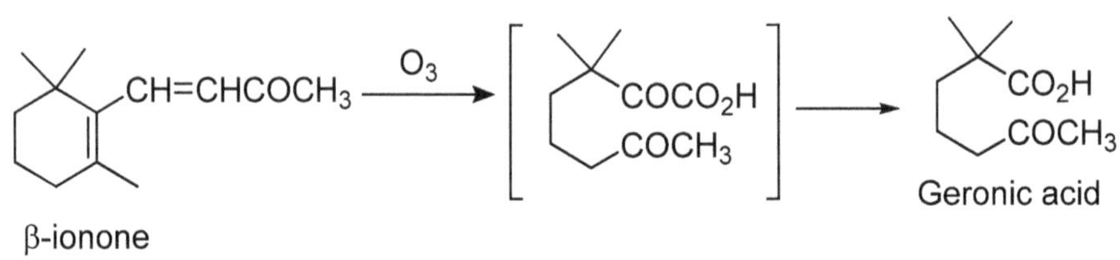

15 **From Progesterone Synthesis**

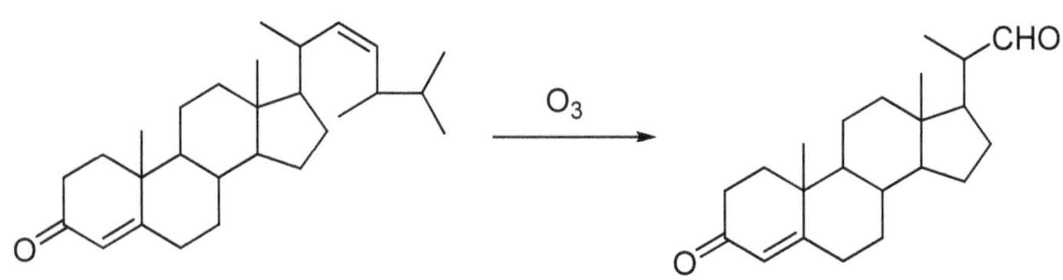

2.9 Sandmeyer reaction

The Sandmeyer reaction was first discovered in the year 1884 by Traugott Sandmeyer, a Swiss chemist. When he was carrying out a reaction to prepare phenylacetylene from benzenediazonium chloride and cuprous acetylide, he obtained phenyl chloride as the main product. This is widely used for the synthesis of aryl halides from aryl diazonium salts. In this reaction the amino group attached to an aromatic ring is converted into a diazonium salt by the treatment with nitrous acid in the presence of mineral acids (HCl or H_2SO_4) at low temperatures (0-5°C). The diazonium salt can be transformed into various functional groups. The diazonium salt is decomposed by heating with CuCl or CuBr in the presence of excess HCl or HBr resulting in aryl chlorides or bromides. In this the diazonium group acts as an excellent leaving group facilitating substitution.

It has wide utility and applicability in the organic transformations. Many variations and adaptations were developed over the original reaction leading to the generation of phenols, aryl thioethers, aryl nitriles and aryl fluorides (the Schiemann reaction). It can be categorized as a substitution reaction and an example of radical-nucleophilic aromatic substitution ($S_{RN}Ar$). Copper salts like Copper chloride, Copper bromide or Copper iodide are used as catalysts. The reaction is a two-step process, a). the formation of diazonium salts, b). conversion of diazo intermediates into aryl halides. Here N2 acts as an excellent leaving group. However, presently any reaction displacing diazo group by any nucleophile in the presence of catalytic copper(I) salts can be referred as Sandmeyer reaction. Apart from copper salts other transition metal salts like iron (III) and cobalt (III) have also been used. By virtue of the wider applicability, variations and importance this reaction is treated as complementary to electrophilic aromatic substitution.

General reaction:

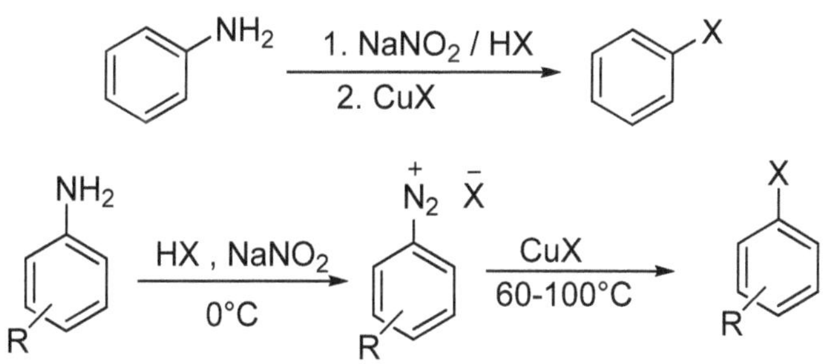

X= CN, Br, Cl,SO_3H

Mechanism:

Copper has the ability to reduce the diazonium salt into aryl radical by oxidation-reduction sequence involving single electron transfer. It first reduces and then oxidizes. The formation of aryl halide by cupric ion may proceed either through carboniumion or organocopper compound.

Step I - Formation of diazonium salt.

Step II – Decomposition of diazonium salt and substitution.

Extensions of the reaction

Gattermann reaction

It uses copper bronze or copper powder in place of cuprous chloride.

Schiemann reaction

Aryl fluorides can be prepared by reacting diazonium salt with fluoroboric acid or fluoroborate salt.

Applications and examples:

1. Preparation of aryl halides.

a)

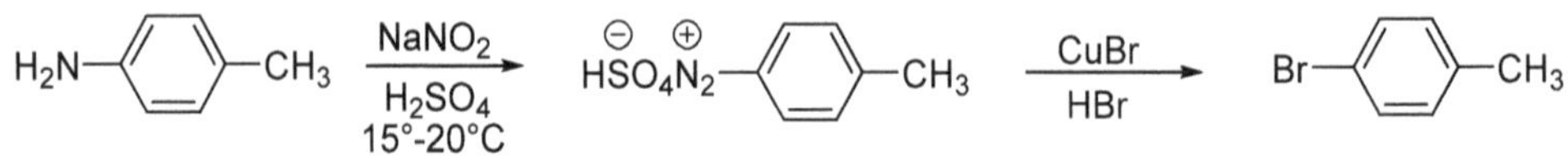

b)

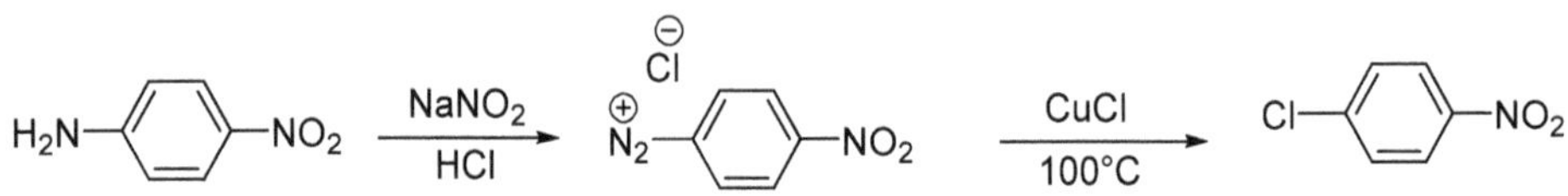

c)

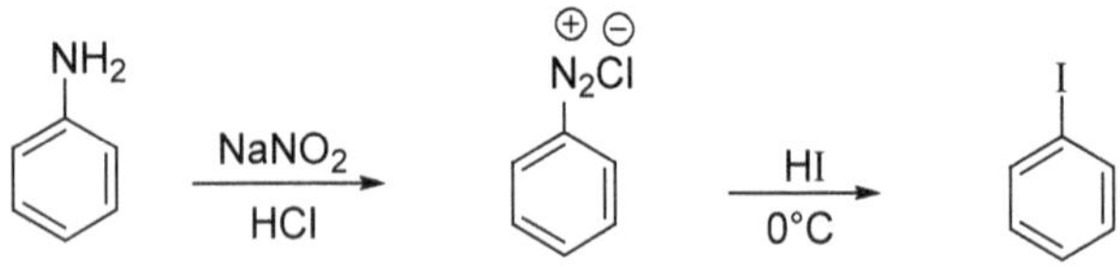

d)

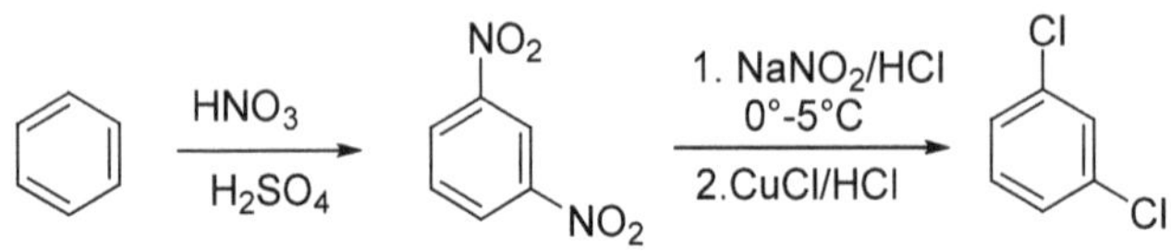

e)

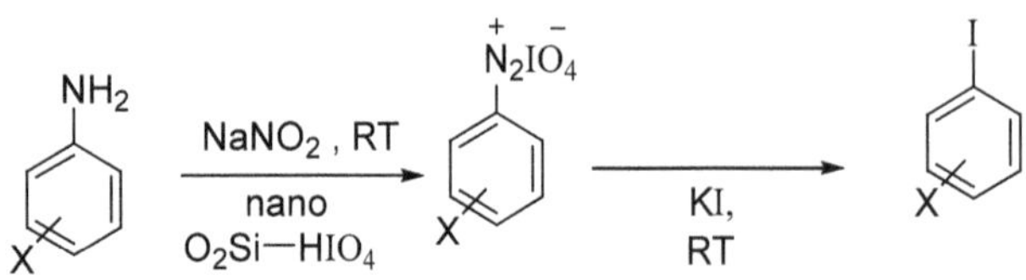

X= Cl; Br; Me; NO_2; H

2. Preparation of phenols[18]

Aryl amines are converted to phenols at room temperature proceeding through the formation of an aryl diazonium salt, in the presence of copper catalyst.

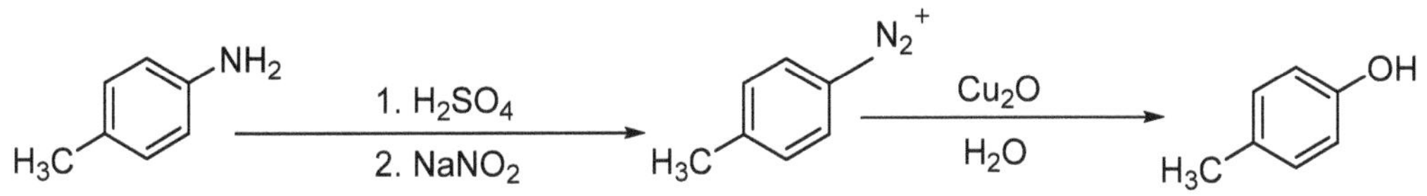

3. Preparation of benzonitriles

a)

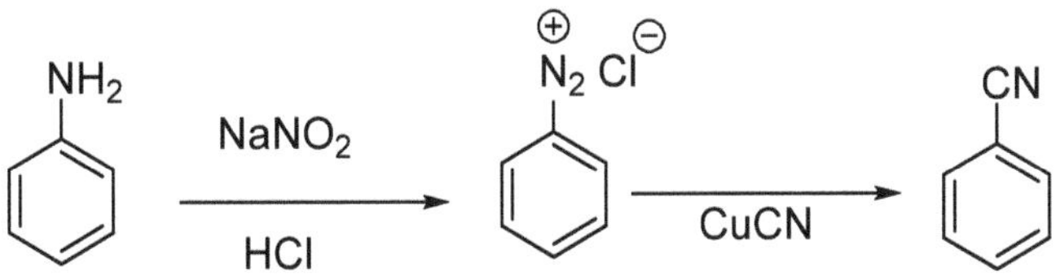

b) A new process was developed for the production of 2-chloro-5-trifluoromethyl-benzonitrile by the Sandmeyer reaction of 2-chloro-5-trifluoromethylaniline employing copper cyanide/sodium cyanide[19].

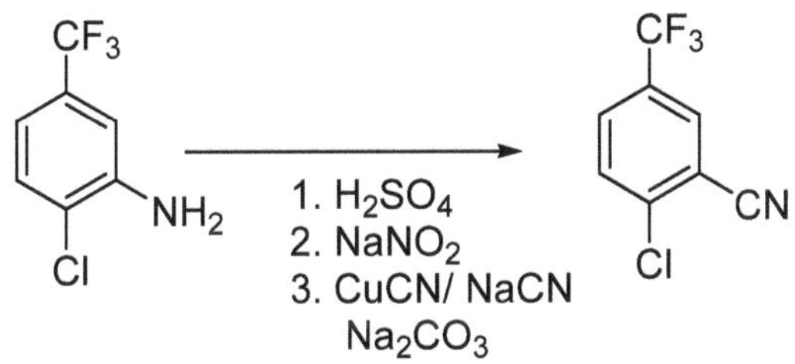

4. Preparation of benzoic acid

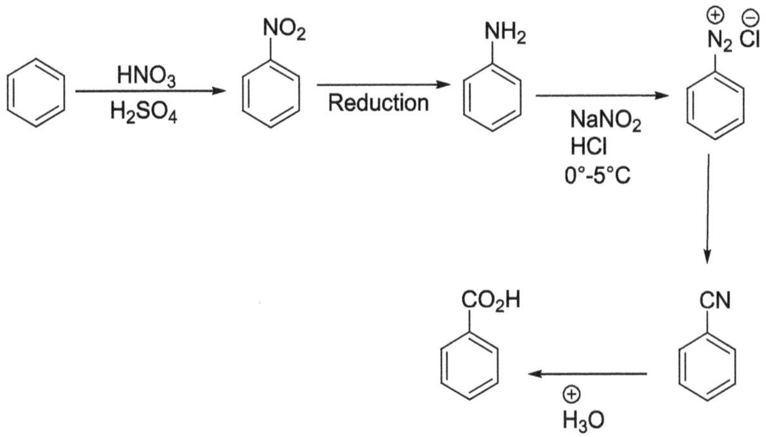

5. Preparation of 3- nitro toluene

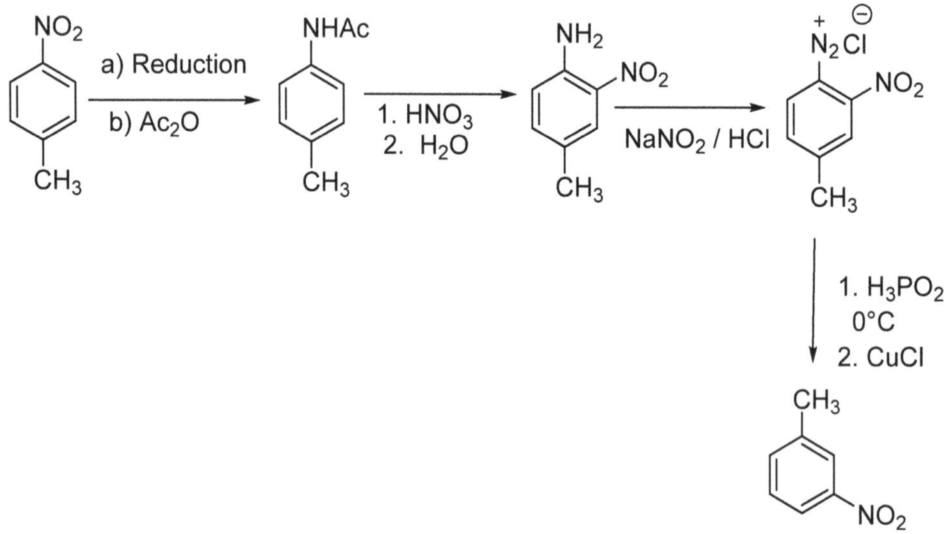

2.10 Shapiro Reaction

The Shapiro reaction, reported by Robert H. Shapiro in 1967 is a variant of the Bamford-Stevens reaction which was first reported in 1952.

These two are convenient methods for synthesizing olefinic compounds from ketones and aldehydes via sulfonyl hydrazones. In Bamford and Stevens reaction strong bases such as NaOMe, NaH, LiH, $NaNH_2$, etc. are used, whereas in the Shapiro reaction the bases like alkyllithiums and Grignard reagents are used. Both the reactions have similar mechanistic pathways. Highly substituted olefins are produced as thermodynamic products in the Bamford Stevens reaction. But in the Shapiro reaction less substituted olefins are generated because kinetic products are formed preferentially. These reactions are of interest as from simple molecules to biologically active complex molecules with double bond can be produced with the application of these reactions. Thus, Shapiro reaction involves the conversion of aryl sulfonyl hydrazones of aldehydes and ketones into olefins by reacting with alkyl lithium reagent, Grignard reagent, or alkali metal amide i.e. the basic decomposition of tosyl hydrazones. This reaction was applied in the total synthesis of Taxol reported by Prof. Nicolaou.

Shapiro suggested that the Shapiro reaction proceeded by a carbanion mechanism involving the approach of the alkyl lithium reagent at the least hindered and most acidic proton.

General reaction:

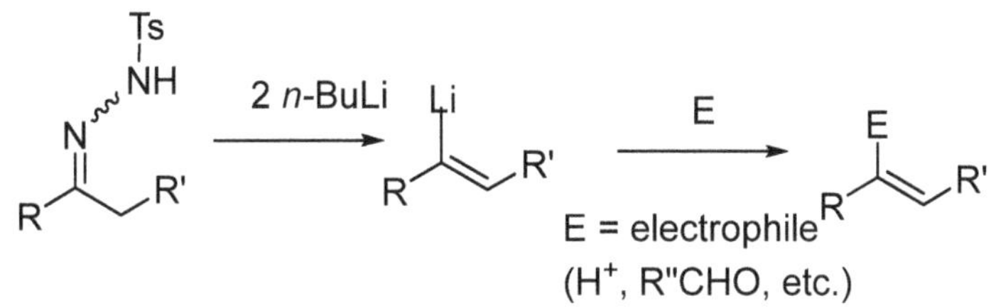

Mechanism:

Initially, a ketone / aldehyde reacts with p-toluenesulfonyl hydrazide generating tosylhydrazone. The proton from the hydrazone is abstracted by using two equivalents of strong base such as n-butyllithium followed by the less acidic proton α to the hydrazone carbon, resulting in a carbanion. This undergoes an elimination reaction affording a carbon–carbon double bond losing the tosyl anion leading to a diazonium anion. This with a loss of nitrogen molecule forms a vinyllithium species, which reacts with an electrophile or simple neutralization with water or an acid.

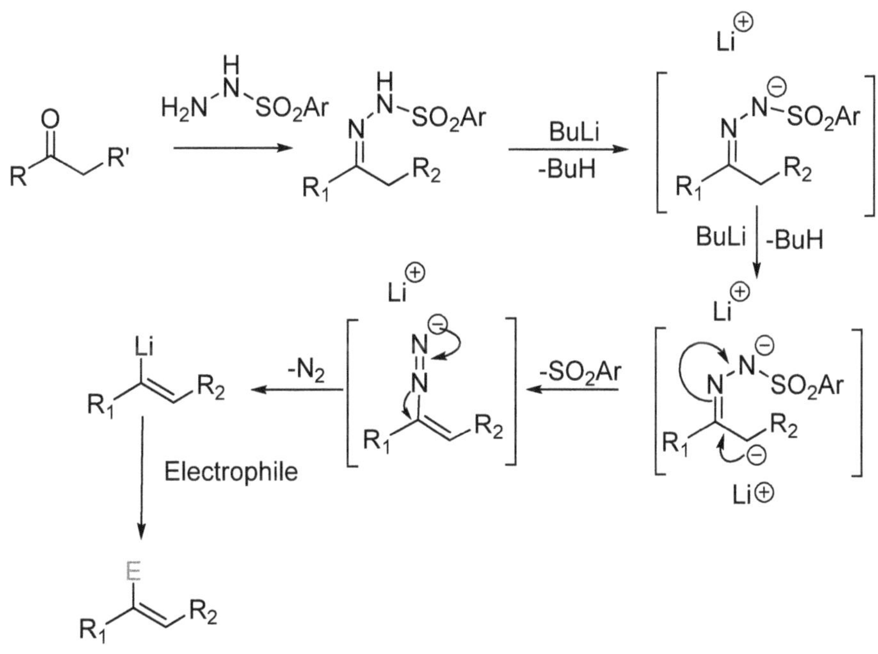

Applications and Examples:

1. **Camphor forms the intermediate hydrazone which on Shapiro reaction gives the Vinyl lithium:** Addition of water results in 2-bornene and with addition of an *n*-butyl bromide affords the alkylated product.

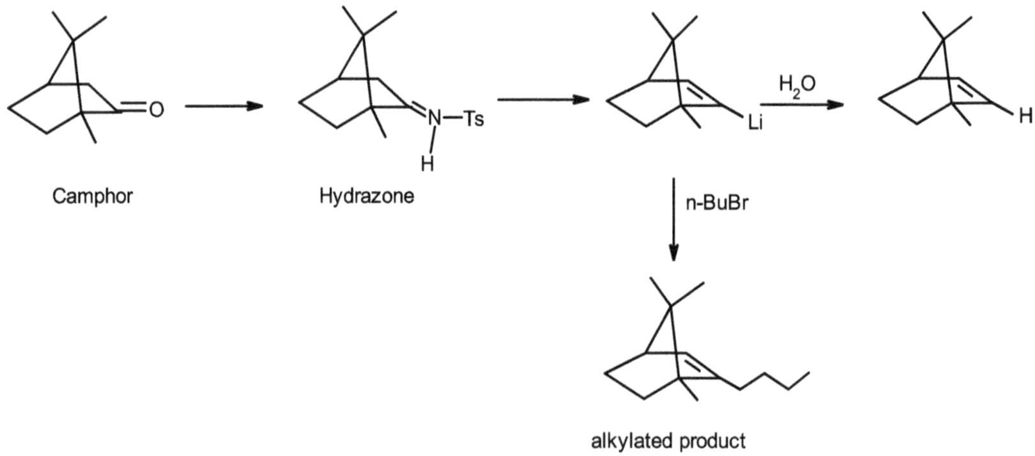

2. **Synthesis of an intermediate of Mequitazine, an antihistamine drug:** The intermediate can be efficiently generated via the Shapiro reaction, from trisylhydrazone with excess n-BuLi followed by reacting the nucleophilic vinyl lithium reagent with paraformaldehyde.

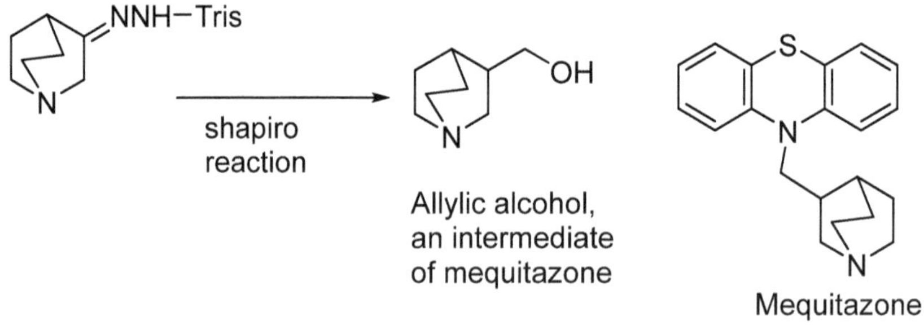

3. **A structurally challenging polycyclic olefin was synthesized by Maier et al. by Shapiro reaction:** The ketone was converted to hydrazone, which was reacted with n-BuLi in THF affording tricyclic olefin[20].

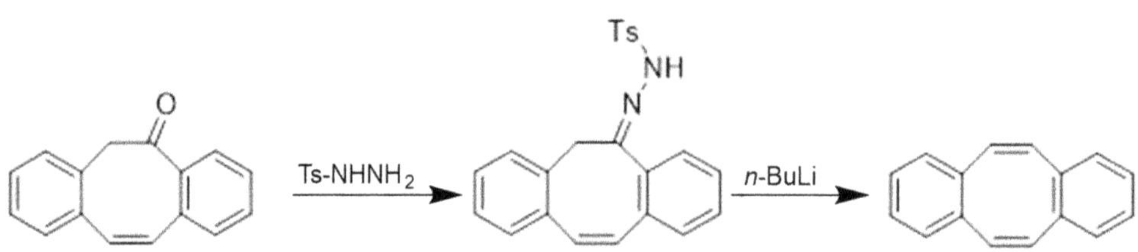

4. **Shapiro-Suzuki reaction:** The Shapiro reaction can also be combined with the Suzuki reaction to generate different olefin compounds. Keay and co-researchers developed a methodology combining both Shapiro reaction and Suzuki reaction in a one-pot process avoiding the isolation of the boronic acid. This application has a broad scope, substrate tolerance for a wide spectrum of tosylhydrazones and aryl halides, as well as several solvents and Pd sources.

2.11 Sharpless Asymmetric Epoxidation

When a reaction occurs between two achiral agents, the chiral product formed consists of both enantiomers in equal amounts and called a racemic mixture. The formation of exclusively one enantiomer is very difficult. Developing enantioselective methods for the synthesis of biologically potent molecules is a challenging task.

William S. Knowles, K. Barry Sharpless, and Ryoji Noyori in their pioneering work developed in 1980-this enantioselective asymmetric epoxidation and 2001 Nobel Prize in Chemistry was awarded to them. When a chiral catalyst is used it temporarily holds the substrate molecule in an unsymmetric environment, as the nature does in case of enzymatic catalysis in biochemical reactions. When the substrate is open to a reaction to only one side, an excess of only one enantiomer is formed. Sharpless epoxidation is most popular and widely applicable to induce asymmetry in synthetic design for chiral target molecules.

General reaction:

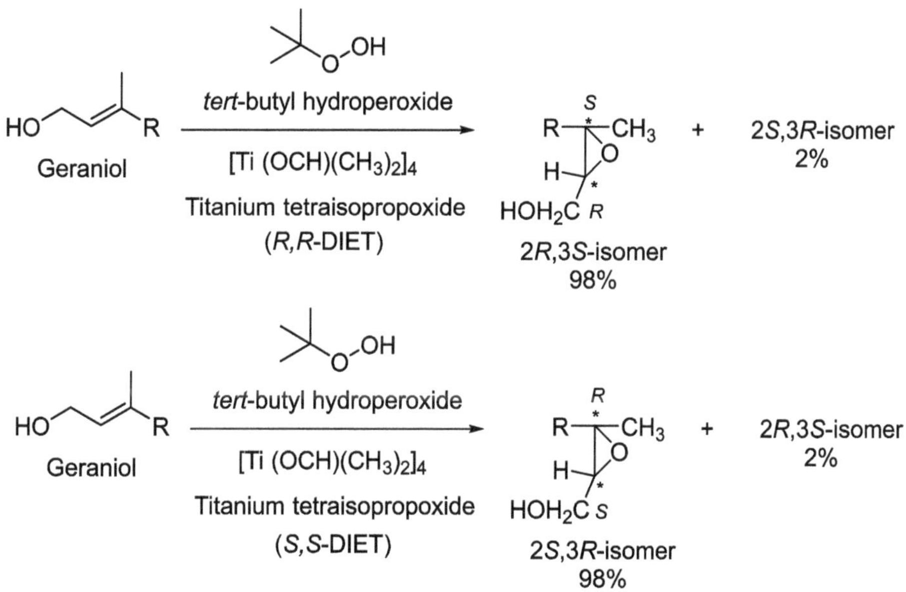

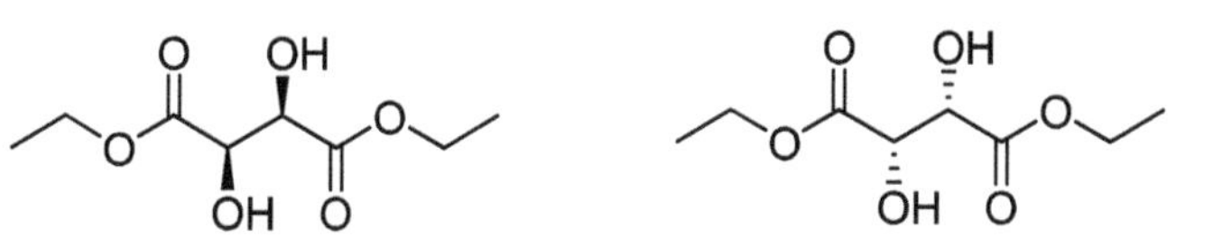

(R,R)-Diethyl tartarate (DIET) (S,S)-Diethyl tartarate (DIET)

2.12 Suzuki Reaction

The Suzuki reaction, first published in 1979 by Akira Suzuki, is a cross-coupling reaction between a boronic acid and an organohalide catalyzed by a palladium(0) complex in the presence of base.

Suzuki shared the 2010 Nobel Prize in Chemistry with Richard F. Heck and Ei-ichi Negishi for the discovery and development of palladium-catalyzed cross-coupling reactions in organic synthesis. It is extensively used to prepare polyolefins, styrenes, and substituted biphenyls. It is also known as the Suzuki coupling or Suzuki–Miyaura reaction. In this reaction a new C-C bond is formed by the coupling reaction of a halide with organoboran compound catalyzed by a palladium catalyst and a base.

The advantages of Suzuki coupling are mild reaction conditions, availability of common less toxic boronic acids, use of wide variety of reagents including water-soluble reagents, as well as economical, eco-friendly, practicable nature and overall flexibility of methodology. The reagents include aryl- or vinyl-boronic acids and aryl- or vinyl-halides, pseudohalides such as triflates (OTf), as replacements for halides, Boronic esters and organtrifluoroborate salts in place of boronic acid. Frequently used solvent systems for Suzuki coupling are toluene, dioxane, THF, and DMF. The most frequently used bases are NaOH, K_2CO_3, KOtBu, K_3PO_4, Cs_2CO_3, and NEt_3. The Suzuki coupling reaction is scalable, cost-effective and widely applicable in the synthesis of intermediates for pharmaceuticals or fine chemicals and also many complex compounds. Various catalytic uses of metals other than palladium (especially nickel) have been developed. Percec and co-workers in 1995 reported the first nickel catalyzed cross-coupling reaction using aryl mesylates and boronic acids.

The use of nickel catalysts made the reaction possible for other substrates such as phenols, aryl ethers, esters, phosphates, and fluorides. Even though initially nickel catalyzed reactions required high catalyst loadings (3-10%), excess ligand (1-5 equivalents) and remained sensitive to air and moisture, many advancements and variations are reported making this reaction a very potential player in the development of synthetic organic chemistry.

General reaction:

$$R^1{-}X + R^2{-}BY_2 \xrightarrow{\text{[Pd]cat., base}} R^1{-}R^2$$

Mechanism:

The reaction is initiated by the formation of an active Pd(0) catalytic species, **A**, which forms the organopalladium intermediate B, by the oxidative addition of palladium to the halide reagent. The oxidative addition step breaks the carbon-halogen bond where the palladium is now bound to both the halogen (X) as well as the R^1 group. Oxidative addition proceeds with the retention of stereochemistry with vinyl halides. But in the case of allylic and benzylic halides it results in the inversion of stereochemistry. Even though, the cis–palladium complex is formed initially, it isomerizes to the trans-complex. This, with base gives intermediate, which via trans metalation with the boron-ate complex (produced by reaction of the boronic acid reagent with base) forms the transient organopalladium species. The product is formed by the reductive elimination, releasing the palladium catalyst. This completes a catalytic circle. Transmetalation is an organometallic reaction where ligands are transferred from one species to another. The base activates the organoboron compound and facilitates the formation of R^1-Pd^{II}-O^tBu intermediate from oxidative addition product R^1-Pd^{II}-X. The phosphine ligand is used in the Suzuki reaction. This increases the electron density at the metal center of the complex and helps in the oxidative addition step.

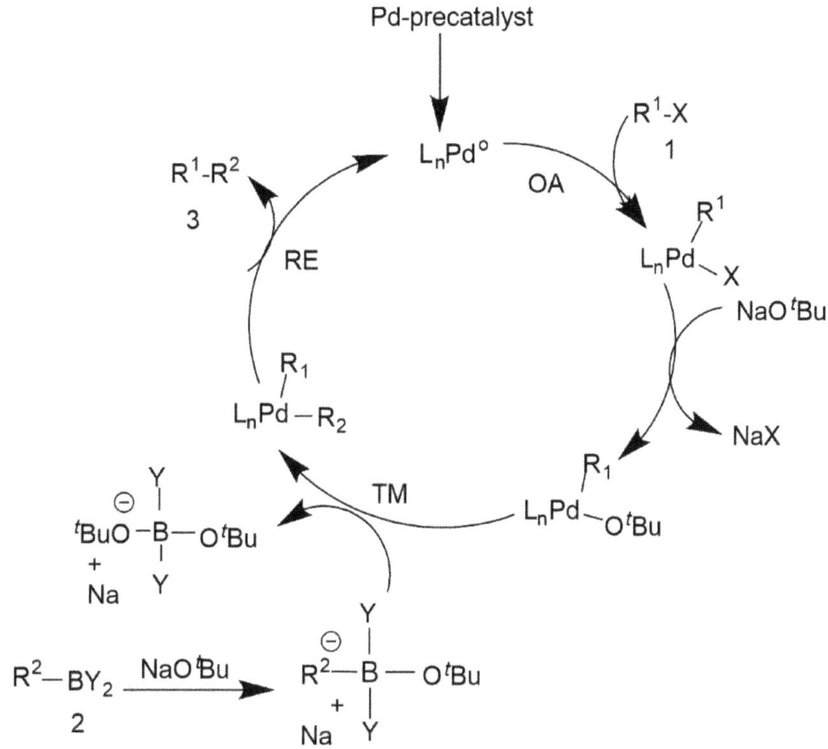

Applications

1. Coupling of 3-pyridylborane and 1-bromo-3-(methylsulfonyl)benzene.

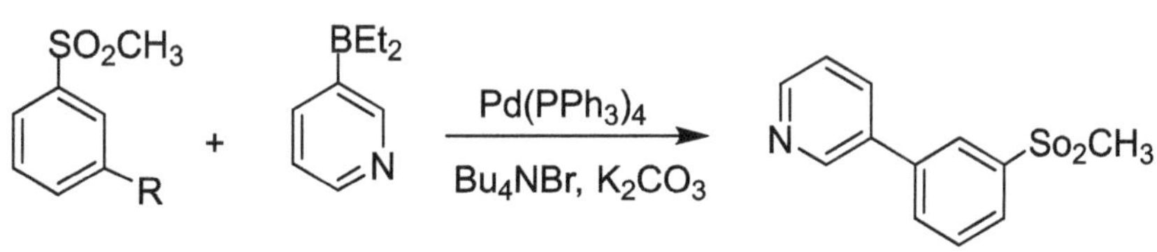

2. **Reaction of 3-chloro anisole with phenyl boronic acid**

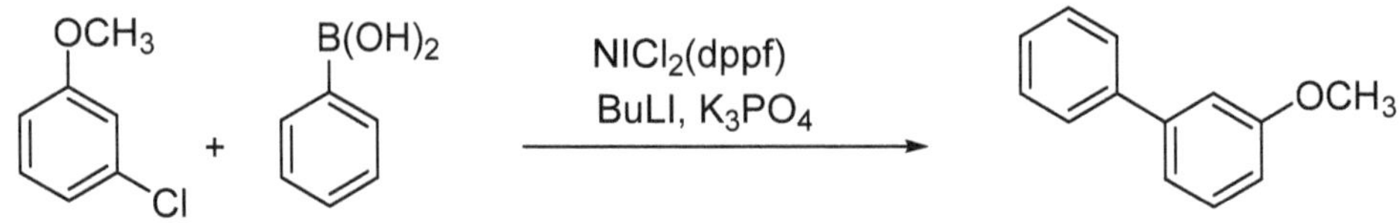

3. **Preparation of Aryltrifluoroborate salts from boronic acids and potassium hydrogen fluoride, followed by the Suzuki coupling reaction.**

a) Aryltrifluoroborate synthesis

$$R{-}B(OH)_2 \xrightarrow{KHF_2} R{-}\overset{-}{B}F_3\ \overset{+}{K}$$

b) Aryltrifluoroborates in Suzuki reaction

$$Ar{-}Br + R{-}BF_3K \xrightarrow{[Pd]\ cat.,\ base} Ar{-}R$$

4. **Synthesis of capparatriene, an active compound against leukemia, from citronellal derivative[21].**

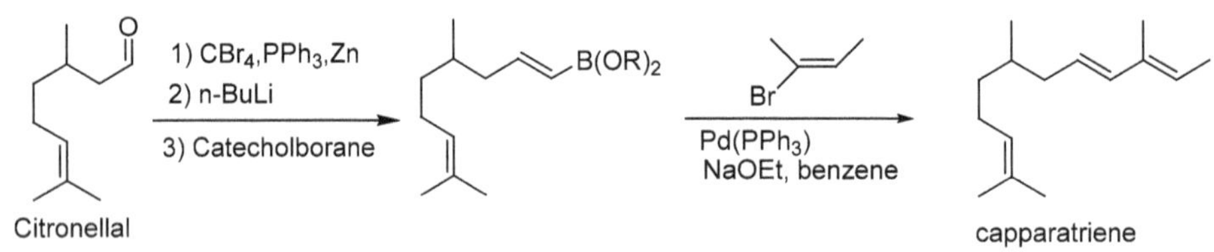

5. **Suzuki-Miyaura Cross–Coupling reactions under ligand-free conditions using Pd $(OAc)_2$/TBAB/PEG-400 system as a reusable system was developed[22].**

$$ArX + Ar'B(OH)_2 \xrightarrow[Pd(OAc)_2;TBAB;\ K_2CO_3/PEG.400]{110°C;\ 4\text{-}24\ h} Ar{-}Ar'$$

6. **Reaction of 5-bromopyrimidine with furanylboronic acid/pyridylboronic acid under microwave conditions.**

a)

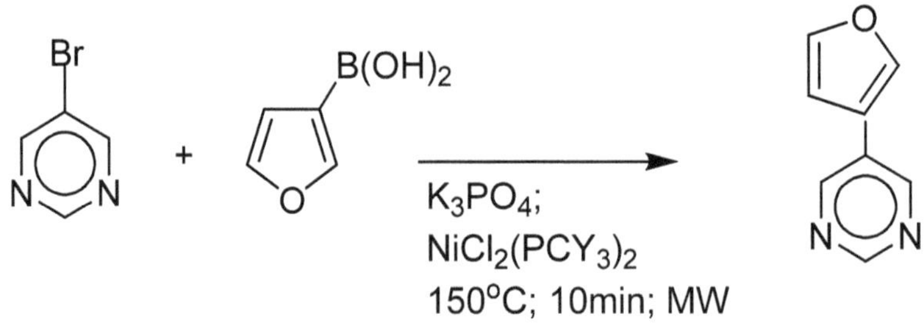

2.13 Ugi reaction

Ivar Karl Ugi first reported this reaction in 1959. It is an important, atom-economical, eco-friendly, four component condensation reaction in which an amine, aldehyde/ketone, a carboxylic acid and an isocyanide react to form a highly substituted bis-amide or α-aminoacyl amide with a loss of water molecule. The products are structurally similar to peptides. These can be called protein mimics or peptidomimetics. This isocyanide-based strategy allows multi-bond formations in a single step with wide applications. Large diversified chemical libraries can be generated using this reaction. By changing the reactants with diversified substitutions on the reactants many new biologically active compounds can be prepared. Ugi reaction can also be conducted combining with other reactions contributing for a broad range of structurally interesting compounds. This reaction is potentially applicable for pharmaceutical domain and combinatorial chemistry. Diversified molecules can be generated in minimum timeframe and energy requirements. It is also suitable to conduct under microwave, ultrasound, solvent- free conditions and also at room temperature as well as on-water. Polar protic solvents such as MeOH, EtOH, 2,2,2- trifluoroethanol (TFE) can be used as solvents. The Ugi as well as Passerini reactions are known to be accelerated in aqueous solutions, with an advantage of direct isolation by precipitation. The reaction can be conducted with high flexibility employing reactants with varied functional groups. Many natural products, macrocyclic molecules, linear and cyclic peptides and drug molecules can be generated employing the Ugi process. Merck applied this in the synthesis of an important HIV protease inhibitor-Crixivan (Indinavir-MK 639). Furanomycin isolated from *Streptomyces threomyceticus* was also prepared using Ugi method.

This reaction can also be applied in combination with other reactions like intramolecular Diels - Alder reaction, Smiles reaction, Heck reaction, Buchwald-Hartwig reaction etc.

The Passerini reaction reported by Mario Passerini in 1921 involving the condensation of aldehyde or ketone, carboxylic acid and isocyanide affording α-acyloxyamide is also related to the Ugi reaction mechanistically. The Passerini reaction is a three-component reaction but does not involve amine component. Many green methods were developed such as microwave assisted and ultrasound promoted protocols for Ugi reaction.

General reaction:

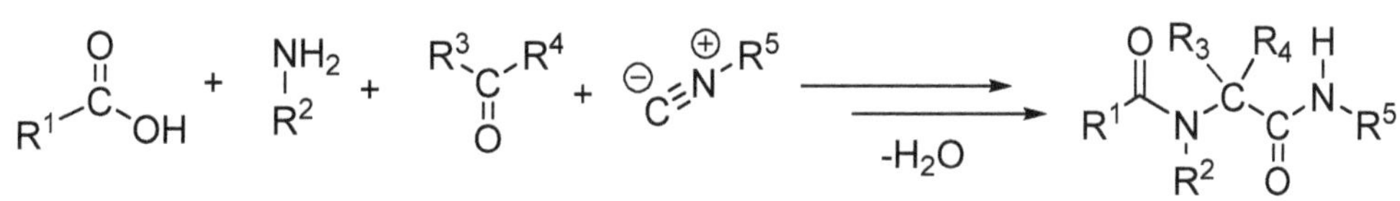

Reaction Mechanism:

Initially, amine reacts with the ketone with a loss of water molecule. An iminium ion is formed by the proton exchange with carboxylic acid. Nucleophilic attack of isocyanide on the iminium ion forms nitrilium ion. Carboxylic acid anion attacks the imino carbon producing acylated isoamide. This rearranges by acyl transfer producing bis-amide.

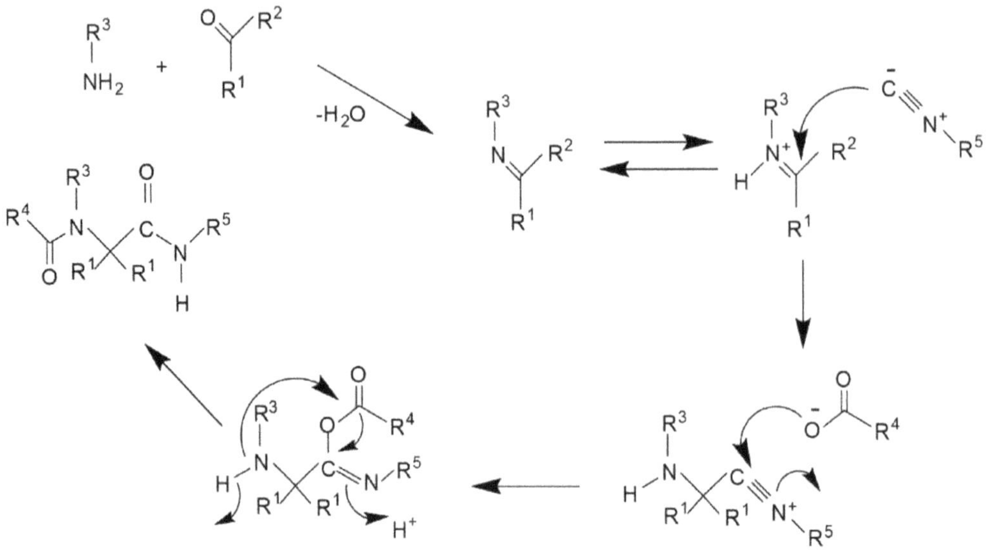

Applications and Examples

1. Ugi-Smiles reaction

The Ugi-Smiles reaction is a powerful and widely applied strategy to get N-arylamines from phenolic substrates. In this reaction amines, carbonyl compounds, isocyanides and phenols with withdrawing groups are used as reactants. Here carboxylic acid of Ugi reaction is replaced by a o-nitrophenol, p-nitrophenol or a salicylate. It is useful in the preparation of N-aryl primary amines. The Smiles reaction takes place in the last step. Different post-condensation strategies of this reaction result in the generation of various fused heterocyclic systems such as quinoxalines, benzimidazoles, benzotriazoles, azepines etc.,

2. Ugi-Diels -Alder reaction

A one-pot, four-component approach involving Ugi reaction followed by an intramolecular Diels–Alder reaction for the preparation of arene-fused iso indolinones is developed[23].

3. Knoevenagel-Ugi reaction

An efficient one-pot multicomponent Knoevenagel-Ugi condensation reaction was carried out by S. Kumar et al. From salicylaldehyde, aniline, benzaldehyde derivatives, isonitrile and 2,2-dimethyl-1,3-dioxane-4,6-dione (Meldrums acid) at 40°c in EtOH affording coumarin based Knoevenagel-Ugi adducts by the sequential reactions. This method offers atom-economic, operationally facile process under mild reaction conditions[24].

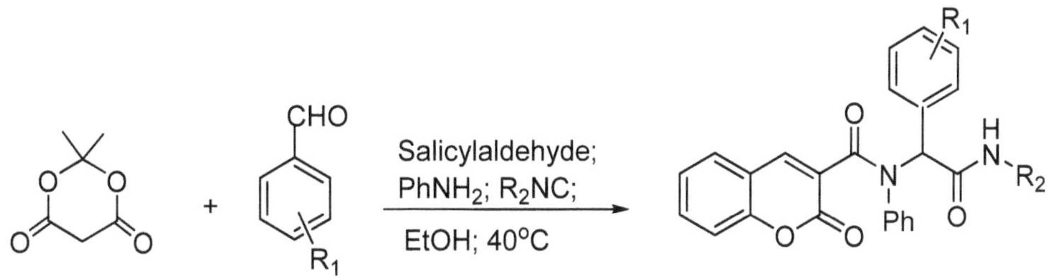

4. Ugi reaction by Microwave irradiation

2-(4-Oxo-4H-1- benzopyran-3yl)-4-thiazolidinones were produced by Zhong-Zheng Zhou et al., using microwave-assisted parallel syntheses following combinatorial approach[25].

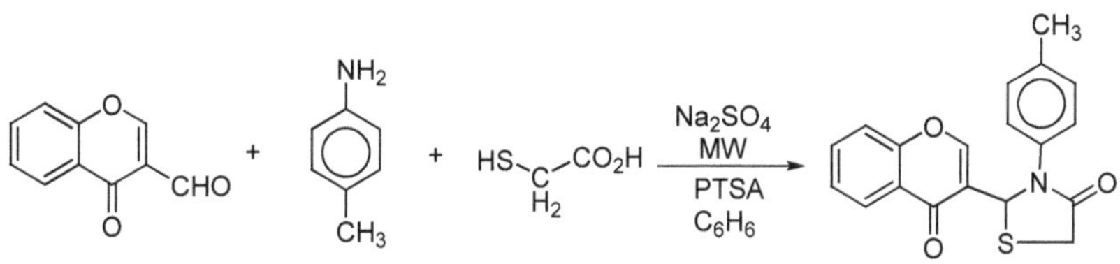

5. Ultrasound-assisted Ugi reaction

Some 2,5-diketopiperazine linked 1,4-disubstituted 1,2,3-triazole derivatives were prepared via the Ugi-4CR/lactamization/click sequence under mild, atom-economical, and ultrasound conditions[26].

6. Synthesis of Praziquantel

With a pyrazonoisoquinoline ring system, the compound is widely used as a drug for schistosomiasis. It is prepared via Ugi reaction under mild conditions[27].

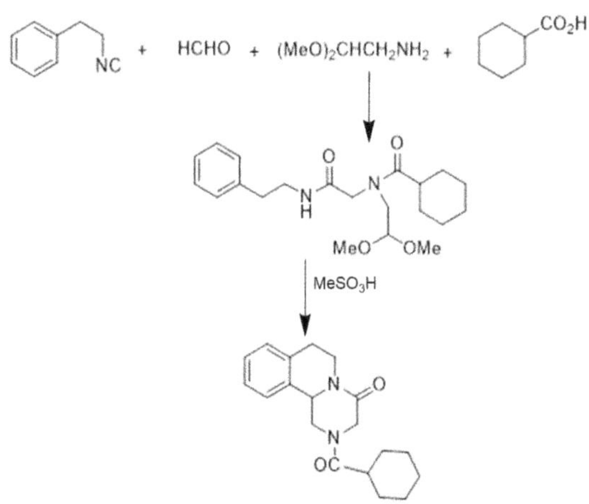

2.14 Ullmann Coupling Reactions

Ullmann cross-coupling reaction, or Ullmann coupling reaction or Ullmann reaction involves the coupling of two aryl halides into a biaryl product in the presence of finely divided copper or copper bronze at elevated temperatures (100-350 °c). It is named after Fritz Ullmann, a German chemist who reported this in 1901. Original Ullmann reaction requires harsh reaction conditions, but over the years many improvements were made and variations of the reaction were reported. Even though traditionally copper was used as catalyst, the use of palladium and nickel as catalysts widened the scope of the reaction. It is the most important and widely applied reaction. The mechanism and reaction conditions of the reaction were extensively studied. Copper-assisted cross-coupling reactions of aryl halides to aryl ethers or aryl thioethers, or aryl nitriles and aryl amines also come under this class of reactions. Generally, the reaction requires higher reaction temperatures and higher boiling polar solvents. Aryl iodides react with ease than aryl chlorides and bromides which require activation by an electronegative group placed on the aromatic ring. In the "classic" Ullmann reaction symmetric biaryls are produced from aryl halides via copper-catalyzed coupling. Ullmann-type" reactions cover the nucleophilic aromatic substitutions between different nucleophiles (e.g. substituted phenoxides) and aryl halides catalyzed by copper. Large number of biaryl and polyaryl compounds can be prepared by this method. Nitro group strongly activates the aryl halides particularly from ortho position whereas alkyl and alkoxy groups activate from any position.

General reaction:

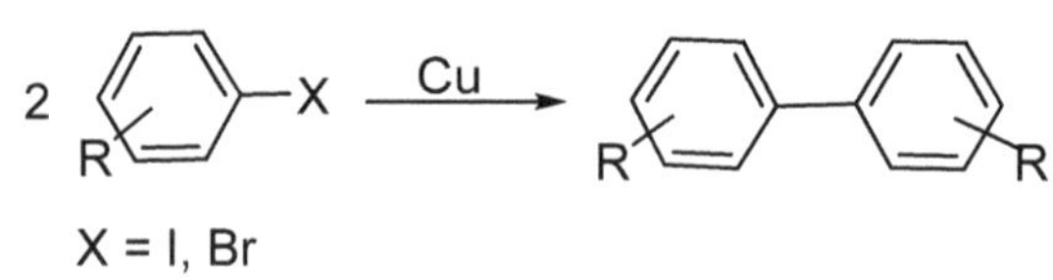

Mechanism:

Copper reacts with aryl halide oxidatively to form Cu(I) compound by the elimination of CuI, which undergoes second oxidative addition with aryl halide followed by reductive elimination affording symmetrical biaryl. The reaction is more similar to Wurtz reaction. In most of the cases the yields are high.

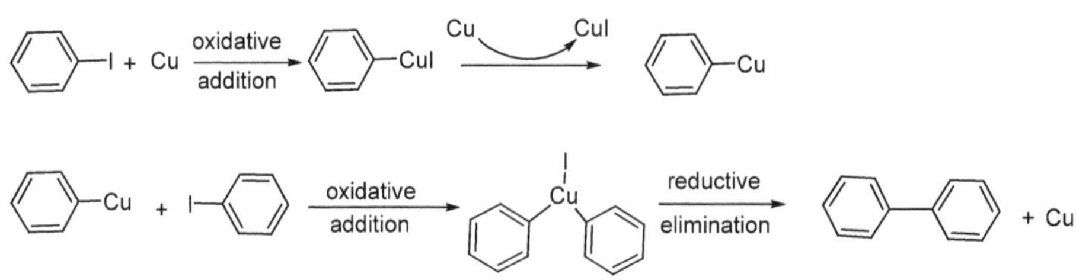

Applications and examples:

1. Preparation of 2,2'-Dinitrobiphenyl

o-Chloronitrobenzene and copper bronze are heated in clean dry sand at 215–225 °C to afford the product.

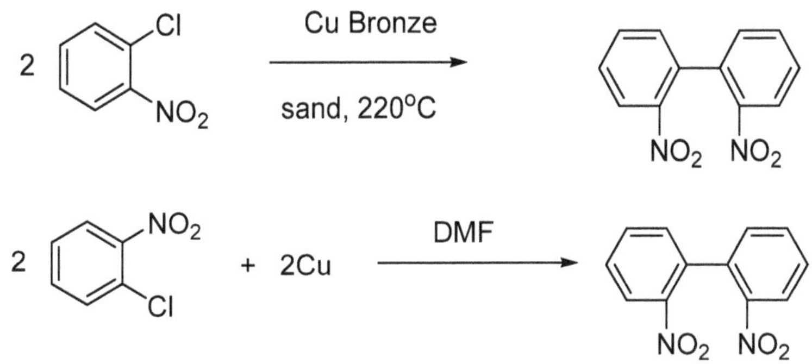

2. Preparation of 2-Methoxy diphenyl ether

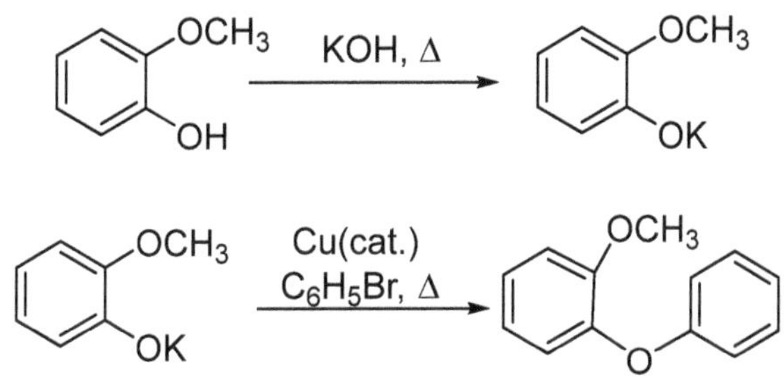

3. Preparation of 4-Nitro diphenyl ether

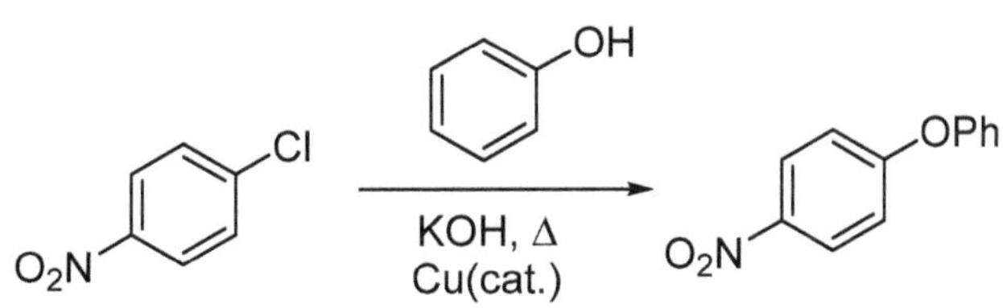

4. Preparation of diphenyl

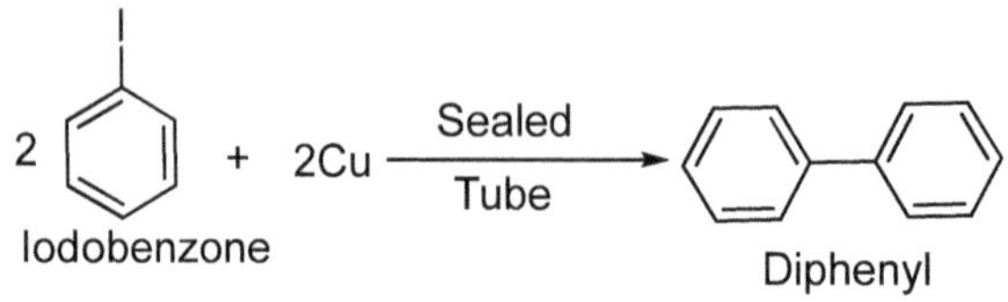

5. Preparation of perylene

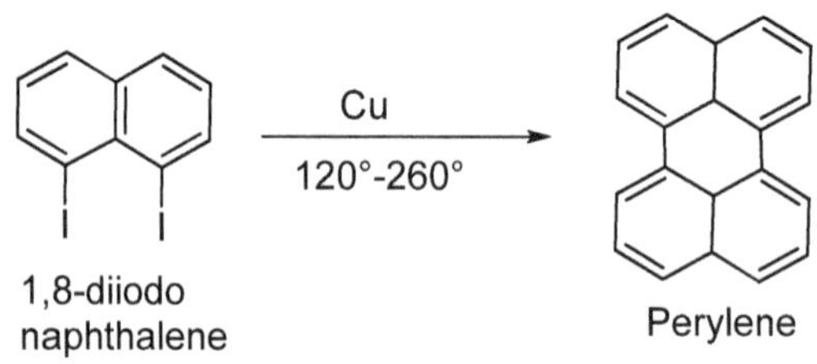

6. Preparation of 4,4- diphenic acid

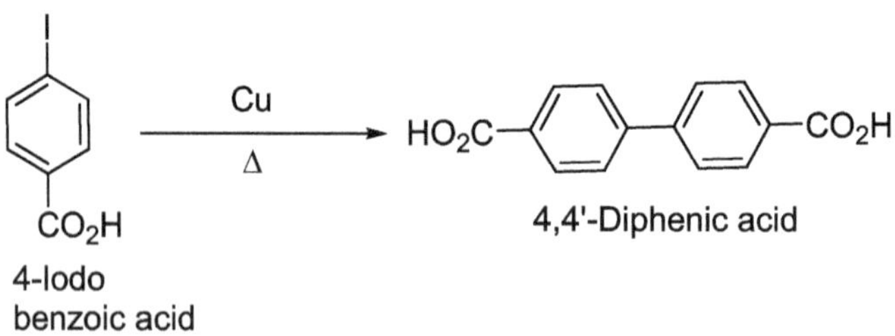

7. Preparation of 4-methoxyphenyl anthranilic acid

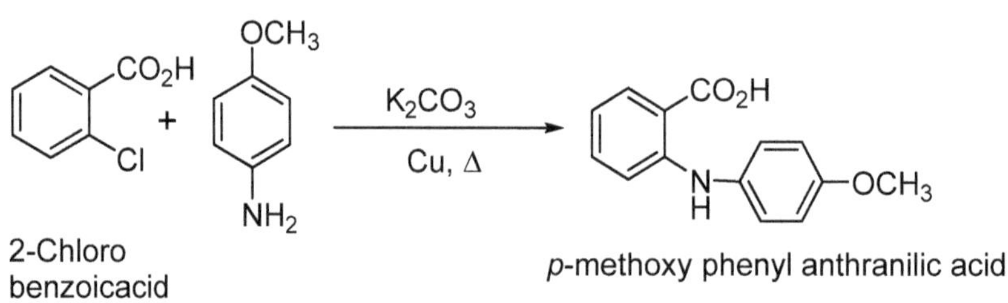

8. Preparation of 2-oxo-1-phenyl tetrahydropyrrole

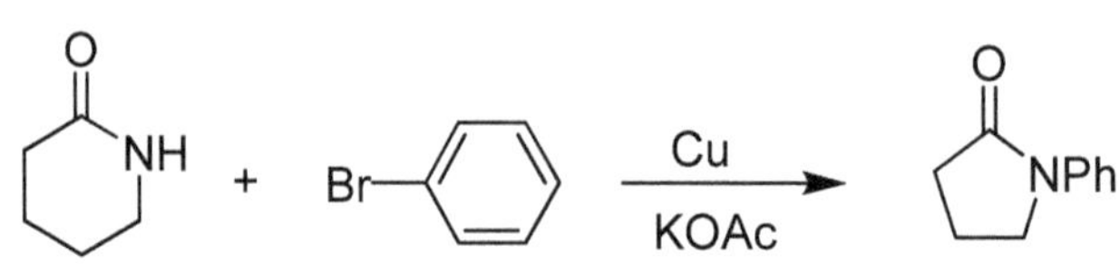

9. **Preparation of 2,4,6- trinitro biphenyl**

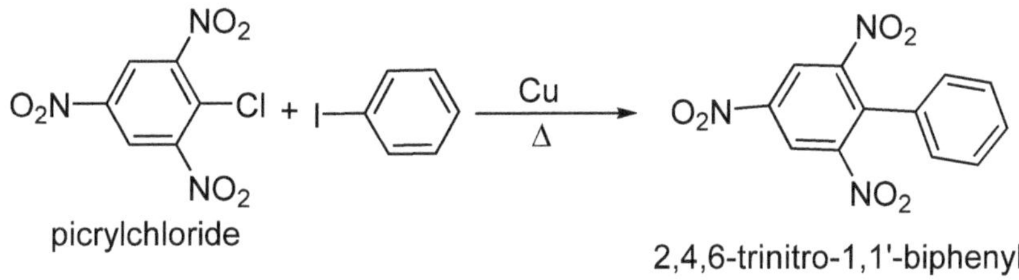

10. **Preparation of 2,2,4,4 –tetramethyl biphenyl**

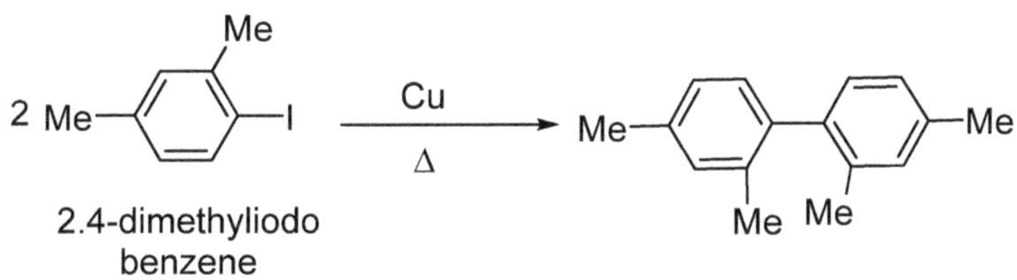

11. **Preparation of 2,7-dimethoxy-9,10-dihydro phenanthrene**

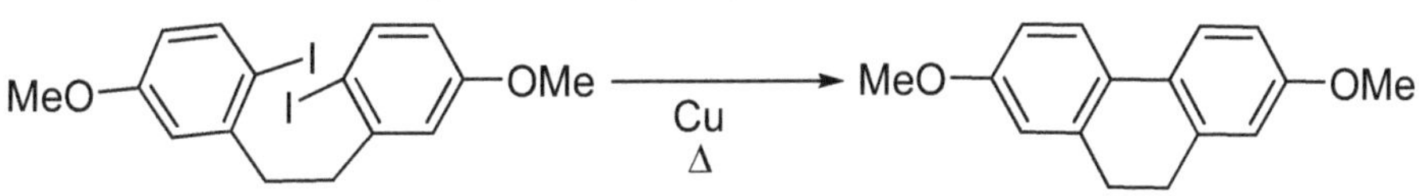

12. **Microwave-assisted Ullmann coupling reaction[28]**

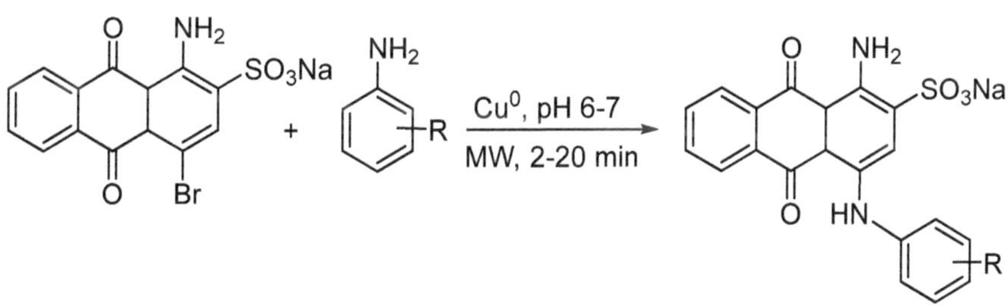

2.15 Vilsmeyer-Haack Reaction

In 1927, Vilsmeier and Haack reported the formylation of electron-rich aromatic or heterocyclic compounds. Dimethylformamide is used as an acylating agent. Activating agents such as phosphorus oxychloride or cobalt chloride are used. The iminium salt complex which is formed between DMF and activating agent is known as Vilsmeier-Haack reagent.

This is very useful reaction for reactive aromatics and heterocycles such as thiophenes, pyrroles, indoles, acridines, carbazoles and ferrocenes. Similar to Friedel-crafts acylation, in this also regioselectivity plays significant role and depends on the electron density of the attacked position in the reactant molecule.

General reaction:

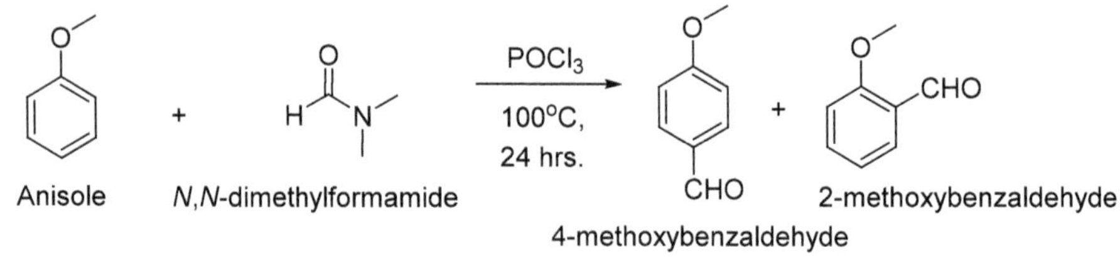

Mechanism:

Step 1: Nucleophilic substitution

Reaction between phosphorus oxychloride and *N,N*-dimethylformamide

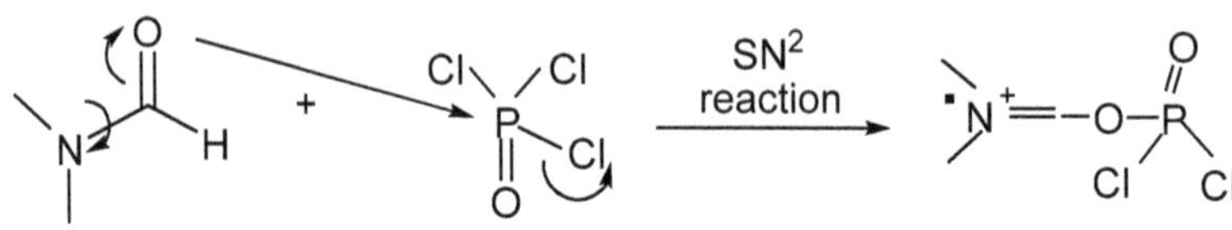

Step 2: Formation of Vilsmeier-Haack reagent

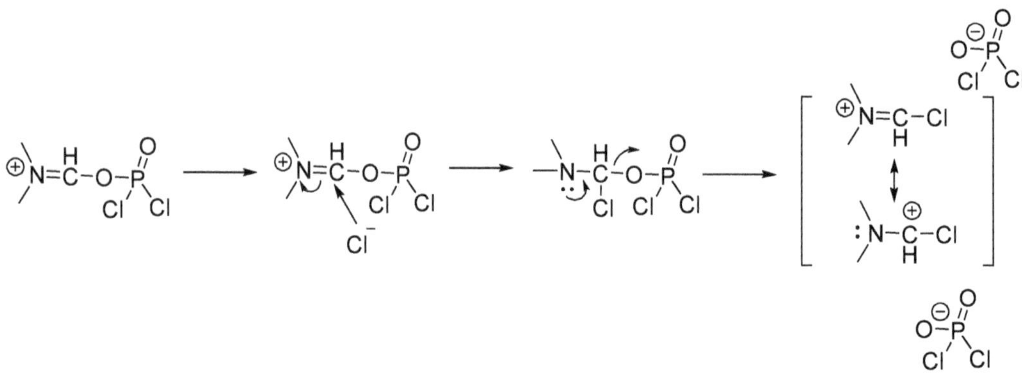

Step 3: Reaction between reactant and Vilsmeier-Haack reagent

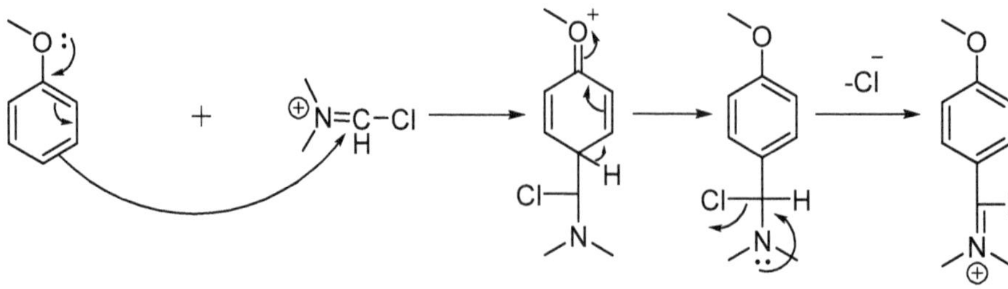

Step 4: Workup

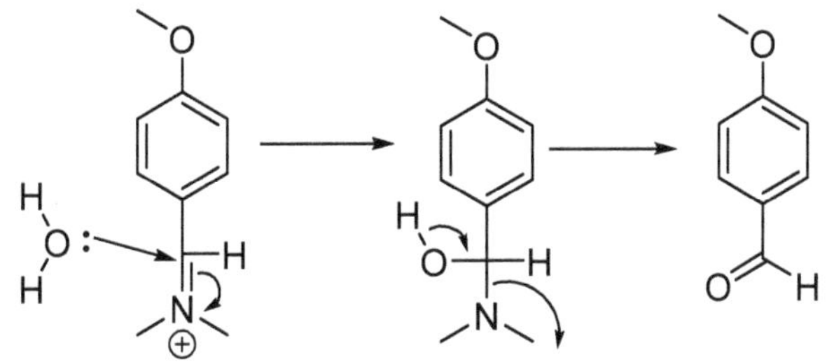

Applications:

1.

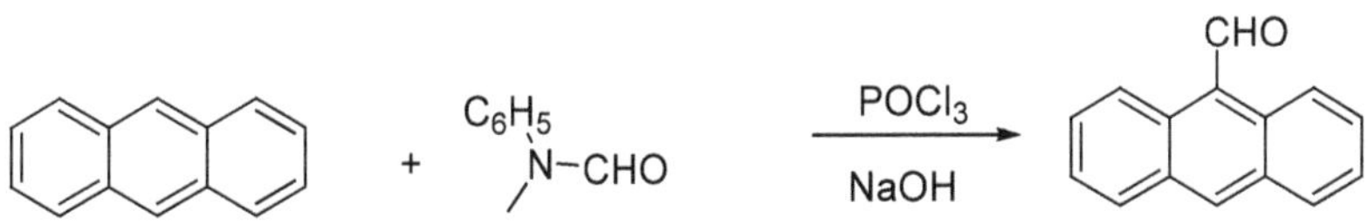

anthracene N-methyl-N-phenylformamide anthracene-9-carbaldehyde

2.

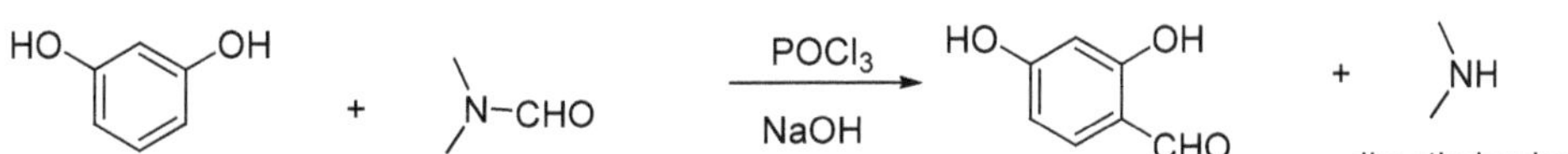

Resorcinol N,N-dimethylformamide 2,4-dihydroxybenzaldehyde dimethylamine

3.

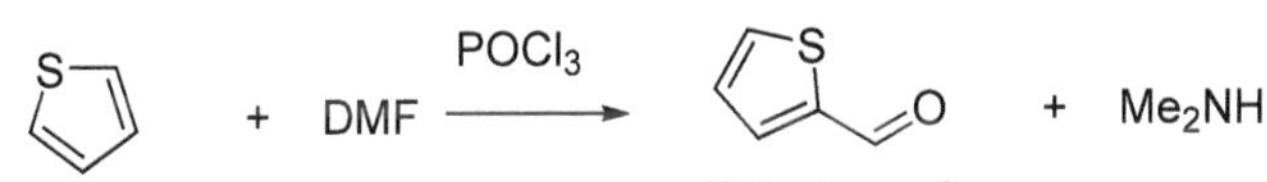

Thiophene Thiophene-2-carboxaldehyde

4.

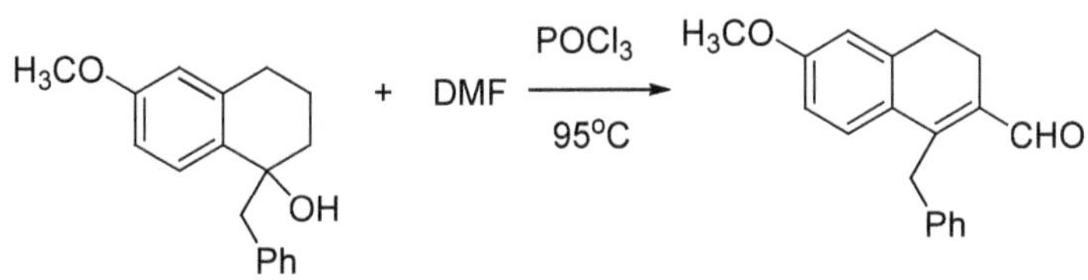

5. **Under the microwave irradiation[29].**

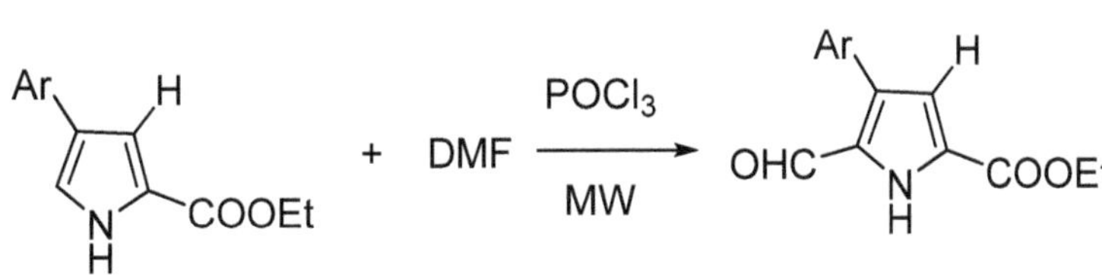

CHAPTER 3

A. Synthetic Reagents and their Applications

Synthetic reagents consist of a broad range of chemicals with many uses in the chemical synthesis and are employed in the transformation of functional groups such as addition, oxidation, reduction, halogenation, alkylation, amination, hydroxylation, phosphorylation, hydrolysis, cycloaddition, dehydration, etc. These chemicals play a crucial role in the field of organic chemistry and synthesis through a novel variety of reactions. These are valuable both in basic as well as industrial research.

1. Aluminium Isopropoxide $[(CH_3)_2CHO]_3Al$

It is a good reducing agent. It acts by the transfer of hydride ions.
It was developed in 1925-26 by Meerwein, Schmidt, Verley and Ponndorf.

Preparation:

It can be prepared from aluminium amalgam taken in anhydrous isopropyl alcohol with a small amount of CCl_4, which acts as a catalyst. The mixture is refluxed till the hydrogen gas generation stops. Aluminium Isopropoxide is obtained as a colourless liquid, after the removal of solvent. It can be obtained by distilling under reduced pressure 140-150°C at 12mm.

$$6Me_2CHOH + 6AlHg \xrightarrow{CCl_4} (Me_2CHO)_3Al + 3H_2$$

The reaction is known as Meerwein-Ponndorf-Verley reduction.

Uses:

It is used to reduce carbonyl compounds to the corresponding alcohols. It will not affect the sensitive groups. It is less polar and does not release alkoxide ions. The reduction is carried out in isopropyl alcohol and acetone is formed as byproduct. The reaction proceeds forward by distilling out the acetone formed. It is a reversible reaction and the reversible oxidation reaction is known as oppenauer oxidation. The same reagent can be applied for oxidation of alcohols. The amount of acetone present in medium controls the course of reaction. The reaction has the advantages: ease of operation, cost effectiveness, chemoselectivity, mild reaction conditions and scalability.

General reactions:

a) $$R_2C{=}O + [(CH_3)_2CHO]_3Al \rightleftharpoons (CH_3)_2C{=}O + R_2CHO\text{-}Al[(CH_3)_2CHO]_2$$

b) $$R_2CHO\text{-}Al[(CH_3)_2CHO]_2 \xrightarrow{(CH_3)_2CHOH} R_2CHOH + [(CH_3)_2CHO]_3Al$$

Reverse of the reaction (Oppenauer oxidation)

$$RCHOHR + CH_3COCH_3 \xrightarrow{Al[OCH(CH_3)_2]_3} RCOR + CH_3CHOHCH_3$$

Mechanism:

Carbonyl oxygen forms a complex with aluminium of the reagent, which transfers hydride ion to the carbonyl carbon by forming a cyclic transition state. The mechanism is proved by labelling experiments.

$$RCHO + Al[OCH(CH_3)_2] \longrightarrow$$

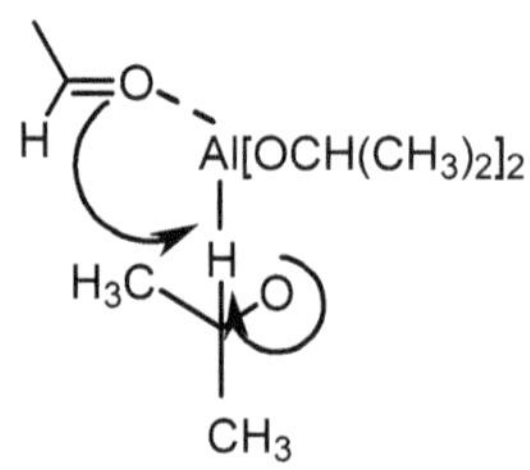

$$\rightleftharpoons R\,CH_2O\text{-}Al[(CH_3)_2CHO] + CH_3COCH_3$$

$$RCH_2O\text{-}Al[OCH(CH_3)_2]_2 \xrightarrow{(CH_3)_2CHOH} RCH_2OH + [(CH_3)_2CHO]_3Al$$

Solvent isopropyl alcohol plays an important role in the progress of the reaction and release of alcohol molecule. In the reaction, one hydrogen comes from reagent and another from solvent.

Applications:

1. $$\underset{\text{2-pentanone}}{CH_3COCH_2CH_2CH_3} + CH_3CHOHCH_3 \xrightarrow[\Delta]{Al[OCH(CH3)2]3} \underset{\text{2-pentanol}}{CH_3CHOHCH_2CH_2CH_3} + CH_3COCH_3$$

2. $$\underset{\text{acetophenone}}{PhCOCH_3} + CH_3CHOHCH_3 \xrightarrow[\Delta]{Al[OCH(CH3)2]3} \underset{\text{1-phenylethanol}}{PhCHOHCH_3} + CH_3COCH_3$$

3. $$\underset{\text{benzophenone}}{PhCOPh} + CH_3CHOHCH_3 \xrightarrow[\Delta]{Al[OCH(CH3)2]3} \underset{\text{benzhydrol}}{PhCHOHPh} + CH_3COCH_3$$

4. $CH_3CH{=}CH\text{-}CHO + CH_3CHOHCH_3 \xrightarrow[\Delta]{Al[OCH(CH3)2]3} CH_3CH{=}CH\text{-}CH_2OH + CH_3COCH_3$

crotonaldehyde → crotyl alcohol

5.

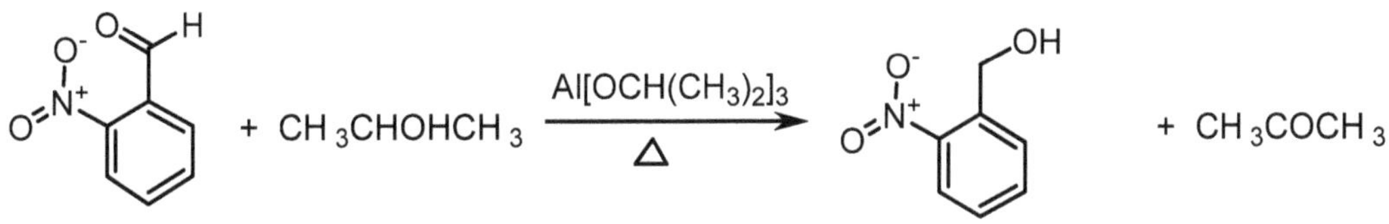

o-nitrobenzaldehyde → o-nitro benzylalcohol

7. $(CH_3)_3CCOCO_2Et + CH_3CHOHCH_3 \xrightarrow[\Delta]{Al[OCH(CH3)2]3} (CH_3)_3CCHOHCO_2Et + CH_3COCH_3$

Ethyl trimethyl pyruvate

8. $Cl_3CCOCH_3 + CH_3CHOHCH_3 \xrightarrow[\Delta]{Al[OCH(CH3)2]3} Cl_3CCHOHCH_3 + CH_3COCH_3$

trichloro acetone → 1,1,1-trichloropropan-2-ol

9.

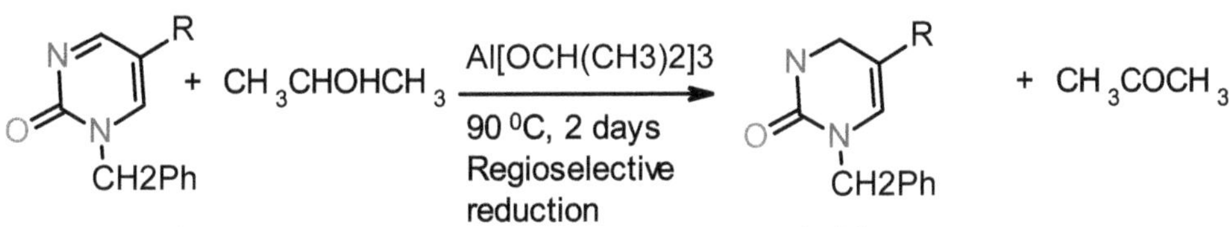

R = H, Halide → pyrimidinone

10.

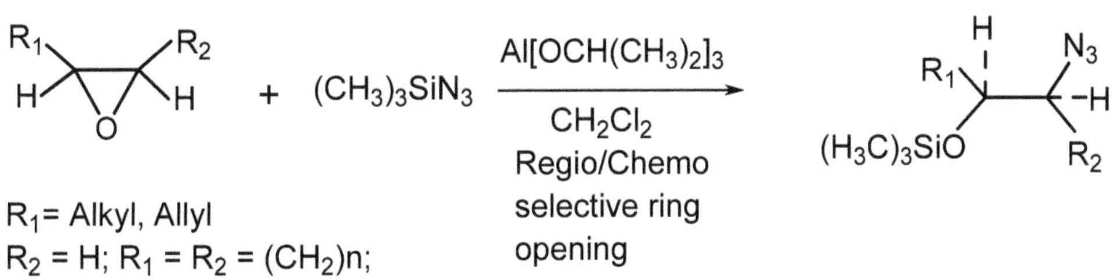

R_1= Alkyl, Allyl

R_2 = H; R_1 = R_2 = $(CH_2)n$;

n = 3, 4, 5

2. *N*-Bromo succinimide:

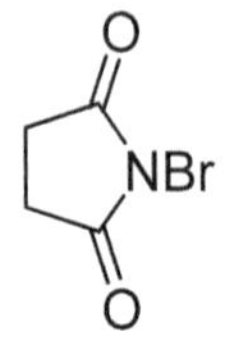

Preparation:

It can be prepared by the bromination of succinimide in alkaline solution at ice-cold temperatures.

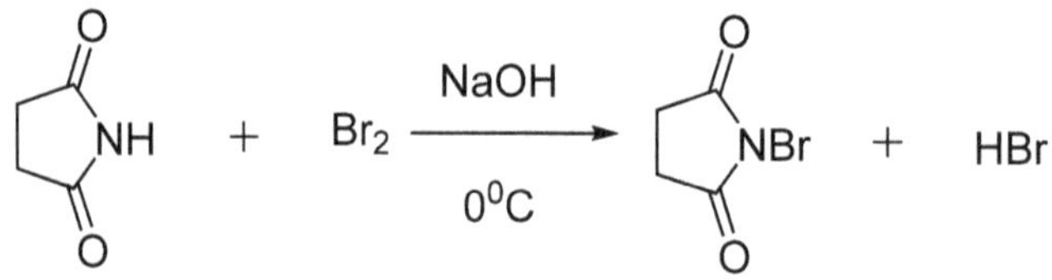

Uses:

It is used for brominating allylic and benzylic positions, particularly α-position of the carbonyl group and triple bonds. The bromination is usually carried out in CCl_4 so that succinimide formed can be easily separated from the reaction mixture on the workup. It can also be used to oxidize primary amines, primary alcohols, and secondary alcohols to the respective aldehydes and ketones. Due to the low dissociation energy of allylic and benzylic C-H and the stabilization by delocalization, these can be easily brominated by NBS. NBS bromination is helpful in the structural determination of molecules. It is used in the peptides for degradation of amino acids.

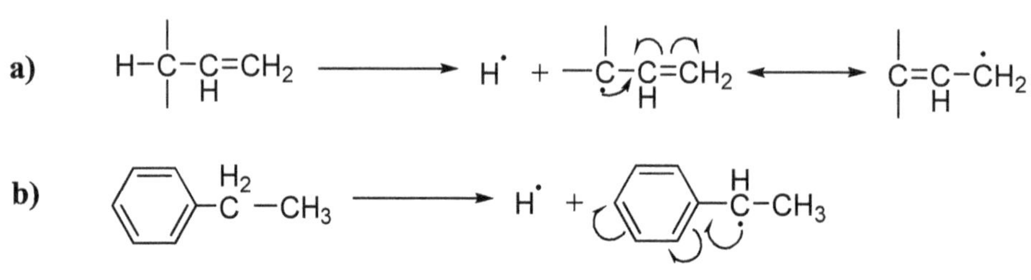

Mechanism: The reaction goes by free radical mechanism, initiated by a small amount of Br• formed.

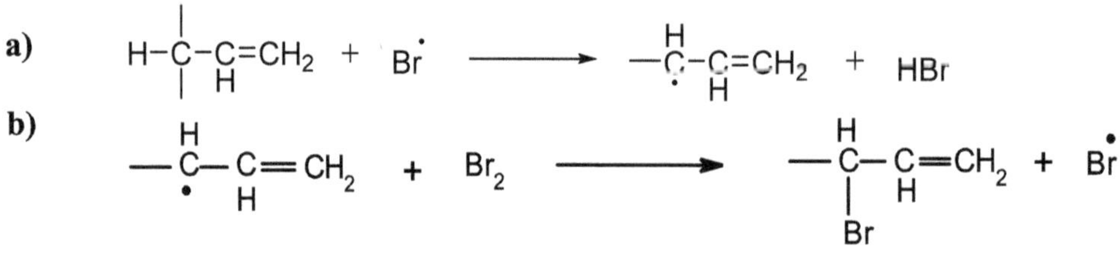

c)

Applications:

1. Allylic bromination

a)

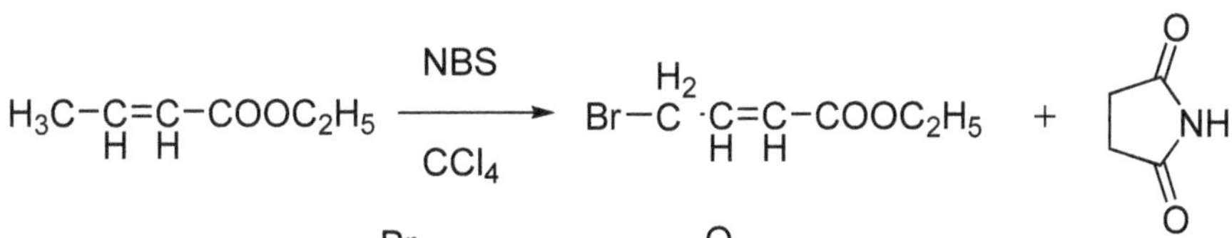

b)

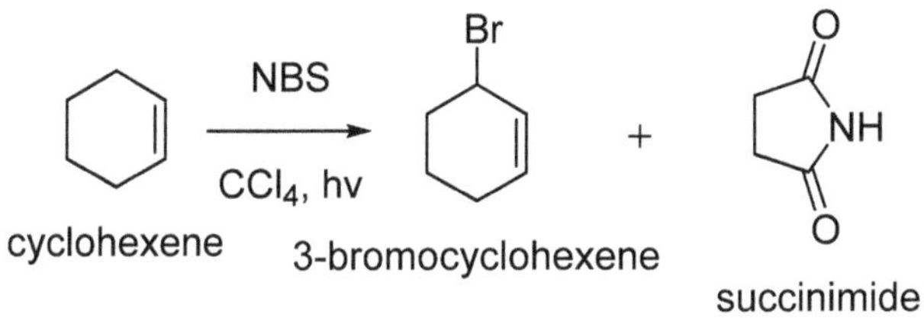

c)

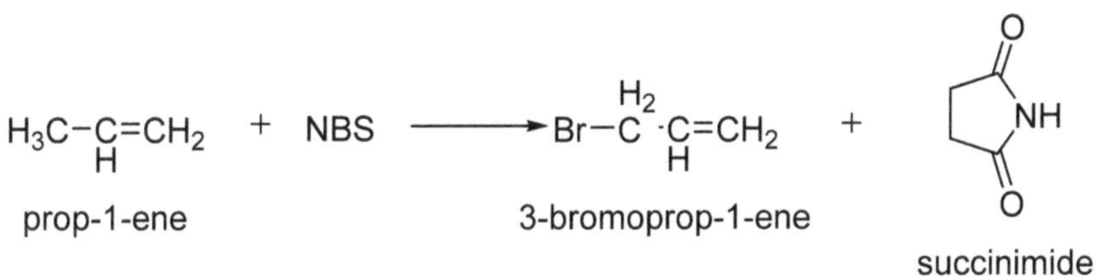

2. Addition reaction

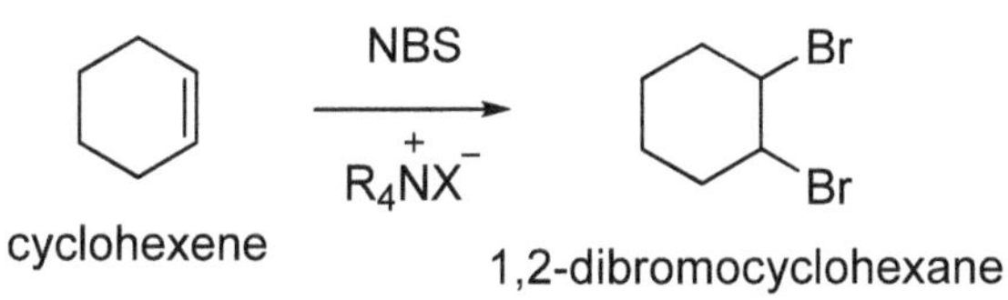

3. Formation of bromohydrin

a)

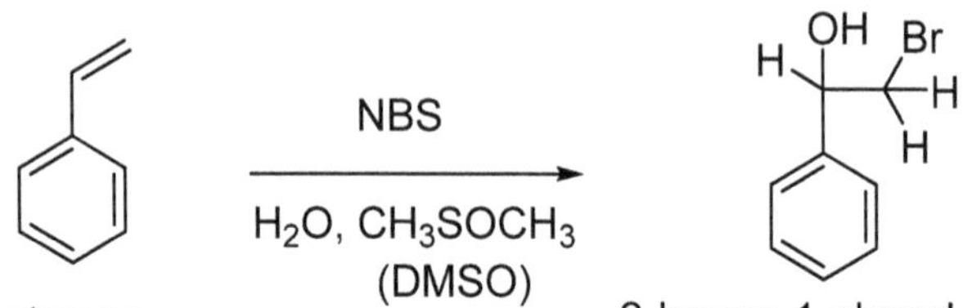

styrene → 2-bromo-1-phenyl ethanol

b)

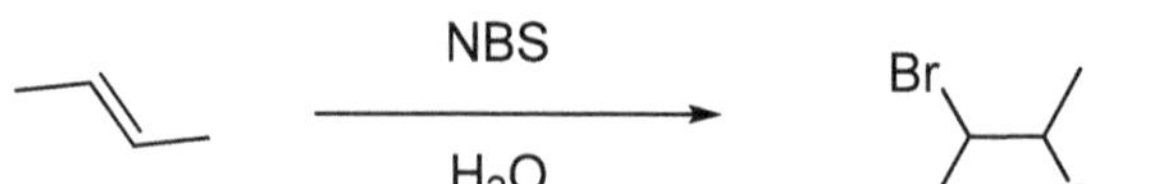

(*E*)-but-2-ene → 3-bromo-2-butanol

4. Oxidation

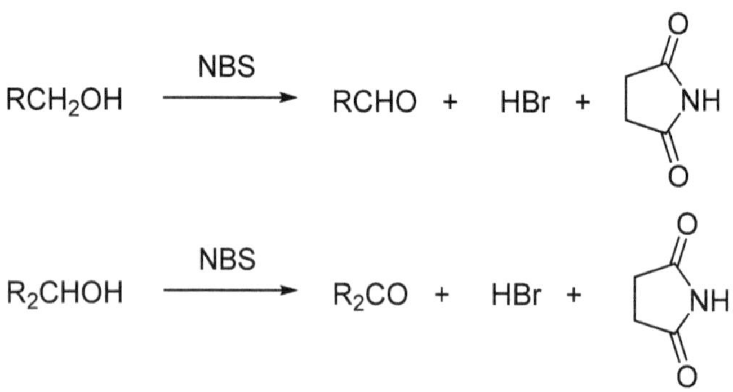

5. Decarboxylation

$$\underset{\alpha\text{-Alanine}}{CH_3CH(NH_2)COOH} \xrightarrow{\text{NBS}} CH_3CHO + NH_3 + CO_2$$

6. Conversion of Vitamin. A_1 to Vitamin. A_2

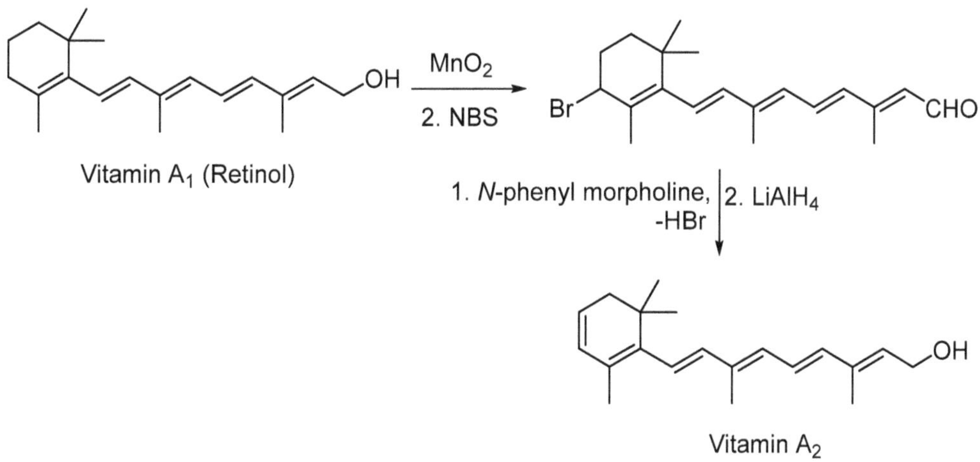

7.

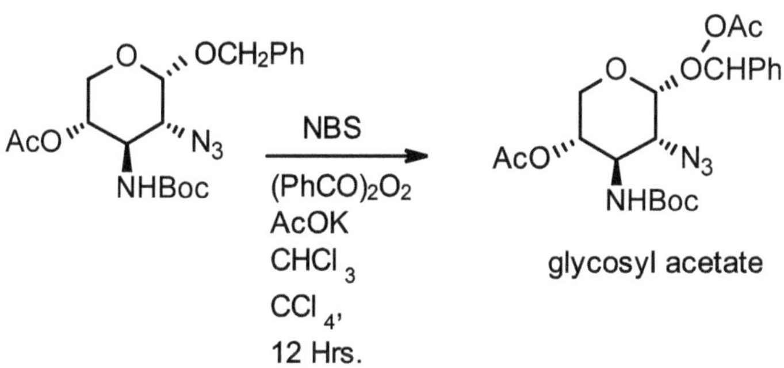

3. Diazomethane

Preparation:

Diazomethane is prepared from several *N*-nitroso-*N*-alkyl amides in the presence of base with an elimination reaction.

General reaction:

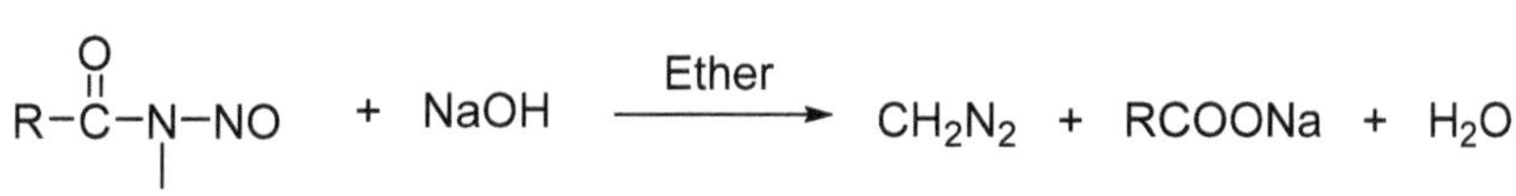

a)

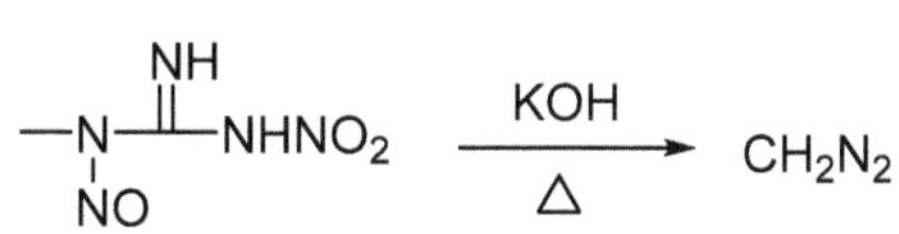

1-methyl-3-nitro-
1-nitrosoguanidine

b)

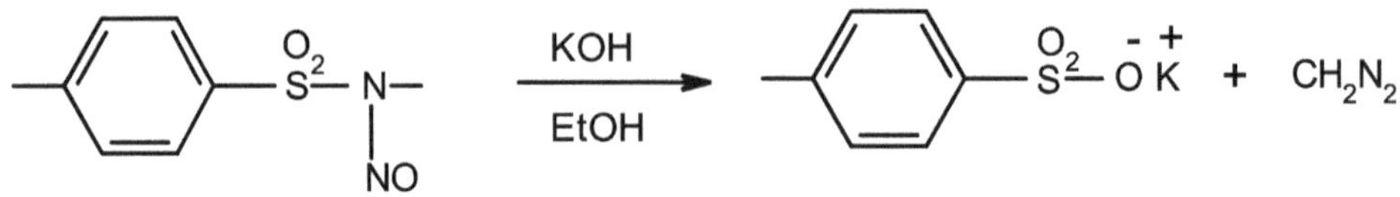

N,4-dimethyl-*N*-nitrosobenzenesulfonamide

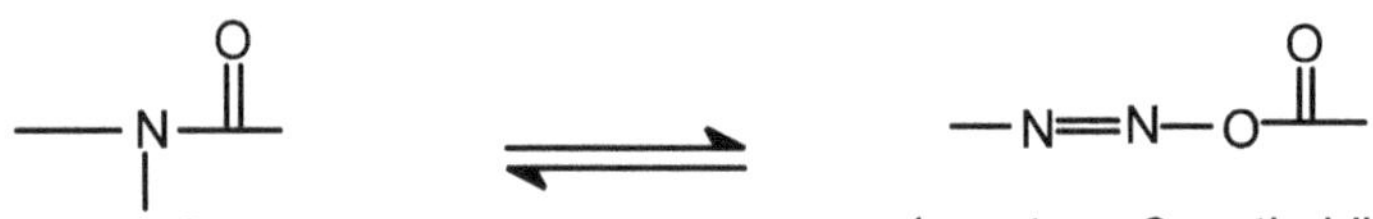

N-methyl-*N*-nitrosoacetamide

1-acetoxy-2-methyldiazene

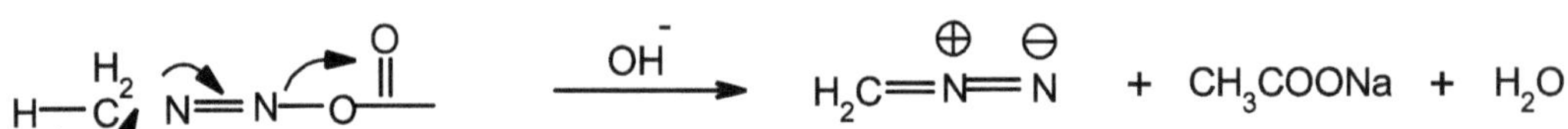

Diazomethane

It is highly explosive and toxic, capable of exploding in gaseous state also. It is stored in ether at 0°C for a period of 24 hours. It decomposes rapidly.

Uses:

It is used as a powerful methylating agent, reacting **rapidly**, affording high yields. Methylation is carried out in ether solution adding diazomethane in ether to the reactant and the reaction occurs with an evolution of N_2.

$$H_2C=\overset{\oplus}{N}=\overset{\ominus}{N} \longleftrightarrow H_2\overset{\ominus}{C}-\overset{\oplus}{N}\equiv N \longleftrightarrow H_2\overset{\oplus}{C}-N=\overset{\ominus}{N}$$

It can react with wide range of reactants like alcohols, phenols, enols, amines, sulphonic acids, carboxylic acids, aldehydes, ketones, ethylenic and acetylenic compounds. Aldehydes provide higher ketones, ketones provide epoxides, cyclic ketones undergo ring expansions. Acidic substrate does not require catalyst but less acidic reactants proceed in presence of catalyst like BF_3. Highly reactive carbene is generated from diazomethane in the presence of light which is used for insertion reactions. Carboxylic acids, sulphonic acids yield esters. Alcohols and phenols react to give corresponding ethers.

Applications:

1. Formation of ether

a) $$ROH \xrightarrow[SiO_2,\ RT]{CH_2N_2} ROMe$$

R= alkyl or aryl

b) $$PhOH \xrightarrow[-N_2]{CH_2N_2} PhOMe$$

c) 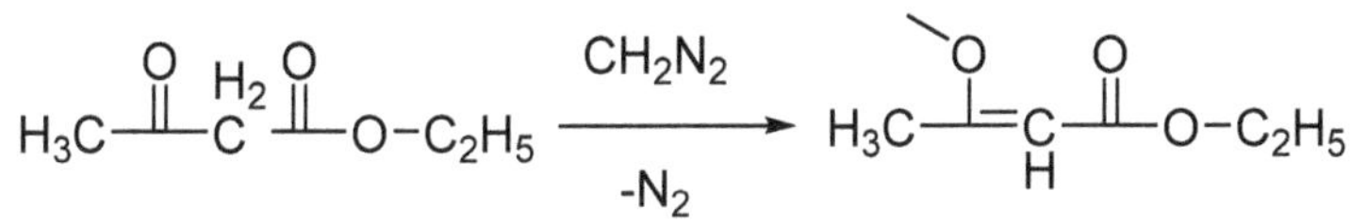

2. Formation of esters

a) $$Ph{-}CH{=}CH{-}COOH \xrightarrow[-N_2]{CH_2N_2} Ph{-}CH{=}CH{-}COOCH_3$$

b) $$Ph{-}COOH \xrightarrow[-N_2]{CH_2N_2} Ph{-}COOCH_3$$

c) $$R{-}SO_3H \xrightarrow[-N_2]{CH_2N_2} R{-}SO_3CH_3$$

d) 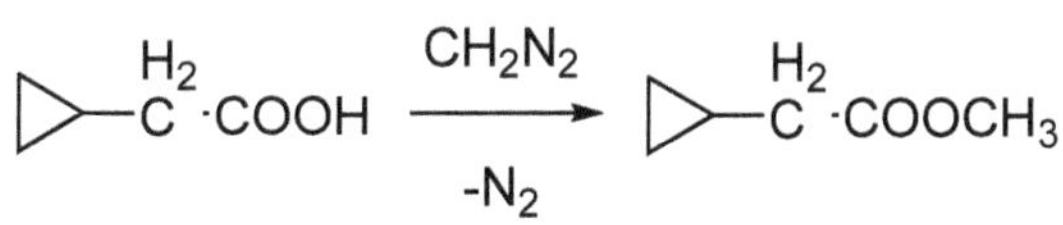

3. Formation of ketones

a) 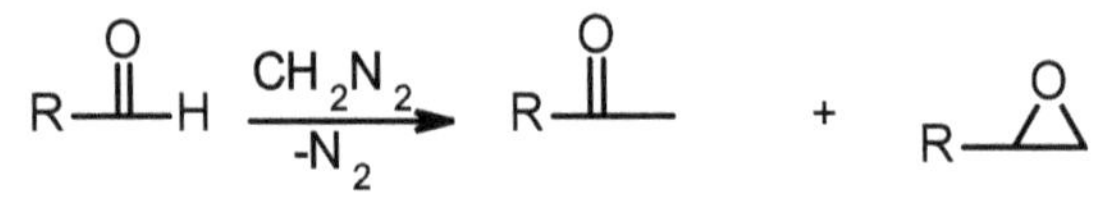

b) 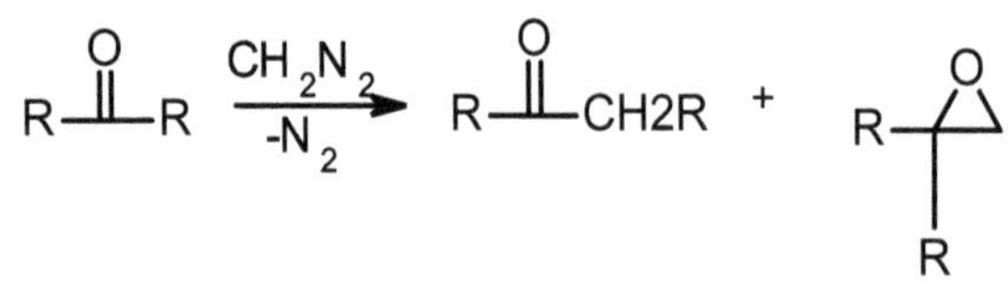

c) 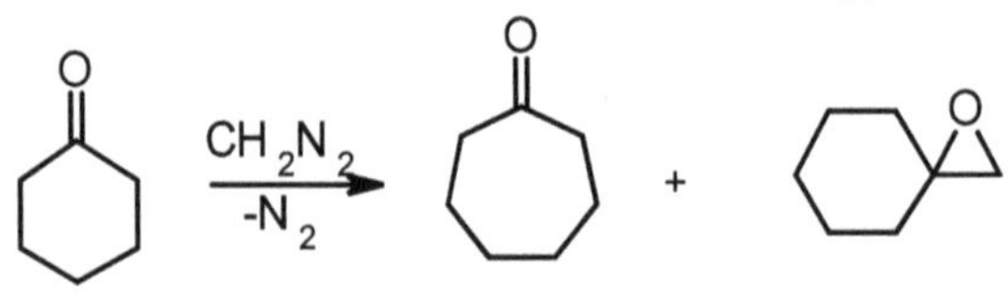

cyclohexanone cycloheptanone

4. Formation of methylamines

$$R_2NH + CH_2N_2 \xrightarrow{BF_3} R_2NCH_3 + N_2$$

5. Formation of heterocyclic compounds

a) 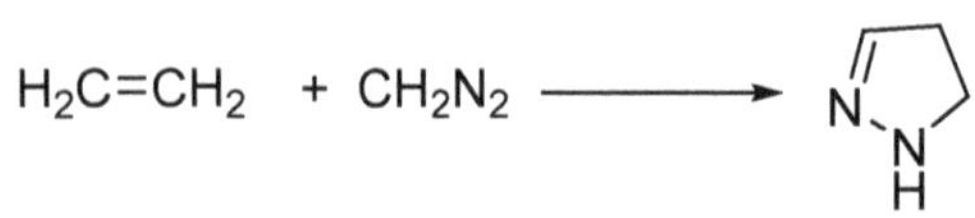

pyrazoline

b) 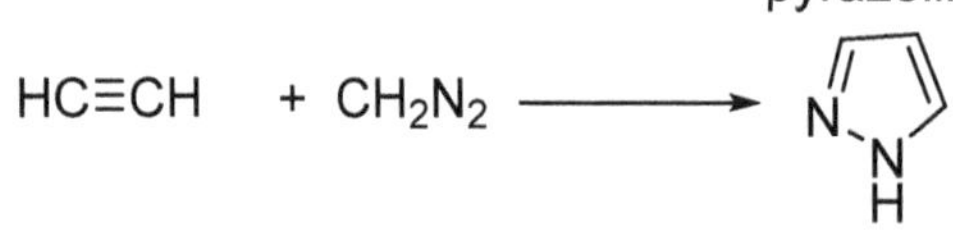

pyrazole

6. Formation of diazoketone and further reactions

Diazoketone undergoes Wolff rearrangement in the presence of Ag_2O, involving homologation reaction.

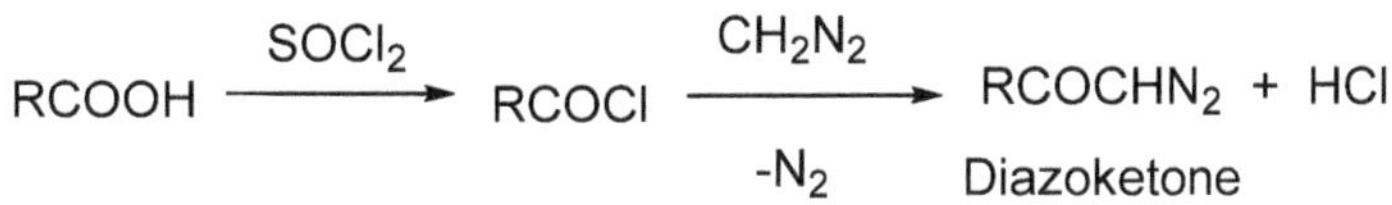

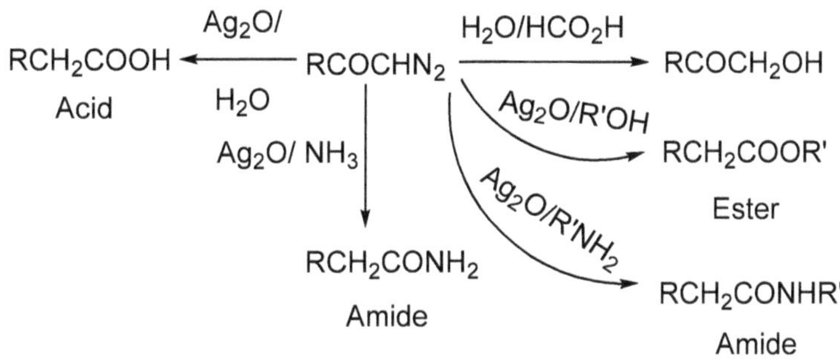

7. Used in (+)-oestrone synthesis

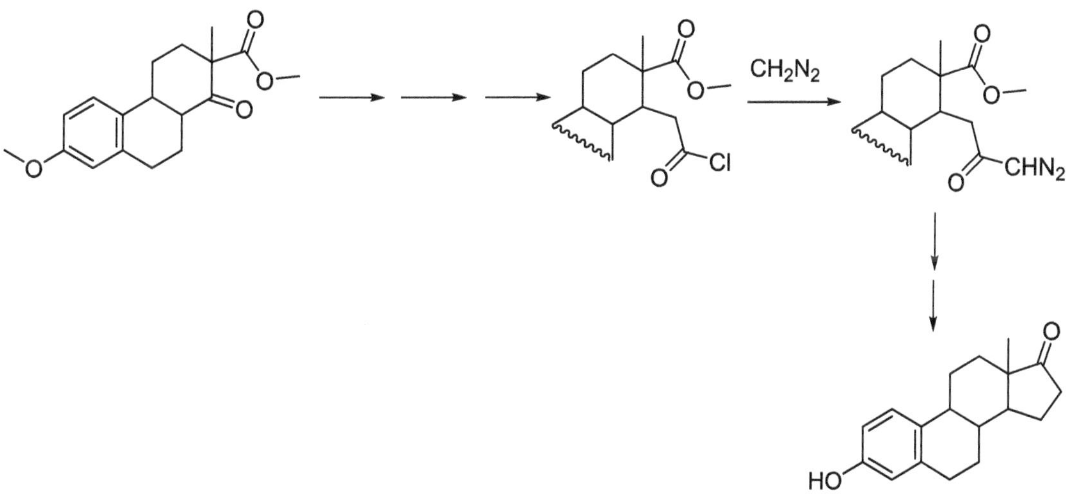

Oestrone

8. Used in deoxycorticosterone: Synthesis (OH group is protected by $-COCH_3$ and $-COCl$ is converted with CH_2N_2)

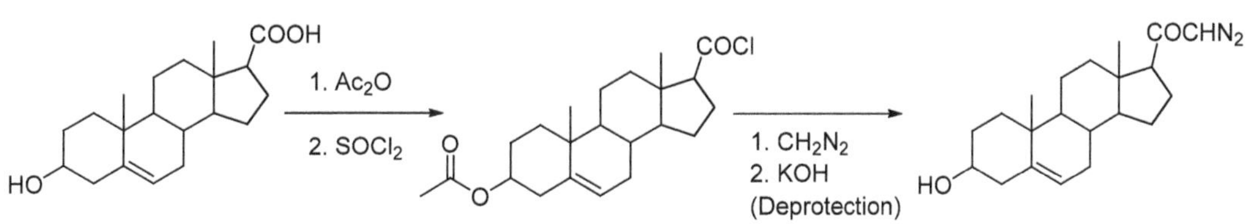

9.

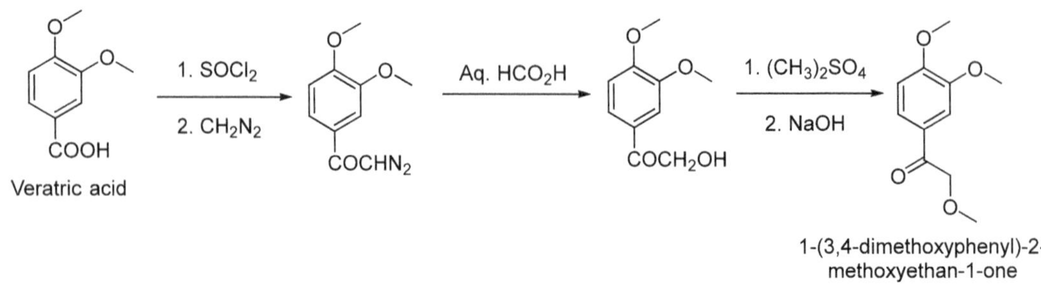

10. A step from the total synthesis of Cholesterol by Woodward (1951)

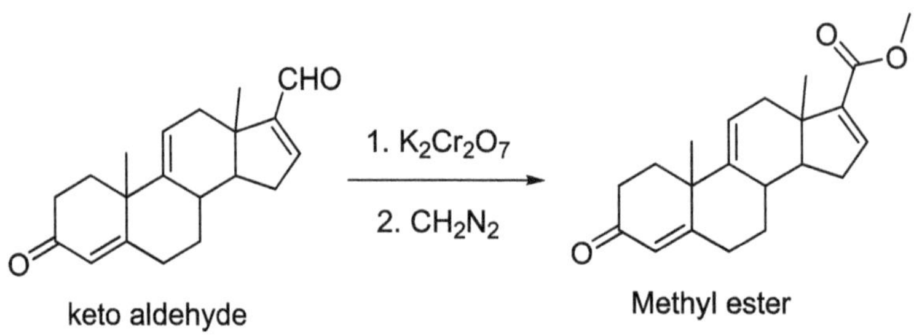

4. Dicyclohexyl carbodiimide (DCC)

Preparation: It can be prepared

a) by the dehydration of dicyclohexyl urea with *p*-toluenesulfonyl chloride

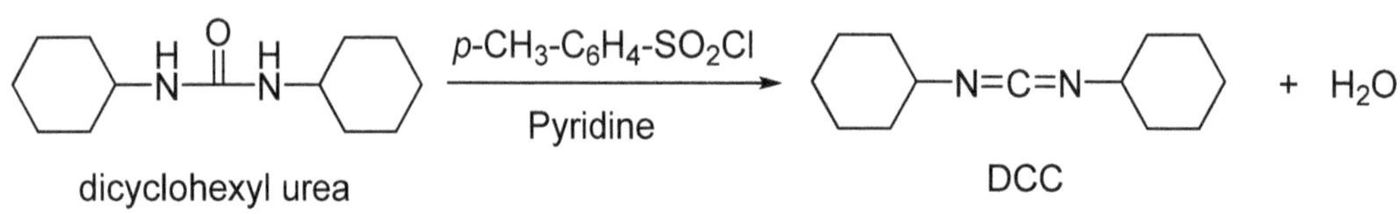

b) by the oxidation of *N,N'*-dicyclohexylthiourea

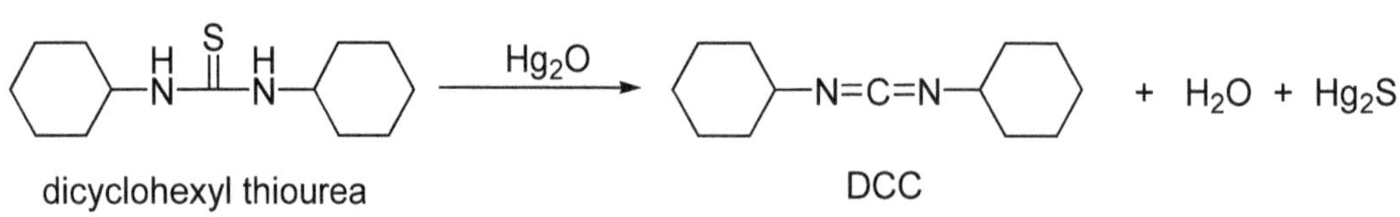

Uses:

It is widely used as a dehydrating agent in the organic synthesis particularly in the preparation of anhydrides, amides, esters, ethers, lactones, lactams and peptides. It is a mild reagent and useful in the formation of sensitive lactams and lactones particularly like in the case of Penicillin V.

Applications:

1. **Preparation of anhydrides**

$$2RCO_2H + DCC \longrightarrow (RCO)_2O + \underset{\text{Dicyclohexyl urea}}{C_6H_{11}\text{-NH-CO-NH-}C_6H_{11}}$$

2. **Preparation of amides**

$$2RCO_2H + R'NH_2 + DCC \longrightarrow RCONHR' + RCOOH + \underset{\text{Dicyclohexyl urea}}{C_6H_{11}\text{-NH-CO-NH-}C_6H_{11}}$$

Amide molecule is formed via the anhydride formation. The anhydride further reacts with amine to finally generate amide molecule.

a) $$2RCO_2H + DCC \longrightarrow (RCO_2)_2O + \underset{\text{Dicyclohexyl urea}}{C_6H_{11}\text{-NH-CO-NH-}C_6H_{11}}$$

b) $$(RCO_2)_2O + R'NH_2 \longrightarrow RCONHR' + RCOOH$$

3. **Preparation of esters**

$$RCO_2H + R'OH + DCC \longrightarrow RCO_2R' + C_6H_{11}\text{-NH-CO-NH-}C_6H_{11}$$

4. **Preparation of ethers**

$$PhOH + EtOH + DCC \xrightarrow{\text{Heat}} PhOEt + C_6H_{11}\text{-NH-CO-NH-}C_6H_{11}$$

5. **Preparation of lactones: In the synthesis of reserpine, γ-hydroxy acids are subjected to lactonization using DCC/Pyridine.**

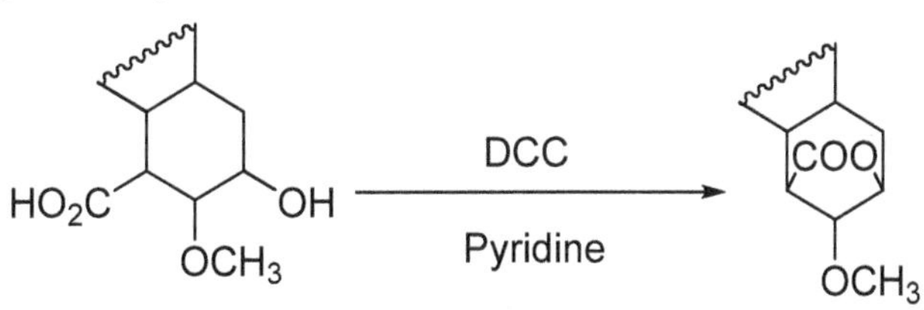

6. **Preparation of lactams**

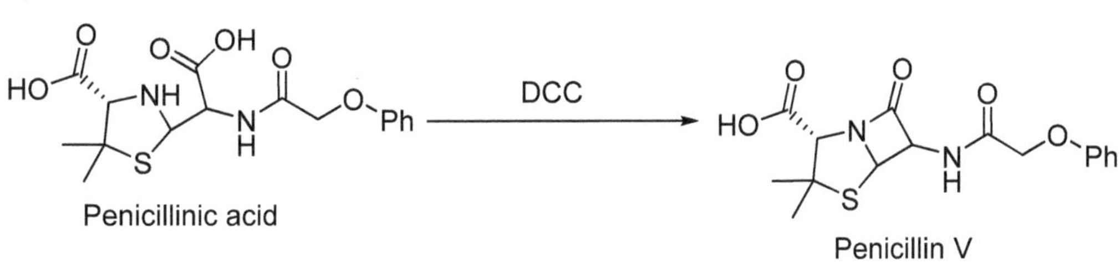

7. Preparation of barbituric acid derivatives

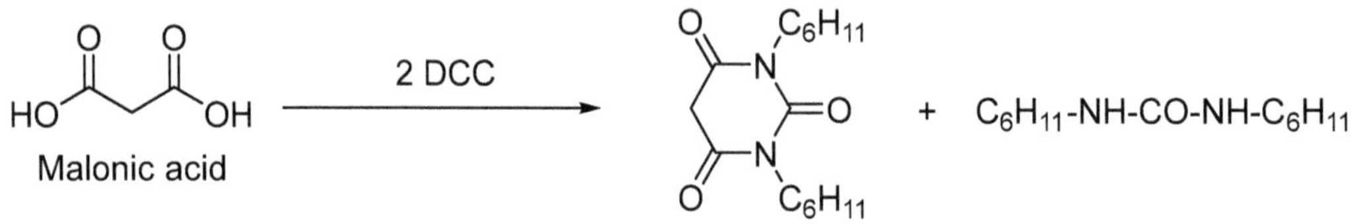

8. Preparation of ketones

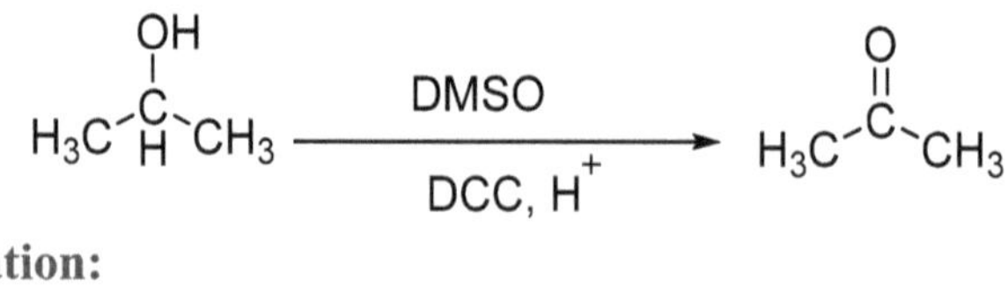

Pfitzner-Moffatt oxidation:

Oxidation of alcohols to ketones or aldehydes with DCC/DMSO

$$p\text{-}NO_2\text{-}C_6H_4\text{-}CH_2OH \xrightarrow{\text{DCC, DMSO}} p\text{-}NO_2\text{-}C_6H_4\text{-}CHO$$

4-nitro benzaldehyde

9. Steglich-Hassner direct esterification

Direct room temperature esterification of carboxylic acids with alcohols, mainly tert-alcohols with 4-dialkylaminopyridine and DCC.

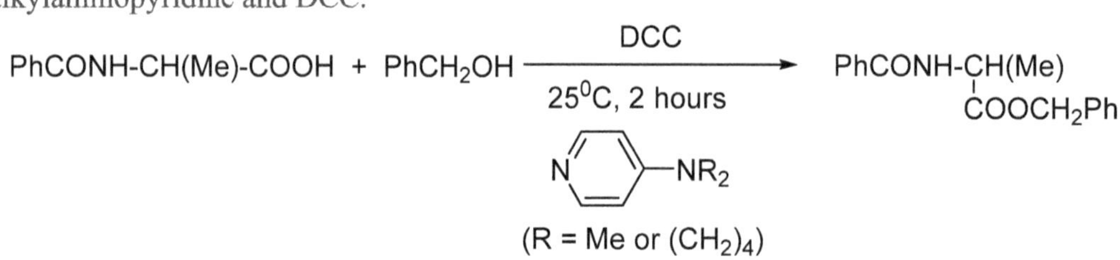

5. Wilkinson reagent

Preparation:

Wilkinson reagent is tris(triphenylphosphine) chlororhodium(I)-$RhCl(PPh_3)_3$, a complex of rhodium, widely used for homogenous hydrogenation. It is named after Sir Geoffrey Wilkinson who popularized its use. It has slightly distorted square planar structure. It can be prepared by reacting hydrated rhodium (III) chloride with excess triphenylphosphine in ethanol. One equivalent of PPh_3 reduces Rh (III) to Rh(I) and the other 3 equivalents of PPh_3 react with Rh to form complex as ligands.

$$4PPh_3 + RhCl_3(H_2O)_3 \longrightarrow RhCl(PPh_3)_3 + OPPh_3 + 2HCl + 2H_2O$$

Mechanism: Due to the vacant coordination sites present in rhodium, initially dihydro complex is formed with the addition of one molecule of H_2 and with the loss of one PPh_3 ligand, followed by formation of a π-complex with the alkene molecule by oxidative addition.

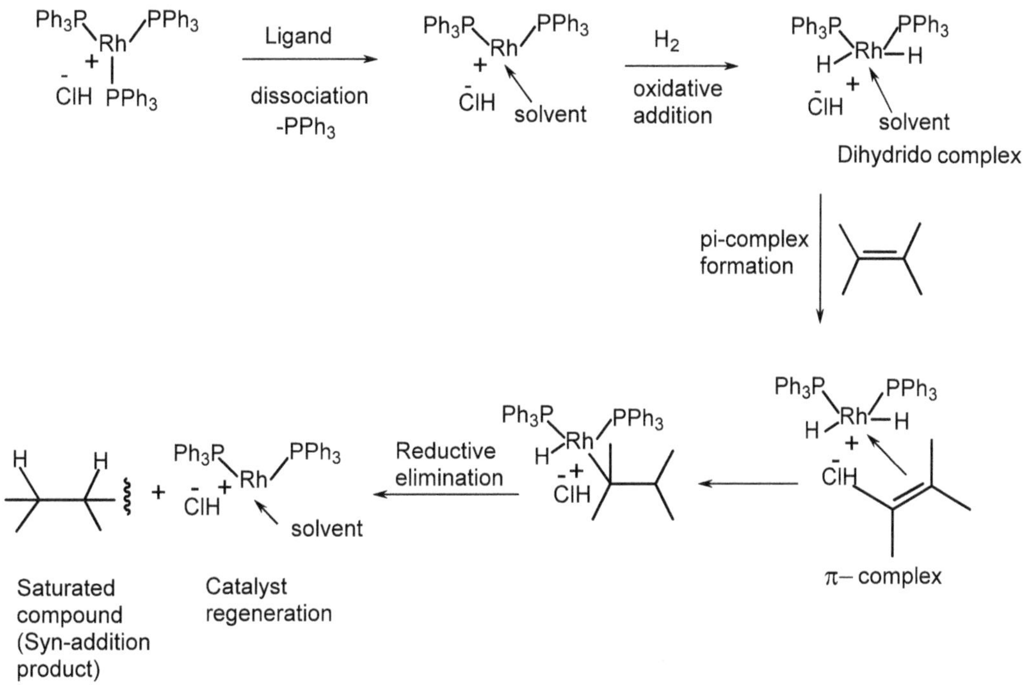

In the next step, hydrogen insertion by migration from metal to the alkene carbons either through intramolecular hydride transfer or through olefin insertion.

Terminal and disubstituted olefins undergo hydrogenation very well with this catalyst.

In the last step, reductive elimination takes place to liberate saturated product and regenerated catalyst. The addition occurs on the same face of the double bond giving Syn-product. The reaction is stereoselective and stereospecific. Insertion of H_2 is the rate-limiting step.
This reaction can be used to produce one or the other enantiomer from optically active ligands by enantioselectivity.

Applications: It is effectively used for faster, energy-efficient selective hydrogenations.

1. Hydroacylation of alkenes: Insertion of alkene into a formyl C-H bond.

a) Cyclization of 4-pentenal to cyclopentanone normalities

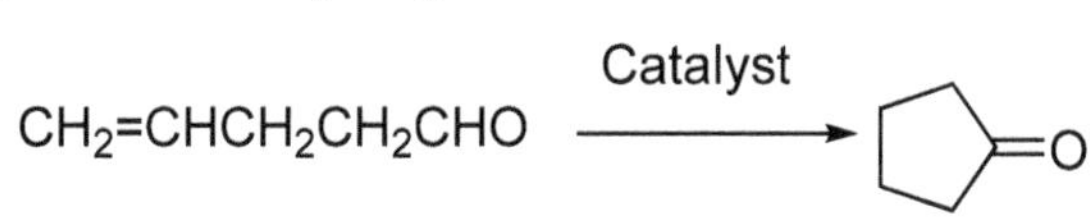

b) $RCHO + CH_2{=}CHR' \longrightarrow RC(O)CH_2CH_2R'$

2. Hydroboration of alkenes

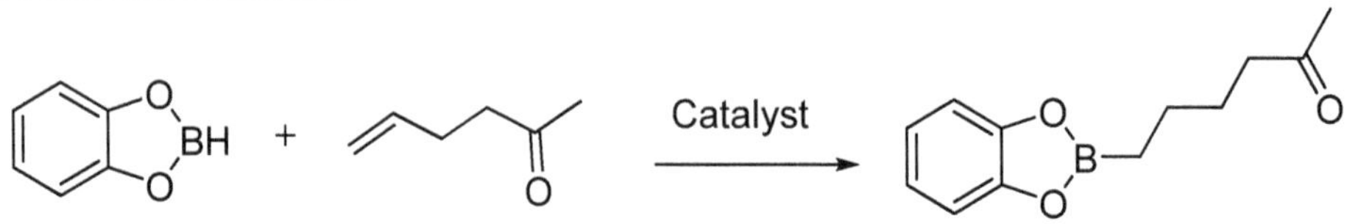

3. Hydrosilylation of alkenes

4. Selective reduction of least hindered olefins

a) Least hindered

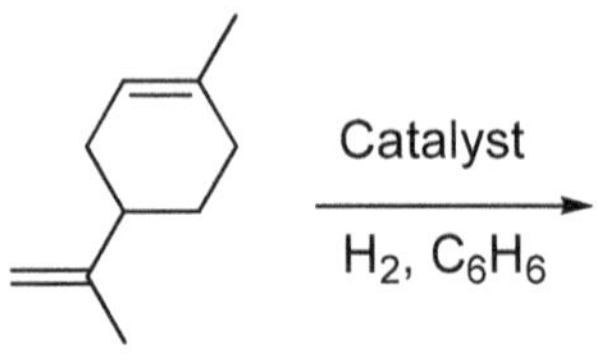

b) Exocyclic reduction

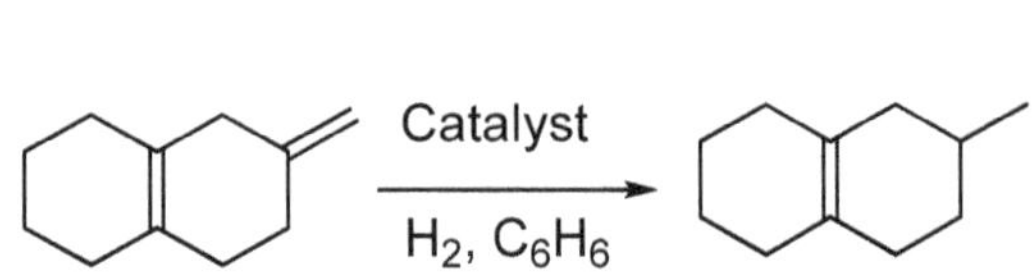

5. Hydrogenation of functionalized trisubstituted alkenes

6. Preparation of L-Dopa, used in Parkinson's disease

7. Cis-alkene reduction

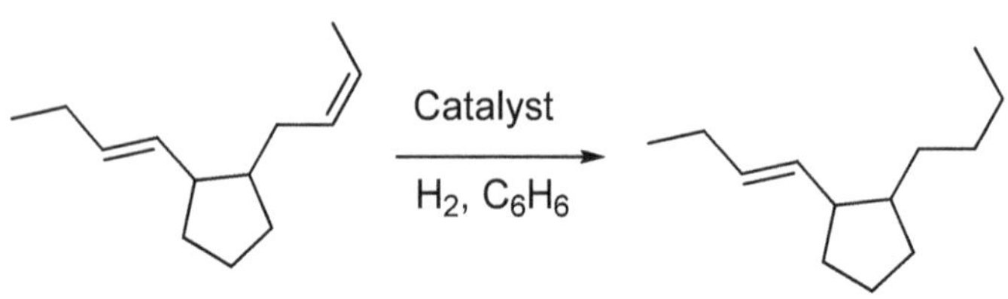

8. Terminal alkynes are reduced faster than terminal alkenes

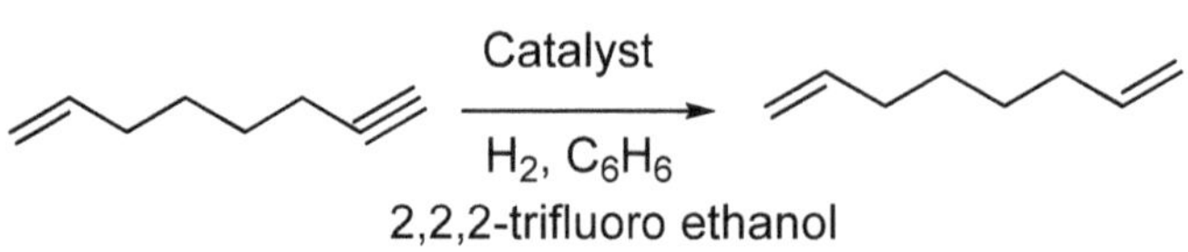

9.

a)

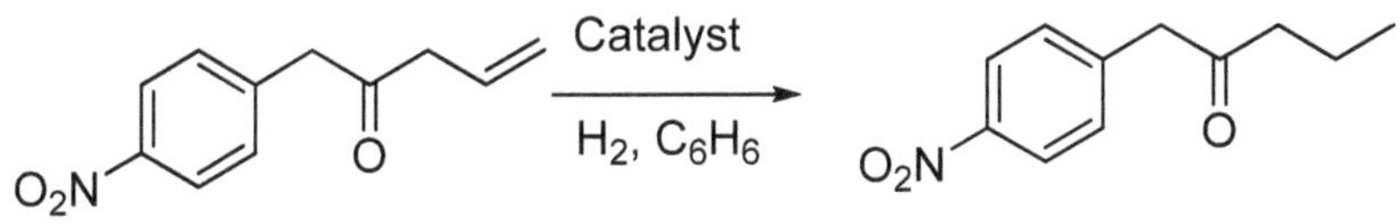

b)

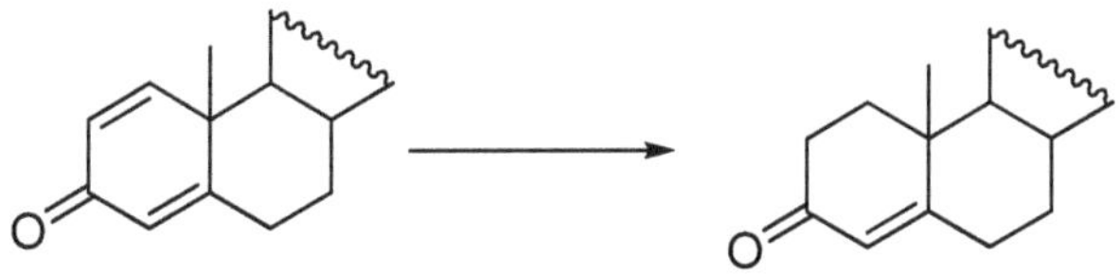

10. Preparation of cis-alkenes from alkynes

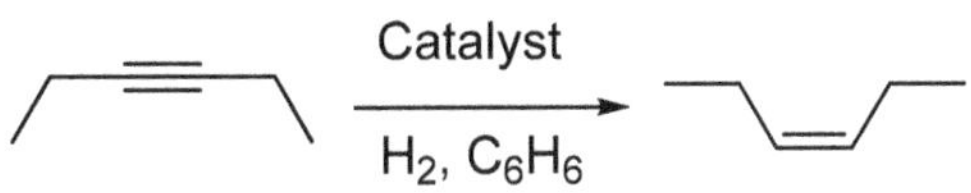

11. Preparation of Ivermectin molecule from avermectin, an anthelmintic compound by the selective reduction of a double bond

12. Wilkinson decarboxylation

Removal of carbonyl groups from aldehydes or acid chlorides with Wilkinson catalyst produce alkanes or alkenes.

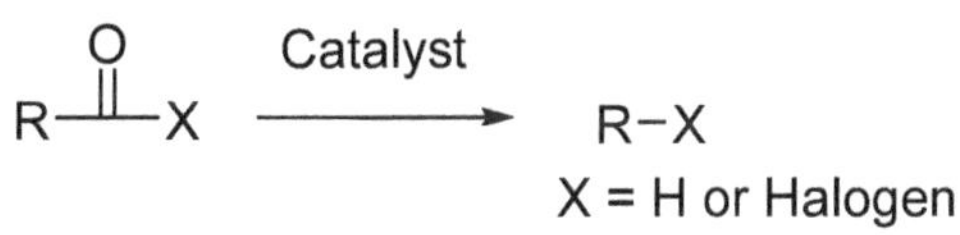

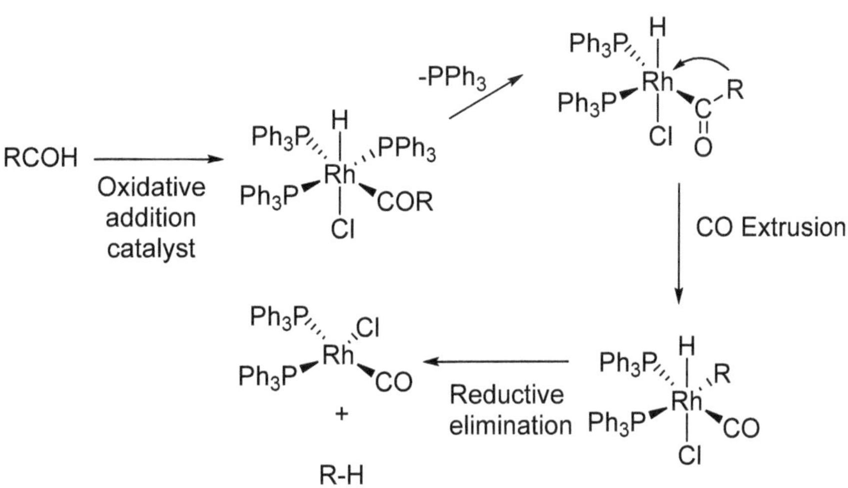

6. Wittig reagent

Wittig reagents are organophosphorus compounds ($R_3P{=}CHR'$), ($R{=}Ph$) and are used to convert ketones and aldehydes to alkenes. This reaction is called Wittig olefination.
The reaction is regularly applied in industries, particularly in the manufacture of drugs and also natural product synthesis.

General reaction:

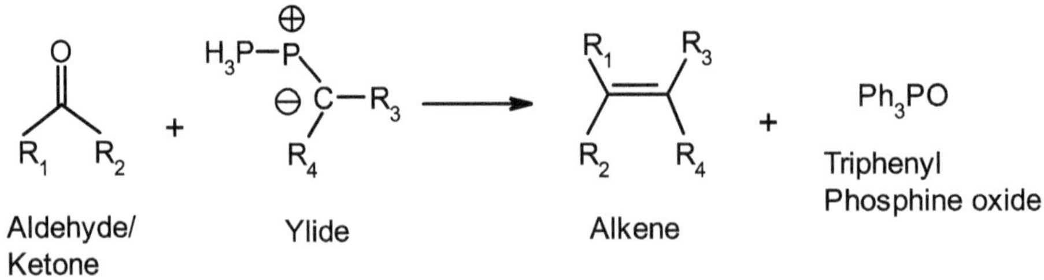

Reagent is known as phosphonium ylide. The reaction was reported by George Wittig and Ulrich Schollkopf in 1954. For this work, Wittig was awarded Nobel Prize in 1979. Methylene group is often introduced into the molecules using $Ph_3P{=}CH_2$, methylenetriphenylphosphorane. The reagent contains a stabilized carbanion capable of attacking an aldehyde or ketone. Phosphorus atom stabilizes the carbanion. These are important reagents and are widely used.

It can also be used to prepare conjugated alkenes from α,β-unsaturated ketones.

Preparation:

These are prepared in air-free environment as these are prone for hydrolysis and oxidation. These are generally generated and used in situ. THF solvent is used. Quaternization of triphenylphosphine with primary alkyl halide gives phosphonium salt which is used for preparing Wittig reagent. The alkyl phosphonium salts are deprotonated with strong bases such as n-butyllithium, sodium or potassium tert-butoxides (tBuONa or tBuOK), lithium, sodium and potassium hexamethylsilazides (LiHMDS, NaHMDS, KHMDS; HMDS = Hexamethylsilazides-N(SiMe3)2 or sodium hydride (NaH). NaOH or K_2CO_3 can also be employed in the case of stabilized Wittig reagents with conjugated electron withdrawing groups. Selection of proper base is crucial for the conduct of reaction.

General reaction:

$$[Ph_3\overset{\oplus}{P}CH_2R]X + C_4H_9Li \longrightarrow Ph_3P{=}CHR + LiX + C_4H_{10}$$

$$Ph_3\overset{\oplus}{P}\overset{\ominus}{C}R_2 \longleftrightarrow Ph_3P{=}CR_2$$

Resonating structures
of the reagent

Wittig reagent examples:

$Ph_3P{=}CHCl$	$Ph_3P{=}CHOCH_3$	$Ph_3P{=}CH_2$
Chloromethylene triphenylphosphorane	Methoxymethylene triphenylphosphorane	Methylene triphenylphosphorane

$Ph_3P{=}CHCOOEt$	$Ph_3P{=}C{=}PPh_3$
Triphenyl carbethoxymethylene phosphorane	Hexaphenyl carbodiphosphorane

Mechanism:

The reaction involves the following steps:

a) Reaction of haloalkane with triphenylphosphine forming phosphonium salt.

b) Formation of phosphorus ylide (phosphorane) from the phosphonium salt by deprotonation in the presence of strong base.

c) The ylide carbon is strongly nucleophilic and attack the carbonyl carbon forming Betaine, containing positively charged phosphorus atom and negatively charged oxygen atom, both forming a very strong bond resulting in four-membered oxaphosphetane ring.

d) The oxaphosphetane ring rapidly transforms to the desired alkenes and triphenylphosphine oxide, a very stable compound.

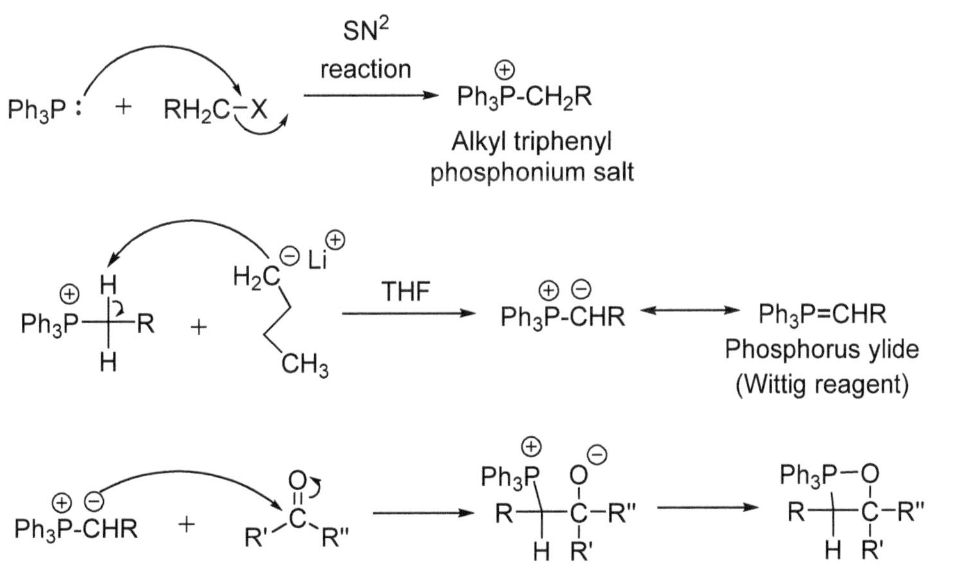

Betaine Oxaphosphetane

The reaction mainly proceeds via the erythron-betaine intermediate generating Z-alkene. When phenyl lithium is used at low temperature, erythron-betaine can be converted to threo-betaine affording finally E-alkene. This modification is called Schlosser modification.

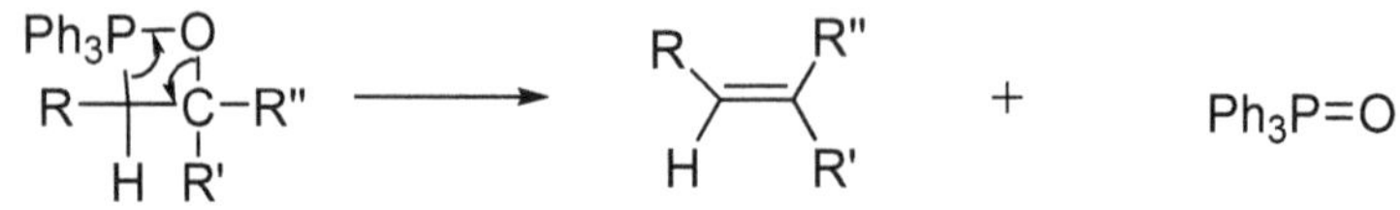

Oxaphosphetane — Alkene — triphenylphosphine oxide

Applications:

1. 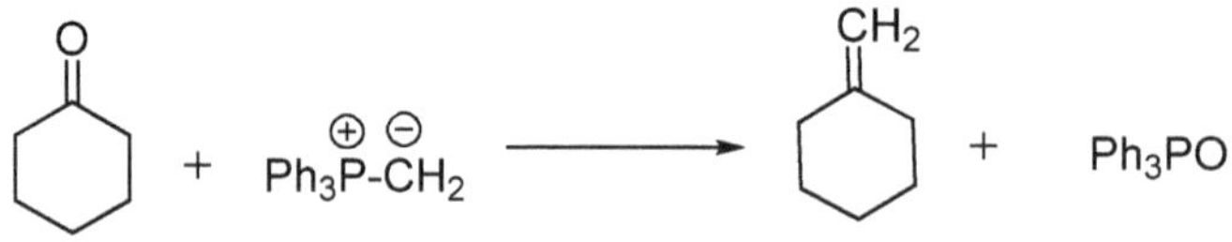

cyclohexanone — Methylene cyclohexane

2. PhCHO (Benzaldehyde) + $Ph_3\overset{\oplus}{P}\text{-}\overset{\ominus}{C}H_2$ ⟶ Ph-CH=CH-Ph ((z)-1,2 diphenyl ethene) + Ph_3PO

3. $PhCOCH_3$ (Acetophenone) + $Ph_3\overset{\oplus}{P}\text{–}\overset{\ominus}{C}H_2$ ⟶ $Ph\text{–}C(CH_3){=}CH_2$ (α–methyl styrene) + Ph_3PO

4. $CH_3CH_2COCH_2CH_3$ (3-pentanone) + $Ph_3\overset{\oplus}{P}\text{-}\overset{\ominus}{C}H_2$ $\xrightarrow{THF}$ $CH_3CH_2\text{-}C(CH_2CH_3){=}CHCH_3$ (3-ethyl-2-pentene) + Ph_3PO

5. 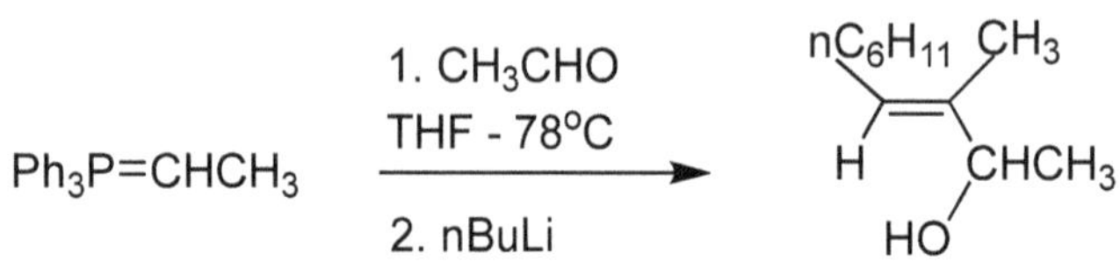

Allylic alcohol

6. 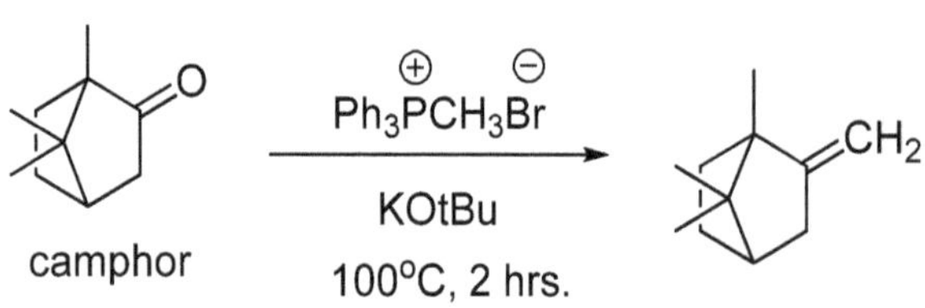

camphor

7. Wittig and Horner reaction-

The reaction of aldehydes or ketones with stabilized phosphorus ylide gives products with E-selectivity.

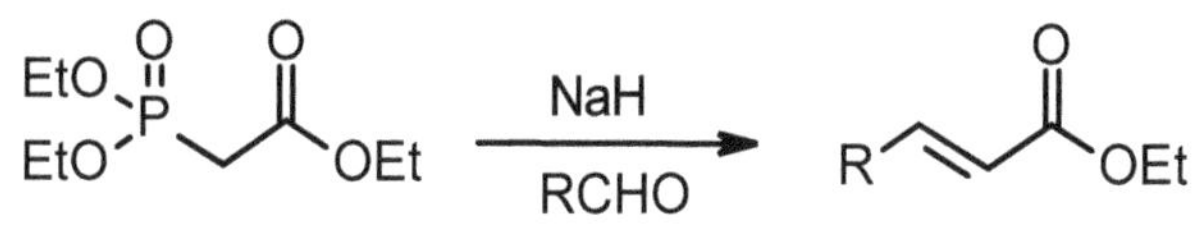

8. Aza and Wittig reaction-

A nitrogen version of Wittig reaction where imines are generated from carbonyl compounds by the reaction of iminophosphorane intermediate.

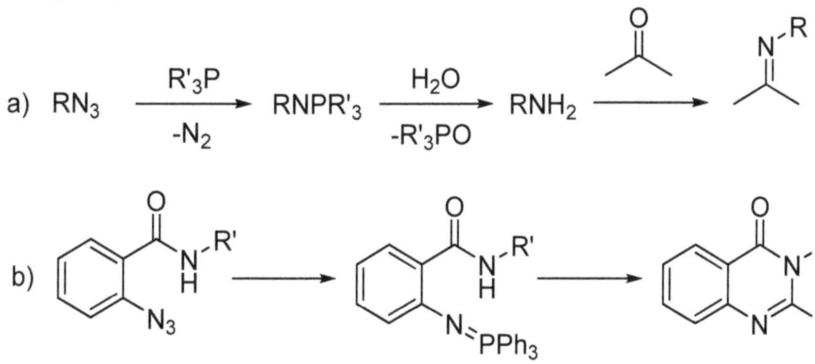

Iminophosphoranes are powerful tools and can be converted to a broad range of products depending on the electrophiles that react with them.

9. Synthesis of Vitamin A acetate

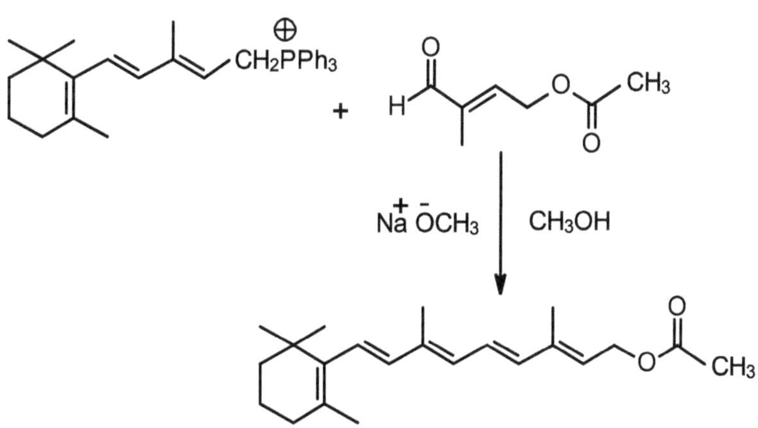

Vit. A acetate

10.

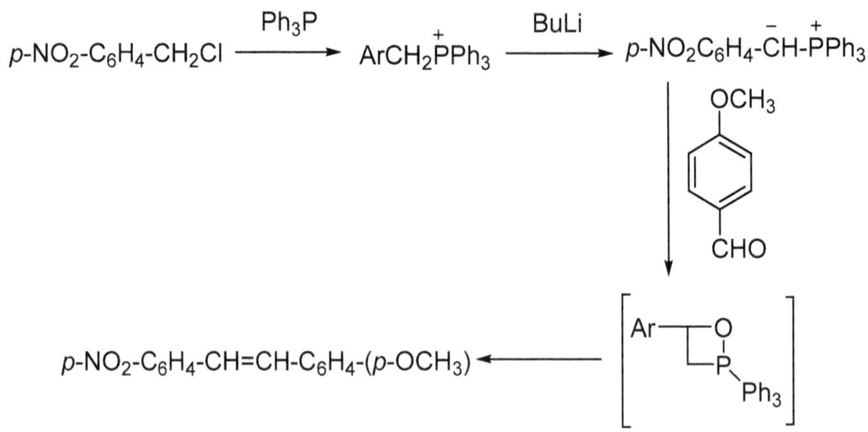

7. Osmium tetroxide:

It is known as osmic acid, a Lewis acid and mild oxidant. Osmium (VIII) tetroxide (OsO_4) is widely used in organic synthesis to oxidize alkenes to vicinal diols (syn-addition) and as staining agent in transmission electron microscopy (TEM) as well as to stain copolymers preferentially.

It is conducted in the presence of ether or tert-butyl alcohol, in presence of base like pyridine. It is toxic, expensive and used in structural elucidation. The compound was discovered by Smithson Tennant in 1803. It was introduced in organic reactions by Palade in 1952.

Preparation:

Osmium powder on oxidation with O_2 at ambient temperature provides OsO_4.

$$Os + 2O_2 \xrightarrow{\text{Red Heat}} OsO_4$$

General reaction:

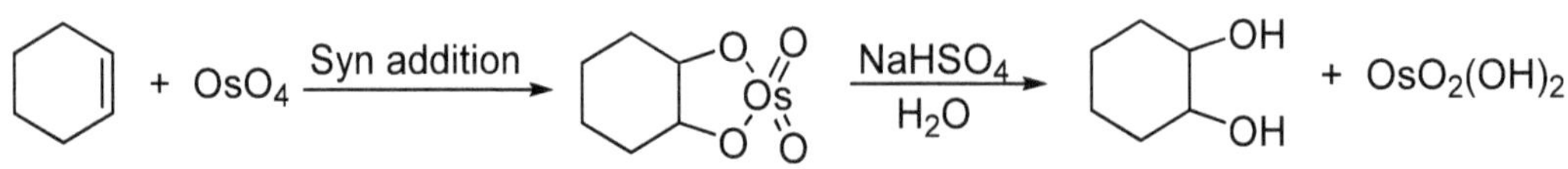

Cis-1,2-diol

Mechanism:

The reaction works by concerted process. via (3+2) cycloaddition. In this two oxygen atoms from OsO_4 interact with same side of the C=C double bond, leading to five-membered osmate ester, which rapidly hydrolyses to generate vicinal diol.

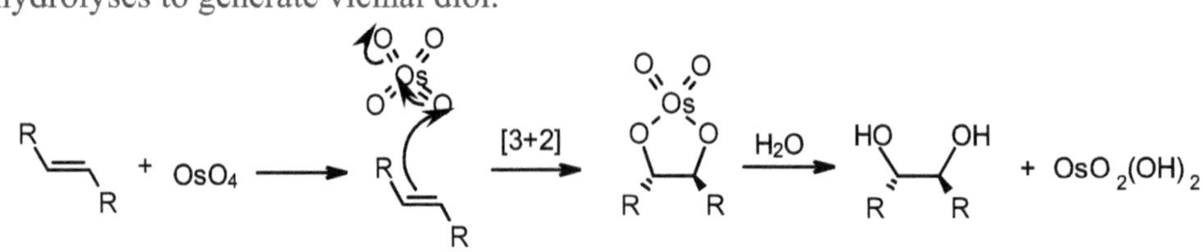

Addition of reoxidants like H_2O_2, *N*-methylmorpholine-*N*-Oxide, and $K_3Fe(CN)_6/H_2O$ reoxidize the Os (VI) to Os (VIII). Lemieux-Johnson oxidation uses periodate for cleaving diols to generate two aldehyde molecules.

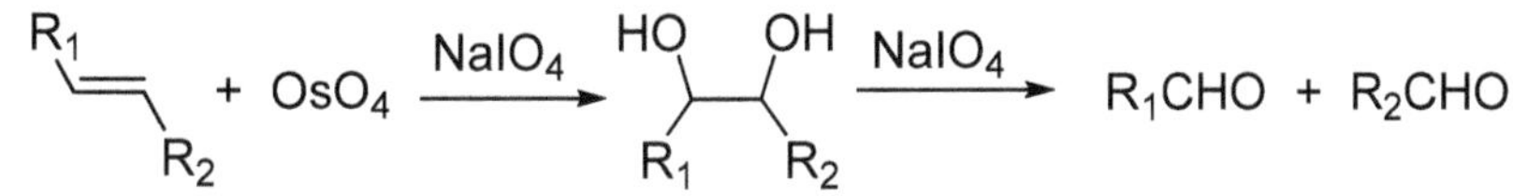

In sharpless oxyamination, OsO4 is used to generate vicinal amino alcohols. It is related to Sharpless dihydroxylation.

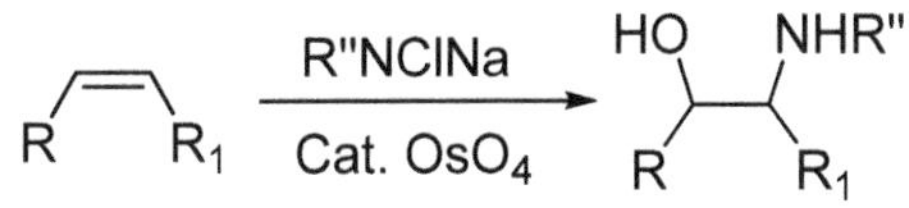

Applications:

1.
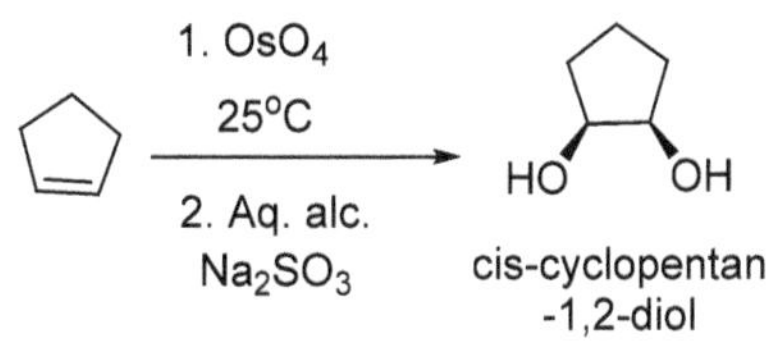

2.
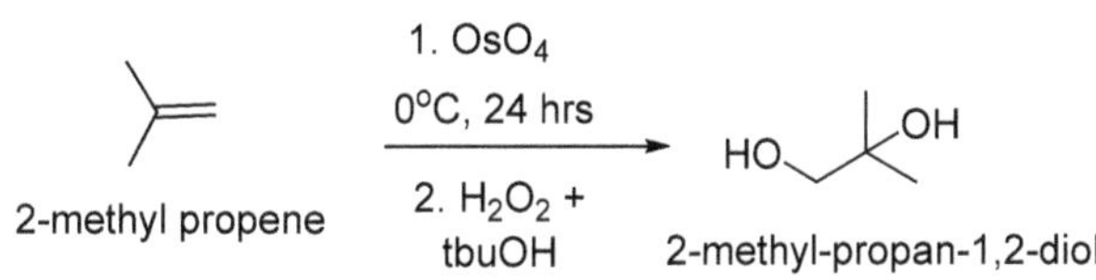

3.
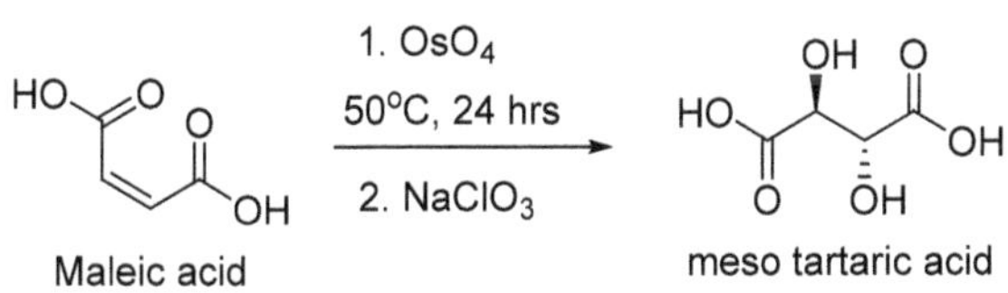

4.
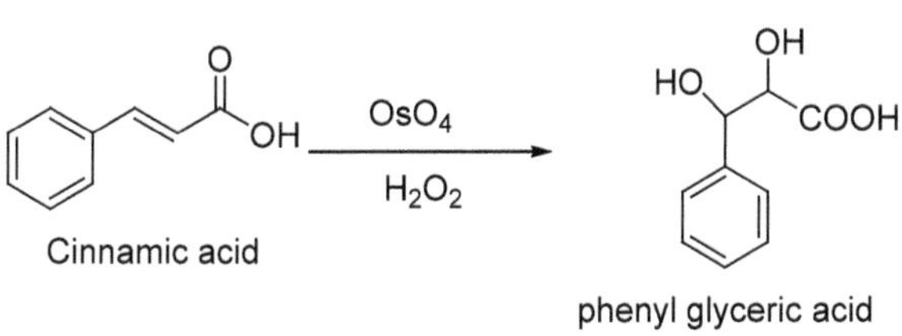

5.
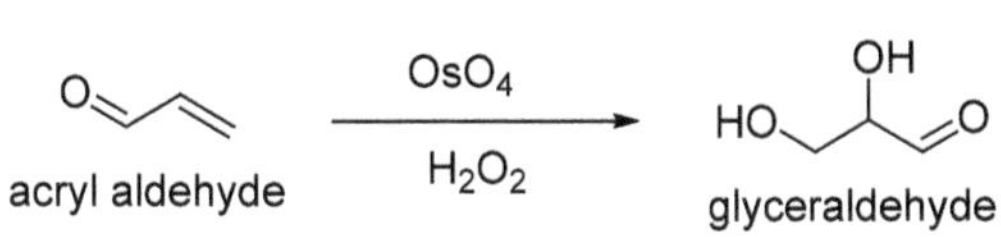

6.

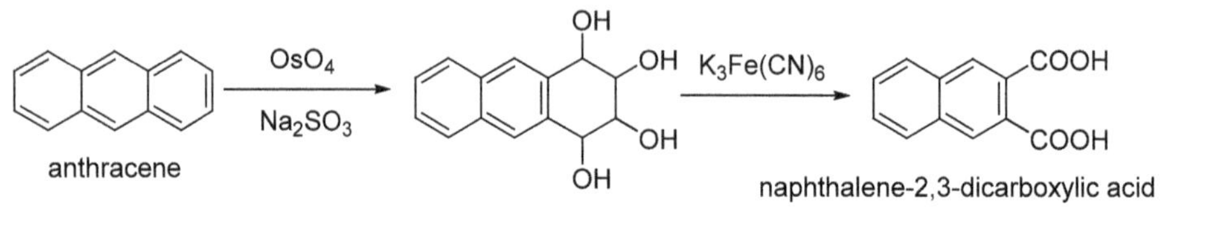

(Indicates linear fusion of 3 rings of anthracene and *ortho* fusion of 3rd ring)

7.

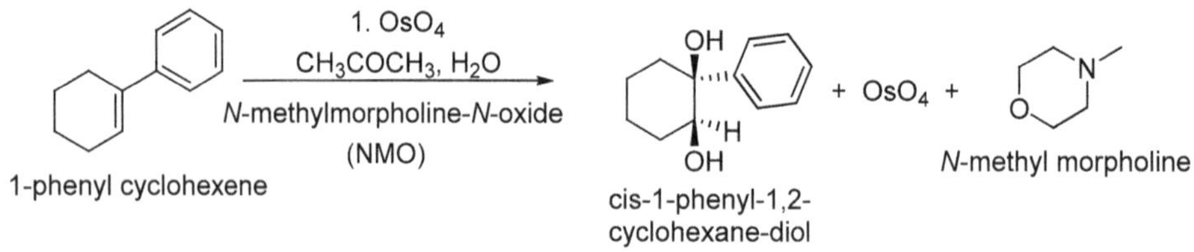

8.

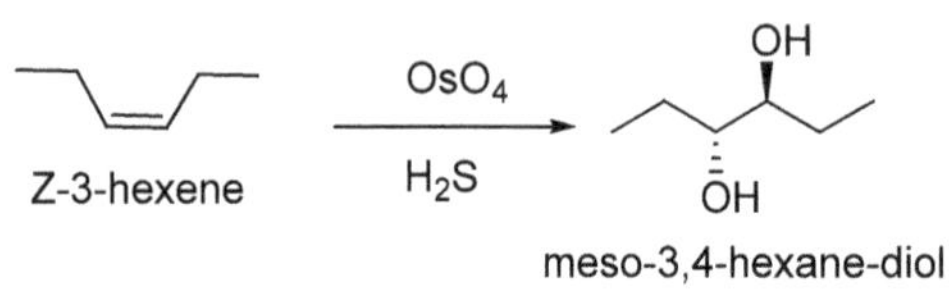

9.

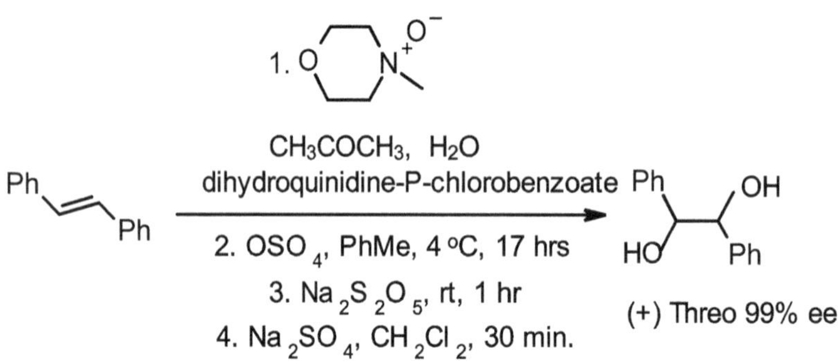

10.

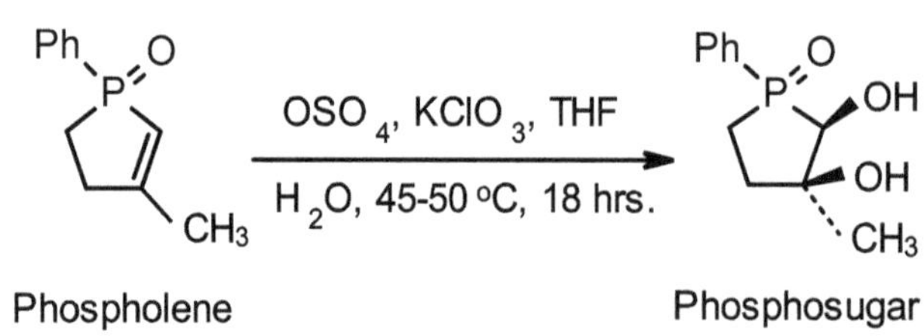

11.

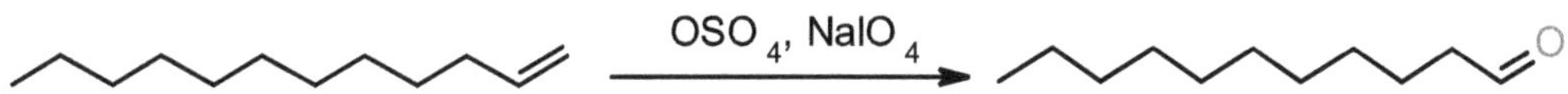

dodecene-1 → undecanal

12. Milas olefin hydroxylation: Hydroxylation of a double bond to 1,2-diol with H_2O_2/OsO_4

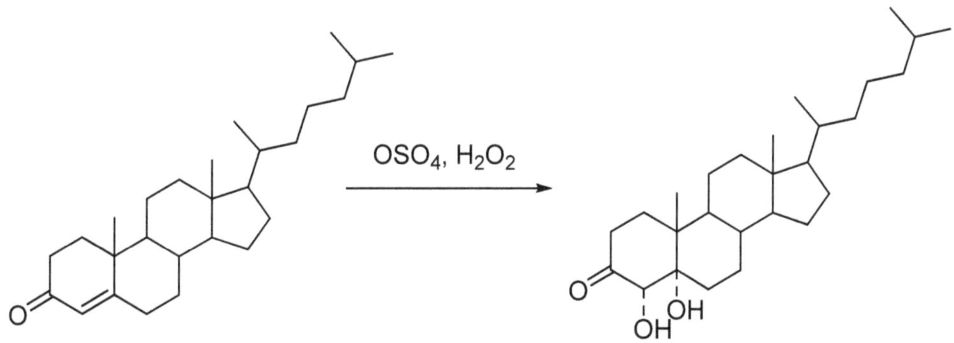

Cholestenone → 4,5-dihydroxy-cholestan-3-one

8. Titanium Chloride: ($TiCl_4$)

It is a dense, colourless, distillable liquid soluble in toluene and chlorocarbons.

Preparation:

It is prepared by the chloride process, involving reduction of titanium oxide ores ($FeTiO_3$), ilmenite with carbon under chlorine gas flow at 900 °C. In this process, undesirable $FeCl_3$ is produced as side product.

a) $$2FeTiO_3 + 7Cl_2 + 6C \longrightarrow 2TiCl_4 + 2FeCl_3 + 6CO$$

In the second method, rutile slag, a crude form of TiO_2 is used. $TiCl_4$ is mainly used for the production of TiO2, an important pigment, by the hydrolysis.

b) $$TiCl_4 + 2H_2O \longrightarrow TiO_2 + 4HCl$$

or

$$TiCl_4 + O_2 \longrightarrow TiO_2 + 2Cl_2$$

Known as "Tickle", $TiCl_4$ is used in smoke machines, and onset smoke effects for motion pictures (earlier to 1980s) due to its property of forming of white, heavy smoke on contact with humid air. Moreover, it is powerful, versatile reagent which can form diverse derivatives in a variety of chemical reactions. It acts as Lewis acid in organic synthesis.

Applications:

1. 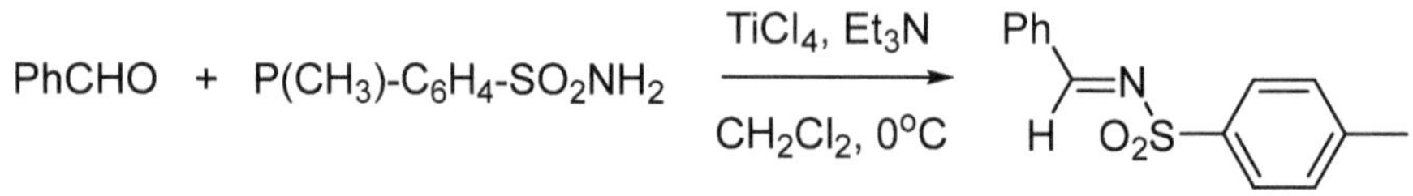

N-sulphonyl imines

2. 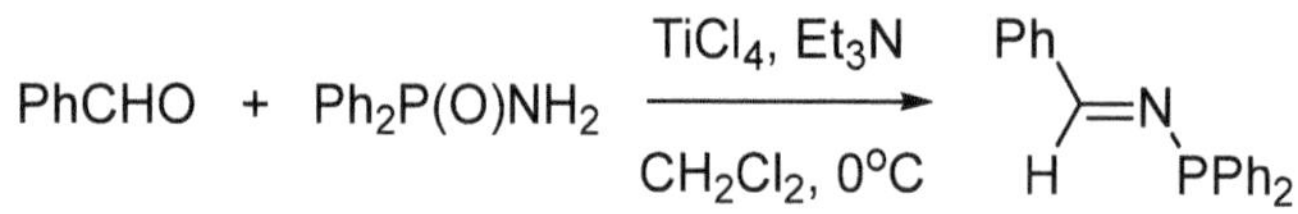

N-phosphinoyl imines

3. 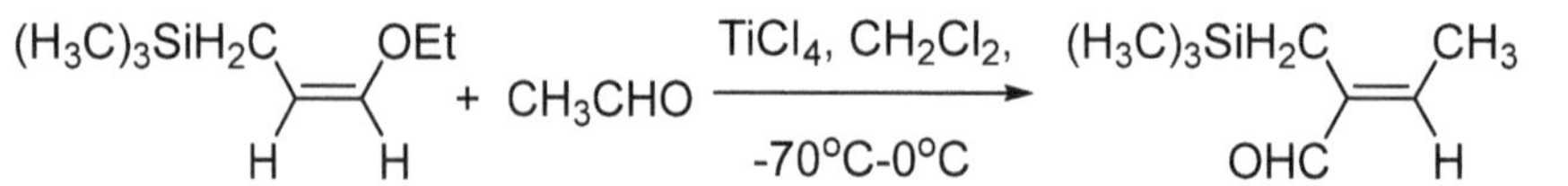

Allyl trimethyl silane

4. 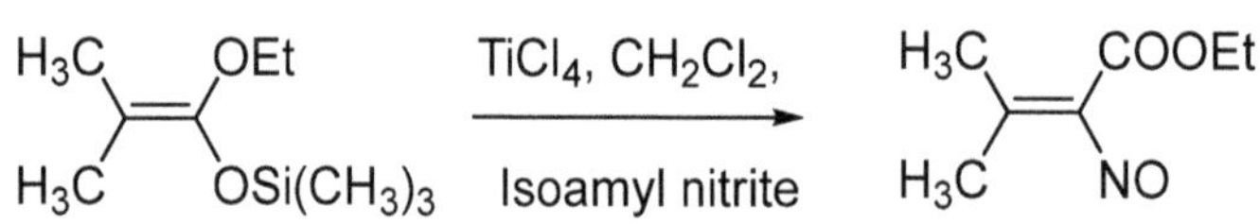

alpha-nitroso ester

5. 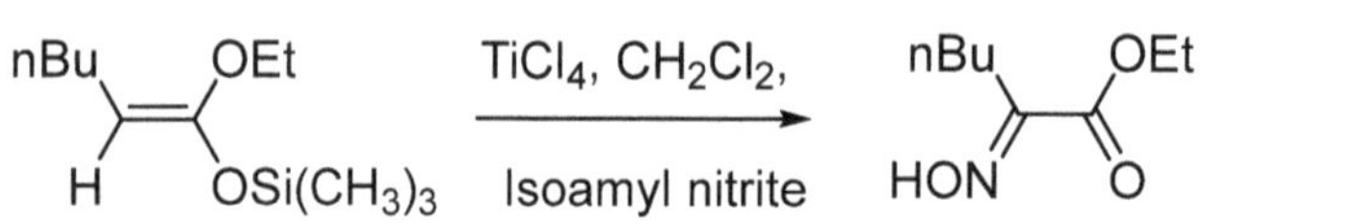

alpha-ketoester oxime

6. Blanc-Quellet chloroalkylation

Lewis-catalyzed aromatic chloromethylation

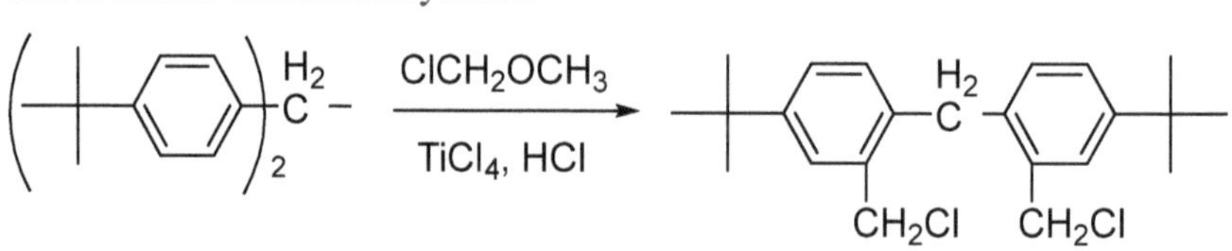

7. Cooper-Finkbeiner hydromagnesiation

Ti-catalyzed reaction of grignard reagents with olefins or acetylenes

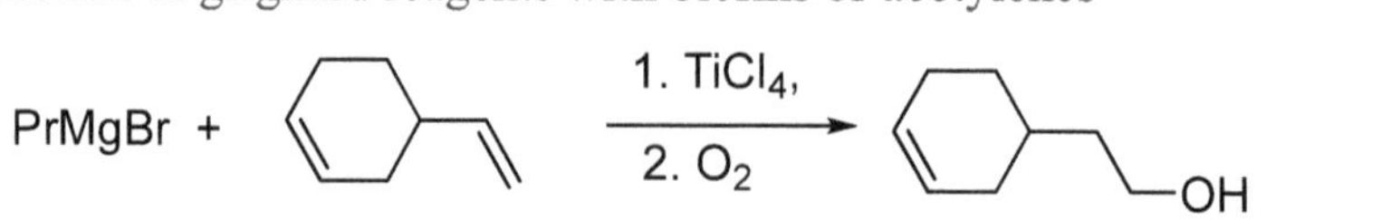

2-(cyclohex-3-en-1-yl)ethan-1-ol

8. Danheiser annulation- Regiocontrolled synthesis of five-membered rings from Silyl allenes and Michael acceptors in the presence of $TiCl_4$.

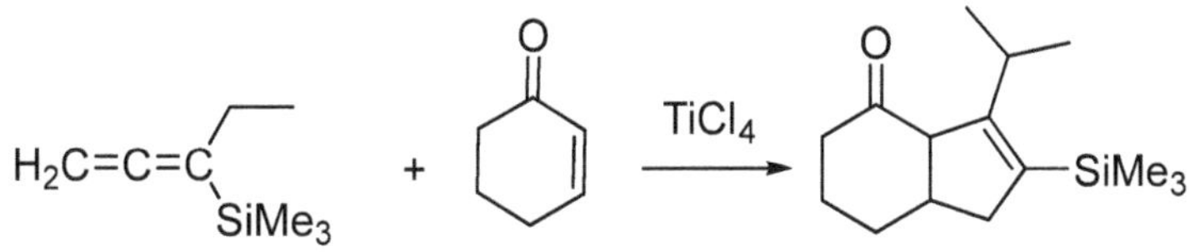

9. REPPE Acetylene reaction

Ni or Ti-catalyzed tetramerization or trimerization of acetylene

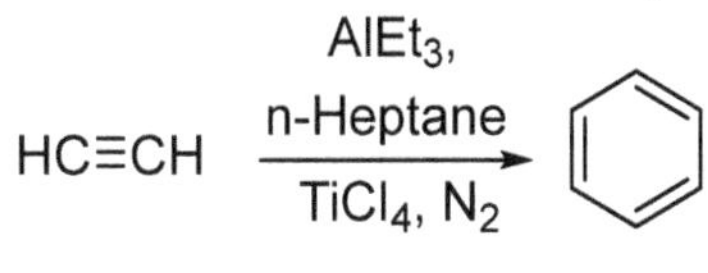

benzene

10. Sakurai Allylation

Ti-mediated intra or inter-molecular addition of allylic silanes to α, β- unsaturated ketones or aldehydes.

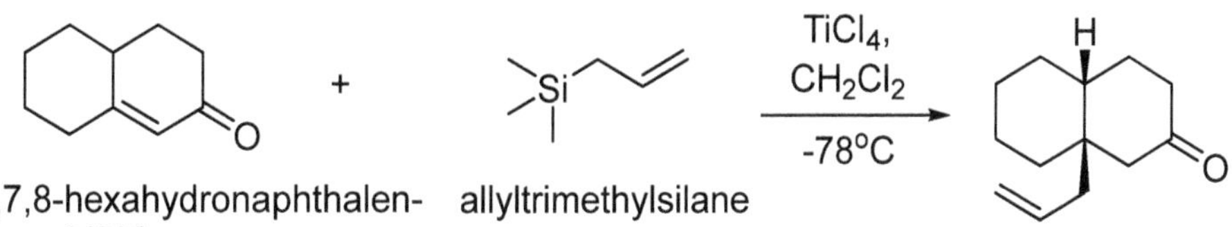

4,4a,5,6,7,8-hexahydronaphthalen-2(3*H*)-one   allyltrimethylsilane   9-allyl-2-decalone

9. Diethylazodicarboxylate: $CH_3CH_2OCON{=}NCOOCH_2CH_3$ (DEAD)

It is an explosive, commercially available, orange-red liquid. It is a good electron acceptor, azadienophile and dehydrogenating agent. It is a most commonly used reagent, particularly in Mitsunobu reaction. DEAD is employed for conversion of alcohols to aldehydes, thiols to disulphides, and hydrazo groups to azo groups. It is widely used in the synthesis of natural products and drug molecules like Zidovudine and Procarbazine (anti-tumor). It dissolves in most of the organic solvents and less soluble in water. It undergoes pericyclic reactions with alkenes and dienes via enes and Diels-Alder mechanism.

Preparation: It can be prepared from hydrazine by alkylation with ethyl chloroformate followed by chlorination.

$$NH_2NH_2 + 2ClCOOCH_2CH_3 \xrightarrow[-HCl]{Na_2CO_3} H_5C_2OOC\text{-}NH\text{-}NH\text{-}COOC_2H_5 \xrightarrow[\text{or } Cl_2]{HNO_3} H_5C_2OOC\text{-}N{=}N\text{-}COOC_2H_5$$

Applications:

1. Preparation of alkyl halides and alkyl cyanides from alcohols

$$ROH \xrightarrow[\text{DEAD, THF}]{\text{LiX, } PPh_3} RX \quad R = \text{Alkyl, Steroidal; } X = \text{Halide, CN}$$

2. Preparation of diethyl (phenyl thio) alkyl phosphonates

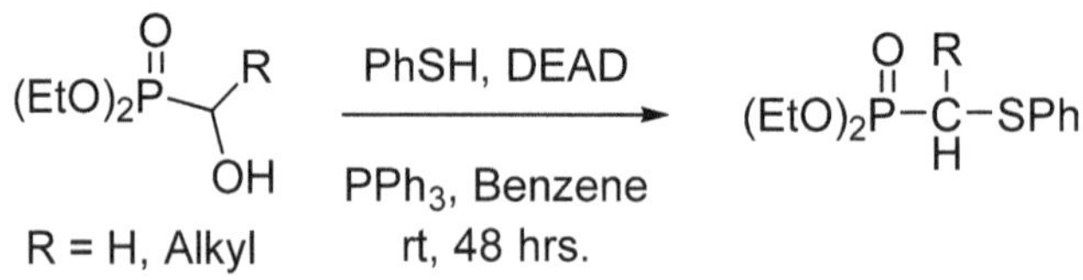

3. Preparation of 2-oxazolines

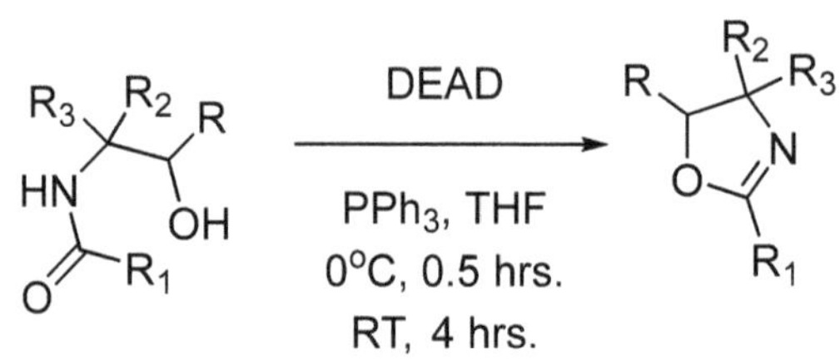

R, R_2, R_3 = H, Alkyl, Aryl

R_1 = Alkyl, Aryl

4. Preparation of pyrazoline compounds

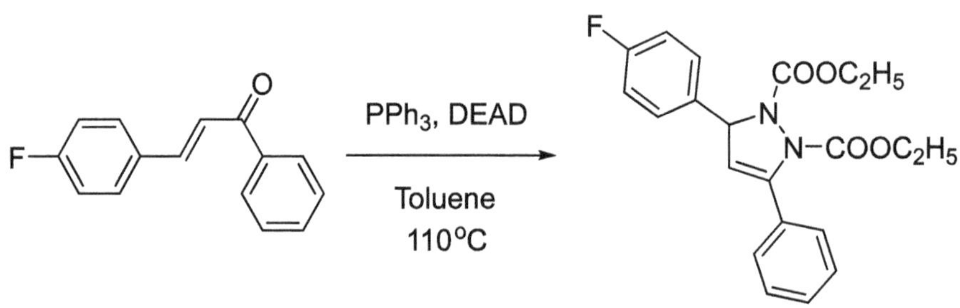

5. Ene reaction

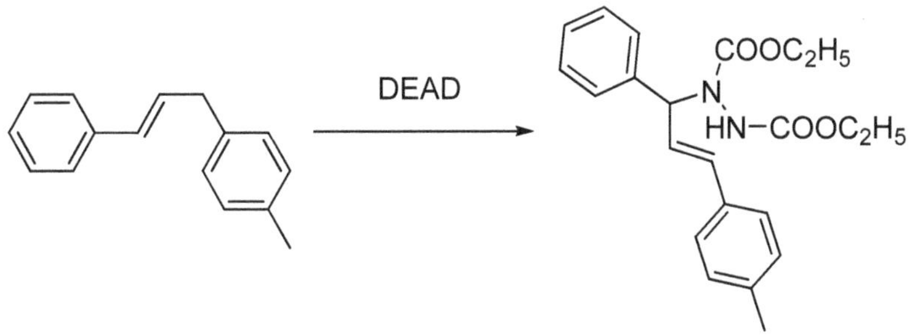

6. Michael reaction

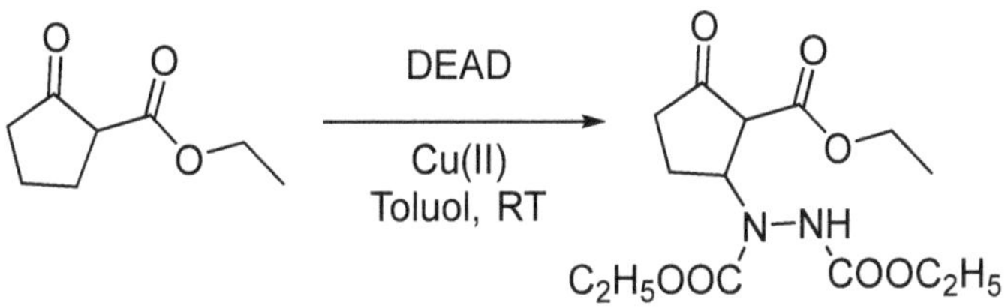

7. Substitution of Boronic acid esters

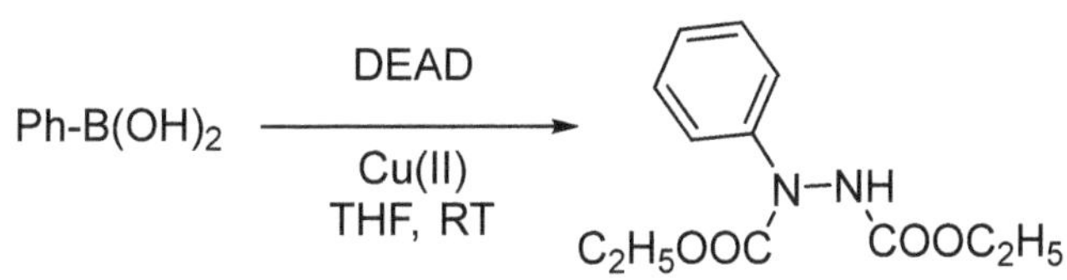

8. Mitsunobu reaction

$$RCOOH + R'OH \xrightarrow[\text{PhI(OAc)}_2\text{, THF, 25°C, 16 hrs.}]{\text{DEAD, PPh}_3} RCOOR'$$

10. Triphenyl phosphine: (PPh_3)

It is an air-stable, colourless compound with solubility in non-polar organic solvents like ether or benzene. It is widely used in the preparation of organic and organometallic compounds.

Preparation:

It can be prepared by the treatment of phosphorus trichloride with phenyl lithium or phenylmagnesium bromide or by the reaction with sodium in chlorobenzene.

$$PCl_3 + 3PhCl + 6Na \longrightarrow PPh_3 + 6NaCl$$

Polymer-anchored PPh_3 derivatives are employed in place of PPh_3 due to ease of separability in many reactions. PPh3 binds to many transition metals forming complexes which find use as catalysts.
Example: $NiBr_2(PPh_3)_2$; $RhH(PPh_3)CO$

Applications:

1. **Formation of phosphanimines**

$$PPh_3 + PhN_3 \longrightarrow PhNPPh_3 + N_2$$

2. **Preparation of vinylglycines via the formation of phosphorane and phosphonate synthons**

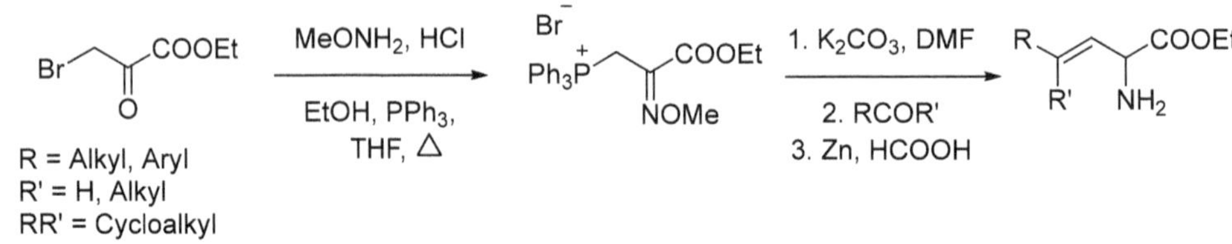

3. **Synthesis of isoquinolines by the condensation of iminophosphoranes**

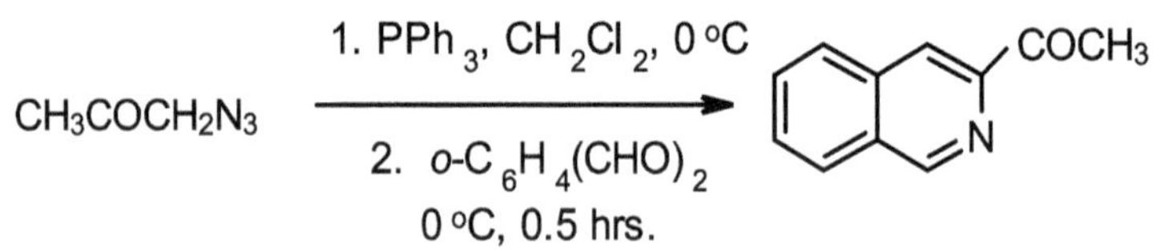

4. **Regiospecific formation of dienes by the inter/intramolecular coupling of vinyl halides**

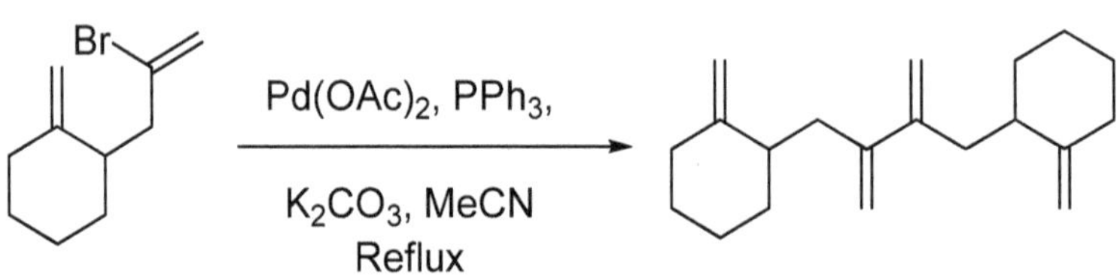

5. **Mitsunobu reaction-synthesis of aryl ethers**

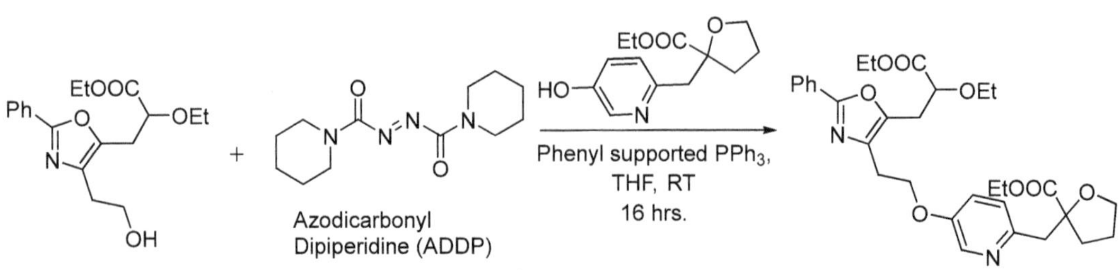

6. Mitsunobu reaction

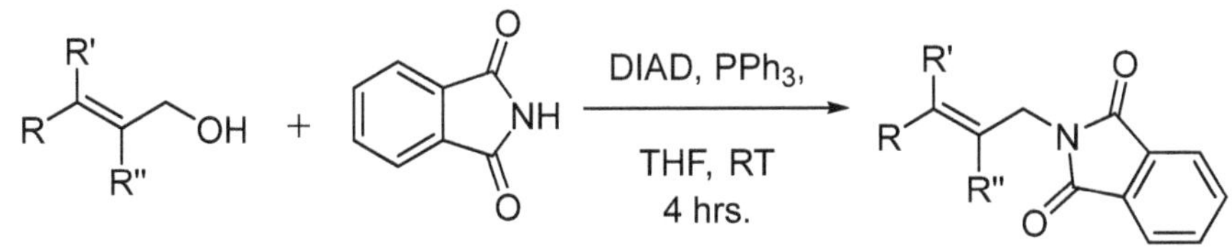

DIAD = Disopropyl Azodicarboxylate

7. Ozonolysis

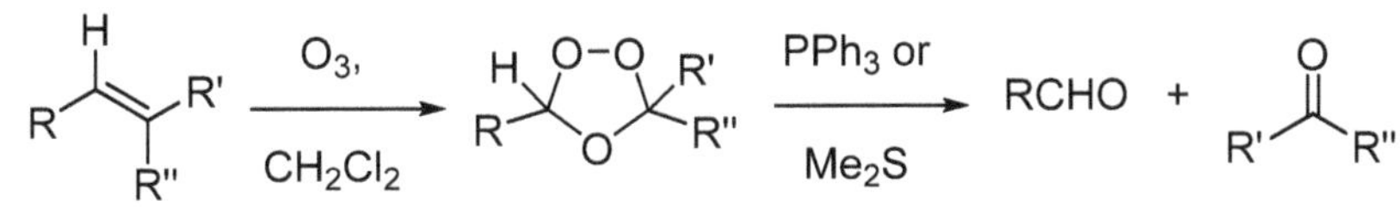

8. Staudinger reaction

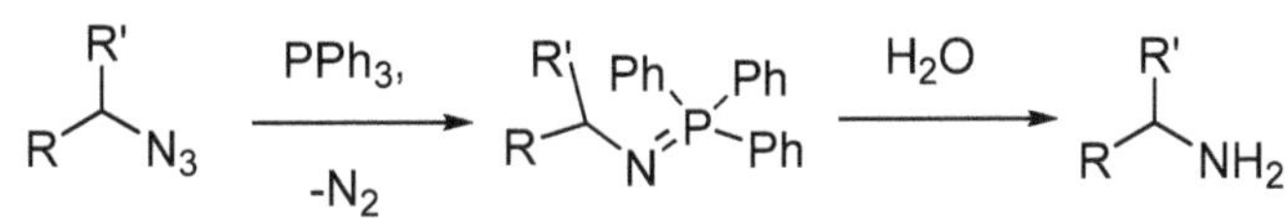

9. Reduction of N-oxides

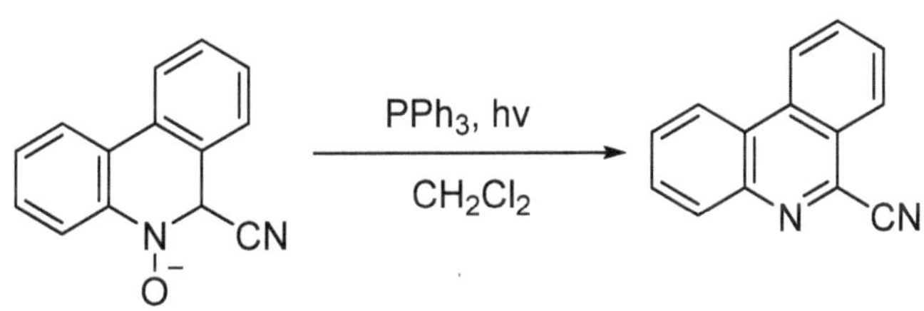

10. Synthesis of cappatriene

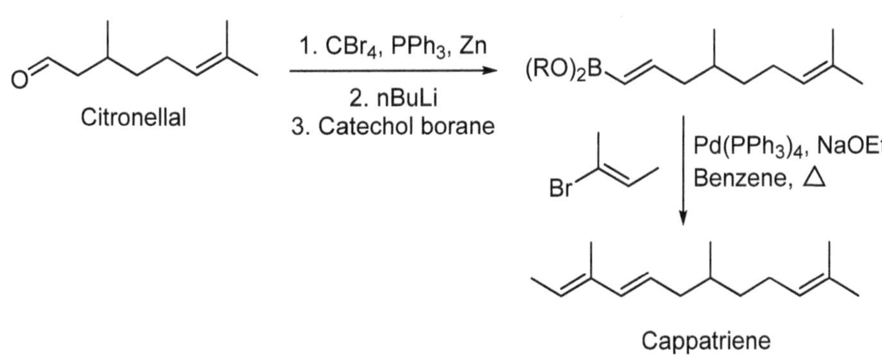

11. Barton-Kellogg Olefination

Olefin synthesis from hydrazones and thioketones

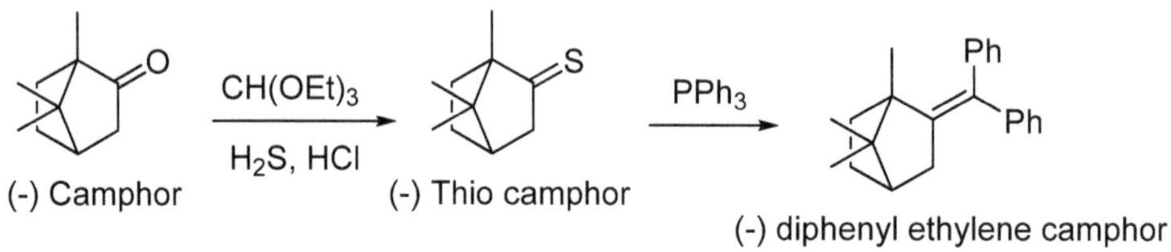

12. Blum aziridine synthesis

Synthesis of aziridines from epoxides via amino alcohols or azido alcohols and reactions with phosphines or phosphites.

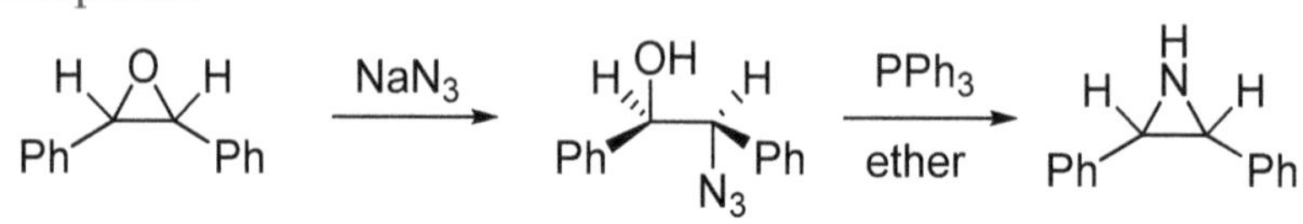

13. Garegg-Samuelsson Olefin synthesis

Vicinal diols conversion to Olefin by I_2/Ph_3P

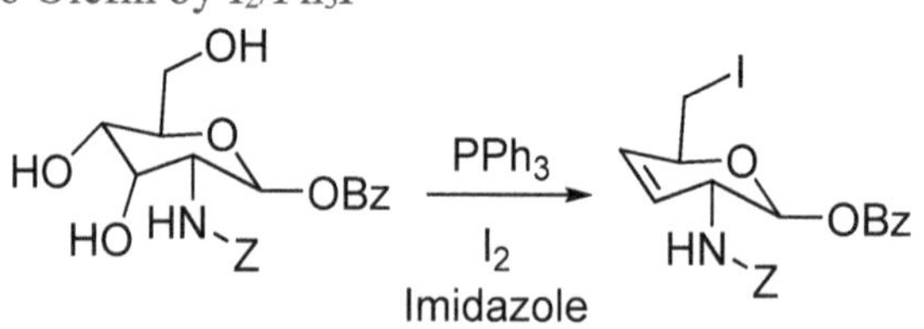

11. Diazopropane or 1-diazopropane:

It is a reagent used for cyclopropanation of alkenes

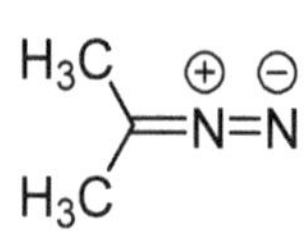

Preparation:

Diazopropane is generally prepared by the oxidation of acetone hydrazone with mercury(II) oxide in the presence of base, carried out in ether. It is unstable and explosive.

General reaction:

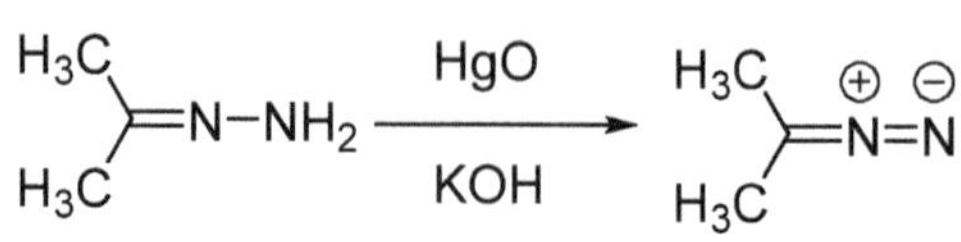

Uses:

It is generally used as potential source of gem-dimethyl groups. It undergoes 1,3-dipolar cycloaddition reaction to olefins, alkenes, acetylenes, affording cyclopropenes, methylene cyclopropanes.

Applications:

1. **Reaction with alkenes- preparation of gem-dimethyl cyclopropyl derivatives**

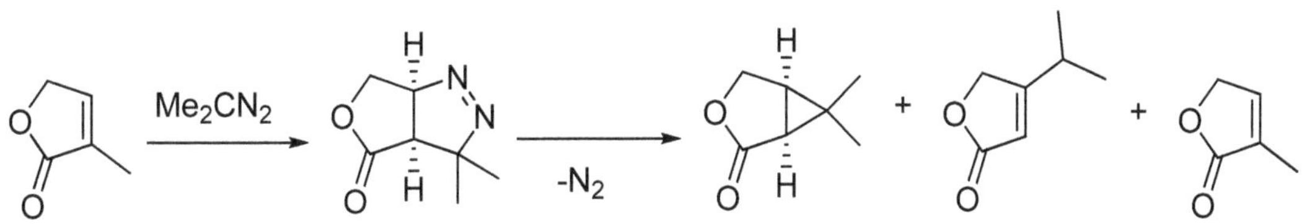

2. **Reaction with Vinylic double bond**

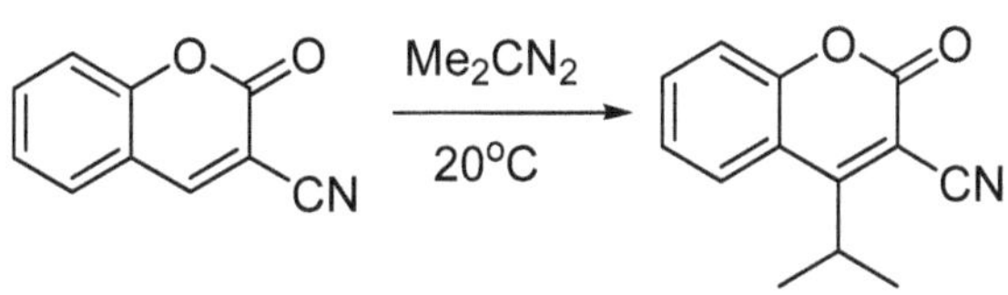

12.Benzotriazol-1-yloxy tris(dimethylamino)phosphonium hexafluoro phosphate (BOP):

BOP, also known as Castro's reagent is used in peptide synthesis.

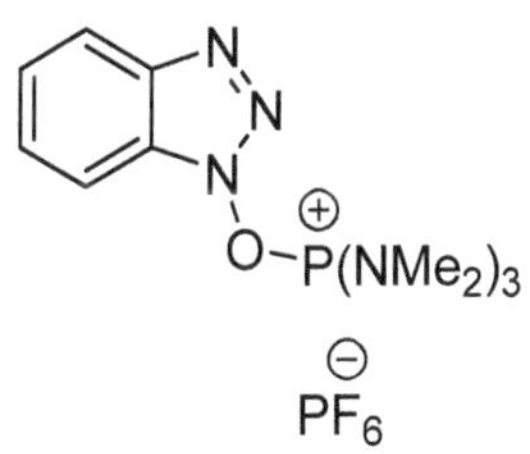

It is generally employed in peptide coupling, esterification of carboxylic acids and reduction of carboxylic acids. It is not much suitable for large-scale synthesis, since it generates HMPA, a carcinogen. It was introduced by Castro et al. and is ideally suited and successfully employed for solid-phase synthesis of peptides. When compared to DCC or DCC/HOBt methods, BOP procedure is favourable with rapid rate of coupling. It is used with selective coupling of Methotrexate to peptide hormone carriers through γ -carboxamide linkage of its glutamic acid moiety.

Other related agents to BOP:

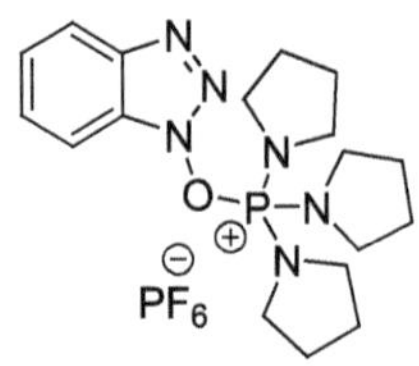

benzotriazol-1-yloxytripyrrolidinophosphonium hexafluorophosphate (PyBOP)

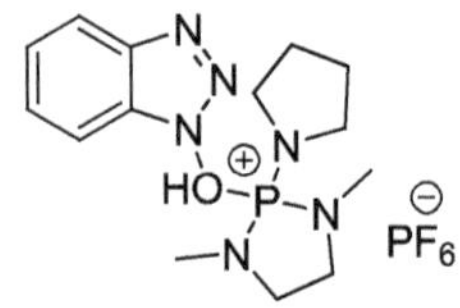

(2-benzotriazol-1-yloxy)1,3-dimethyl-2-(pyrrolidin-1-yl)-1,3-diazaphospholidinium hexafluorophosphate (BOMP)

Preparation:

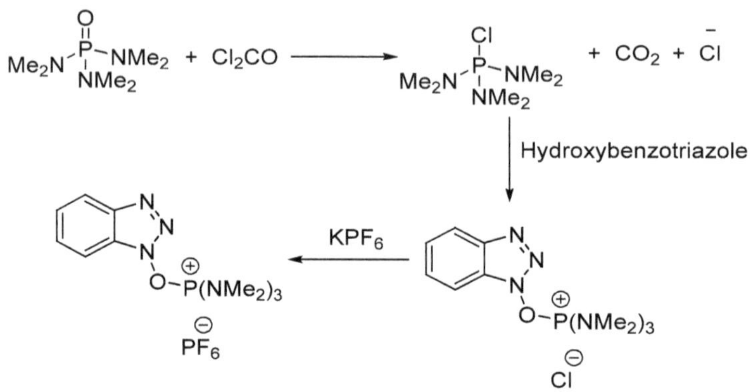

Mechanism:

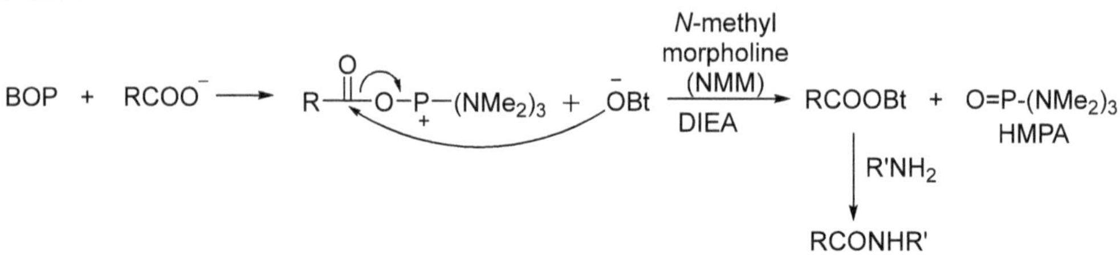

DIEA = Diisopropyl ethylamine

Mechanism of BOP-mediated peptide coupling involves the formation of -OBt ester in the presence of tertiary base such as DIEA.

Applications:

1. Chemoselective reduction of carboxylic acids to alcohols

$$RCOOH \xrightarrow[\text{2. NaBH}_4]{\text{1. BOP, DIPEA, THF}} RCH_2OH$$

2. Synthesis of esters

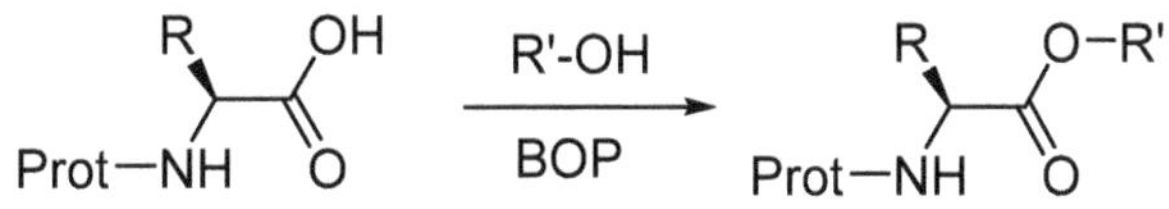

Prot = Protecting groups (FMOC or t-butyl)

3. Schreiber reported the use of BOP in the ring closure of 12 membered tetrapeptides like Trapoxin B.

4. Lactam preparation.

β-amino acids are cyclized to lactams.

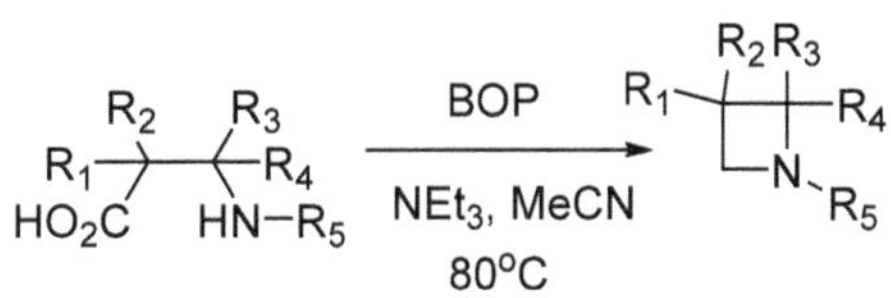

$R_1, R_2, R_3, R_5 = H$

$R_4 = CH_3$

B. Protecting Groups

Protecting groups

A protecting group can be defined as a specific molecular framework which is introduced to block the activity of a functional group in a multifunctional substrate molecule during a multistep synthetic sequence to facilitate changes elsewhere in the substrate. Later the protecting group will be removed to continue further course of the protocol. In general, many natural products, complex organic molecules, or intermediates contain multiplicity of functional groups. During the course of synthetic methods of these molecules some functional groups will be protected, or their activities blocked, for some time, and at a later point of time in the synthesis, the protecting group is released. A good protecting group should have the following qualities.

a) it should be readily available.

b) it should be easily introduced into the molecule particularly under mild conditions.

c) it should not interfere with other functionalities.

d) it should be stable or resistant to the reagents used in further steps.

e) after the purpose of protection is over the group should be labile enough to be removed easily and selectively under mild conditions with readily available reagents.

f) the yields of both protection and deprotection steps are to be excellent.

g) during both the stages the products should be easily separable and purified.

h) both protecting and deprotecting steps should not create additional stereo centres. The selected protecting group must comply with most of the above criteria.

$$\text{R–FG} \xrightarrow{\text{PG}} \text{R–FG–PG} \longrightarrow \longrightarrow \longrightarrow \text{R–FG}$$

FG: Function group.
PG: Protecting group.

However, these steps will be an additional burden both chemically and economically escalating the total cost of the methodology. Moreover, the protection and deprotection reduces the efficiency of the strategy and also decreases the overall yield of the product.

Due to the great importance and significant role played in the total syntheses, a multitude of blocking agents and protecting techniques have been developed in the synthetic organic chemistry over the years. Moreover, many of these reagents require special conditions for attachment as well as removal.

In general, the following functional groups require blocking their activity during a multistep synthesis.

1. alcohols.
2. amines.
3. aldehydes and ketones.
4. carboxylic acids.

The protecting reagents can be broadly categorized into the following-

1. Acylating reagents.
2. Acetalization reagents.
3. Alkoxy methylation reagents.
4. Silylating reagents.
5. Tritylation reagents.
6. Tertiary butoxy carbonylation reagents.
7. Alloc/CBZ/Bn/All- reagents
8. Troc- reagents (2,2,2-Trichloro ethoxy carbonylation).
9. Teoc- [(2-Trimethyl silyl)-ethoxy carbonylation]- reagents.
10. Sulfonylation reagents

Acylating agents: These are stable under oxidative and acidic conditions but can be removed under reductive or basic conditions. Some representative structures are given below.

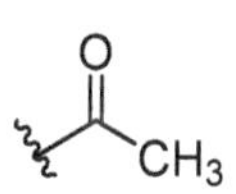

Acyl group (AC)

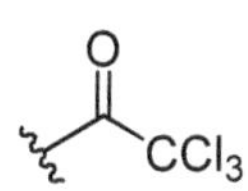

Trichloro acetyl group

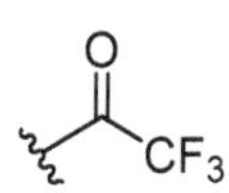

Trifluoro acetyl group (TFA)

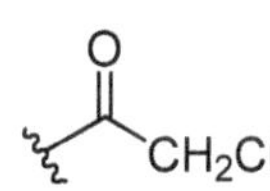

Chloro acetyl group

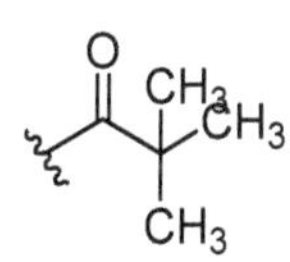

Pivaloyl group (Piv)

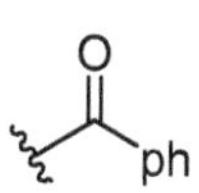

Benzoyl group (bz)

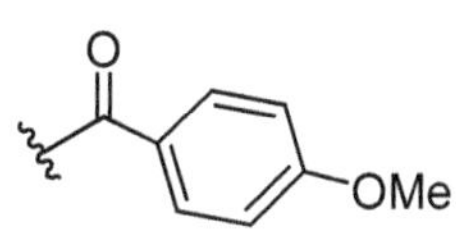

p-Methoxy benzoyl group (pMB)

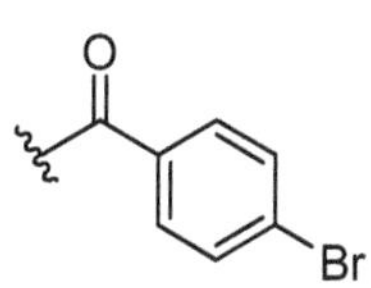

p-Bromo benzoyl group

Acetalization/thioacetalization agents: These are most often used to protect carbonyl compounds such as aldehydes and ketones. These are stable under basic or reductive conditions. Acetals can be removed under acidic hydrolysis but thioacetals require hypervalent iodine or silver or mercury salts for their removal.

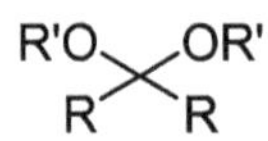

Acetals/ ketals

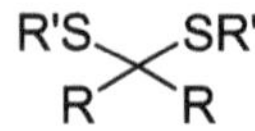

Dithioacetals/ ketals

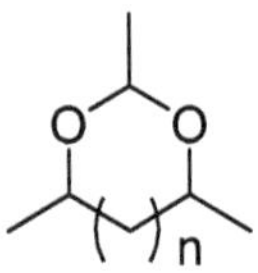

Ethylidene acetal

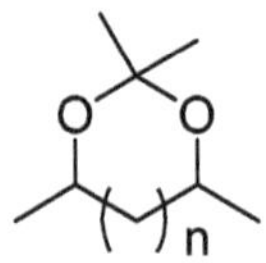

acetonide

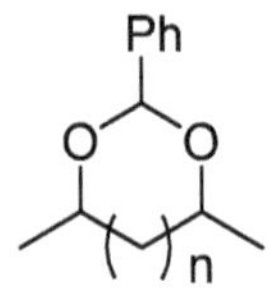

Benzylidene acetal

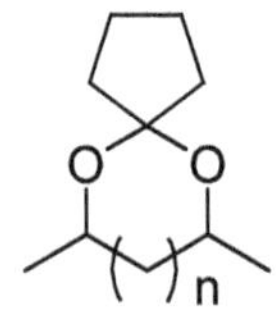

Cyclohexylidene ketal

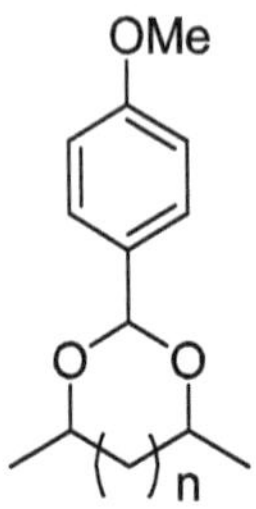

4-Methoxy Benzylidene acetal

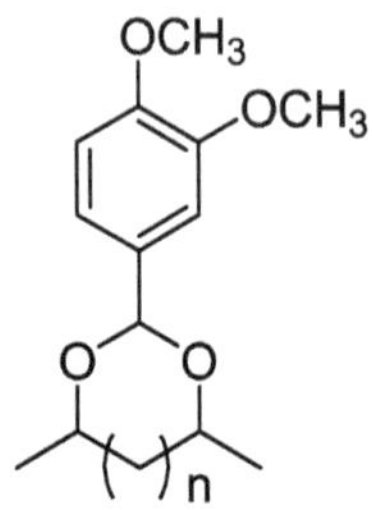

3,4-dimethoxy benzylidene acetal

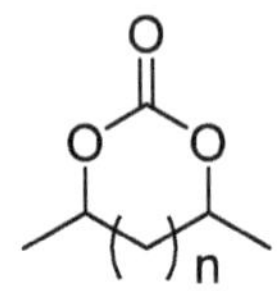

Cycliccarbonate

Alkoxymethylation agents:

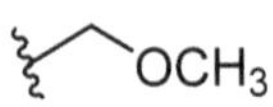

Methoxy methyl group (MOM)

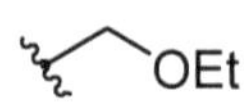

Ethoxy methyl group

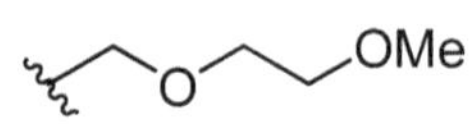

Methoxyethoxy methyl group (MEM)

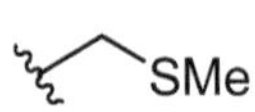

Methyl Thiomethyl group (MTM)

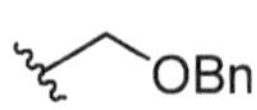

Benzyloxy methyl group (BOM)

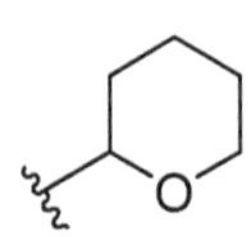

Tetrahydro pyranyl group (THP)

Silylating reagents:

Silylation is the most widely practised protection process to block amino, hydroxy, and carboxyl functionalities. These can be introduced as robust protecting groups, which can be removed using fluoride ions or under acidic conditions. Some representative structures are given below.

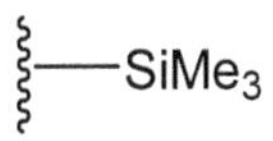

Trimethyl silyl group (TMS)

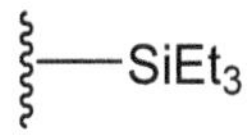

Triethyl silyl group (TES)

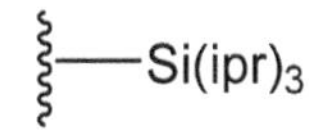

Tri isopropyl silyl group (TIPS)

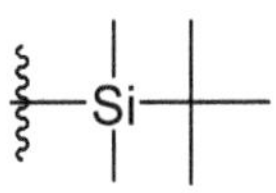

Tertiary butyl dimethyl silyl group

(TBS or TBDMS)

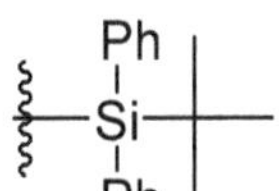

Tertiary butyl diphenyl silyl group

(TBDPS)

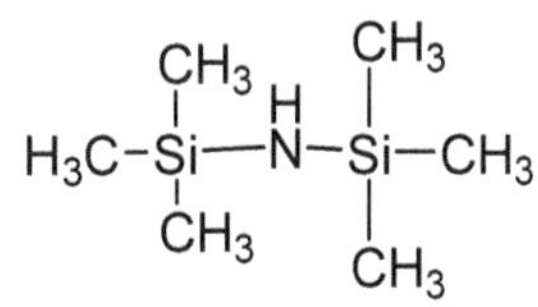

Hexa methyldisilazane (HMDS)

Tritylation agents: can selectively protect the sterically hindered alcohols. These are stable against basic oxidizing, reducing agents and nucleophiles. Trityl ethers can be removed under acid catalyzed hydrolysis. Some representative structures are given below.

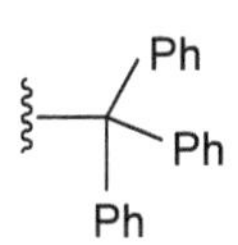

Trityl group (tr)

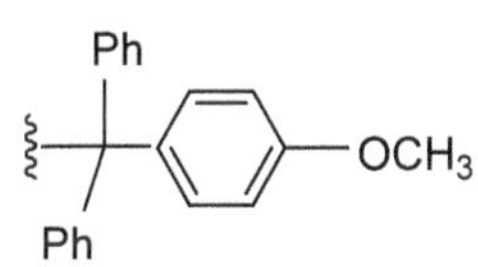

(MM tr)
4-Methyoxy trityl group

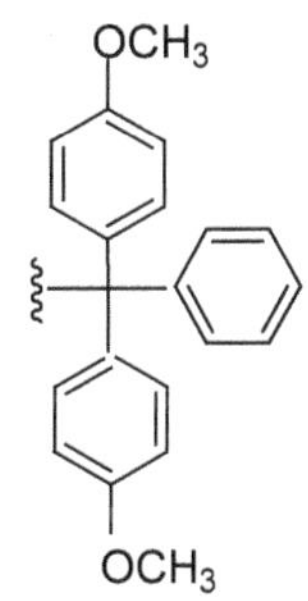

(DM Tr)
4,4'-Dimethoxy trityl group

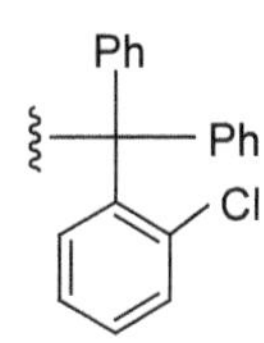

2-Chloro trityl group

Tertiary butoxycarbonylation agents: Tertiary butoxycarbonyl group is frequently used in peptide synthesis to protect -NH2 groups. These are also useful to protect alcohols. These are stable to nucleophilic attacks, catalytic reductions and hydrolyses with bases. BOC group can be removed with CF3 CO2H.

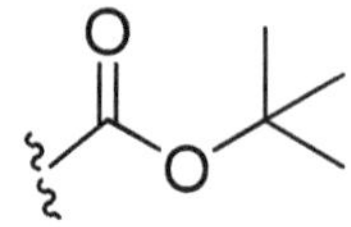

Tert-Butoxy Carbonyl group

Allyloxy carbonylationbenzyloxy carbonylationbenzylation, allylation.

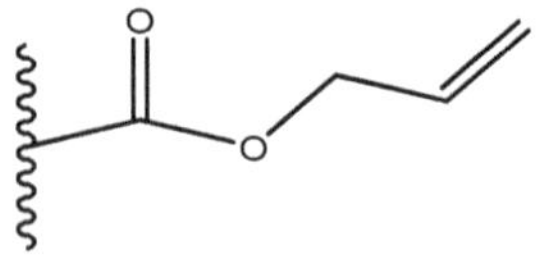

Allyloxy carbonyl group (ALLoc)

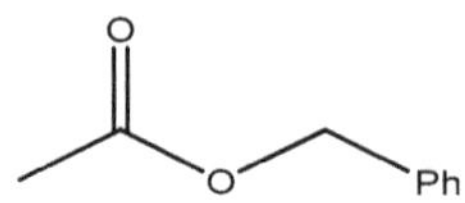

Benzyloxy carbonyl group (Cbz)

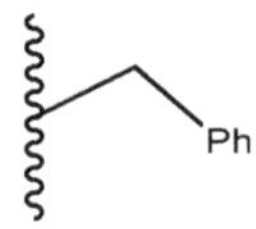

Benzyl group (Bn)

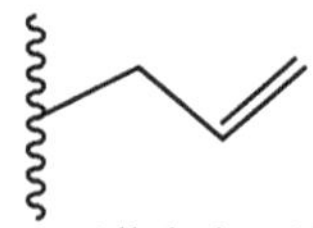

Allylation (ALL)

Troc- group protects both -OH and -NH2 groups. It can be deprotected with zinc powder or electrolysis.

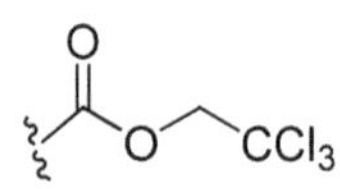

2,2,2-Trichloroethoxy carbonyl group (Troc)

Teoc- group protects amines. These can be removed with fluoride ion containing compounds like TBAF.

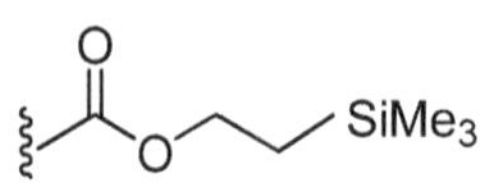

2-(Trimethyl silyl)-ethoxycarbonyl group (Teoc)

Sulfonyl group can be used to protect both -OH and -NH2 groups.

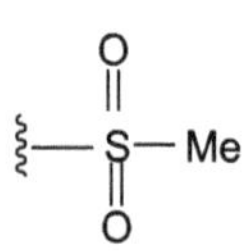

Methane sulfonyl (Mesyl-MS)

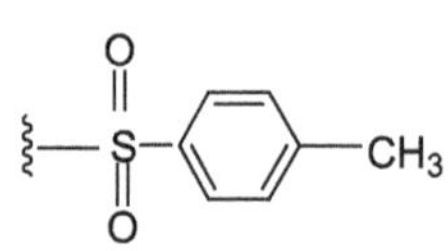

P-Toluene sulfonyl group (Tosyl-TS)

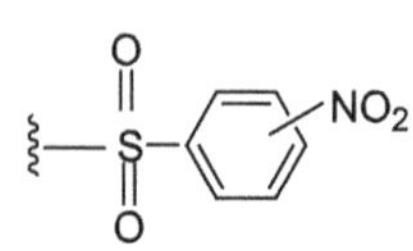

Nitrophenyl sulfonyl group (Nosyl-NS)

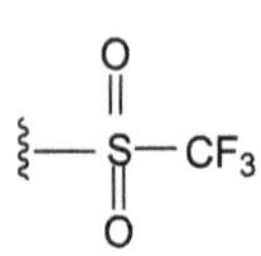

Trifluoro methane sulfonyl group (triflyl-Tf)

Let us examine protecting group information for different functionalities with some examples[30].

Alcohol group protection:

Alcohols, being versatile functional groups can be converted to esters, ethers, carbonates, cyclic acetals, or ketals. During oxidation, substitution, or elimination reactions -OH can be modified to a better leaving group such as tosylates. These must be blocked even in other reactions if they seem to be susceptible.

Esterification, a common process of reacting alcohols with carboxylic acid, is a widely employed strategy to protect alcohol group. The esters can be prepared by reacting carboxylic acid, or acid chloride or acid anhydride. Carboxylic acids can be activated using N,N-dicyclohexylcarbodiimide (DCC), 4-dimethylaminopyridine (DMAP), carbonyl diimidazole (CDI) etc., The introduction of acetoxy or benzyloxy groups into an organic compound is known as acetylation or benzoylation. Acetylation or benzoylation are the most important and frequently employed reactions to block the activities of both hydroxy and amine functionalities. Acetylation is used to protect alcohols, phenols, thiols and amines. Acetylation can be conducted under homogeneous or heterogeneous acid and base catalysis.

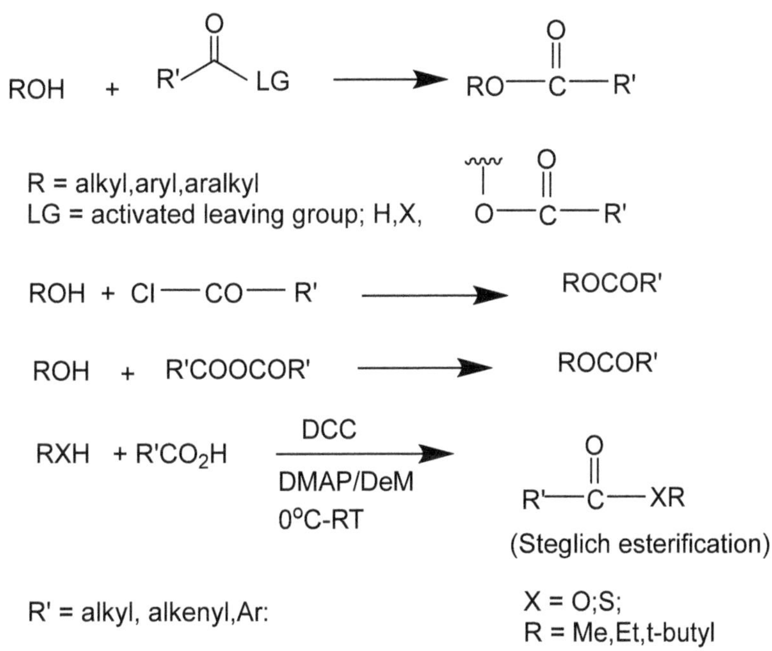

Acid chloride of pivalic acid or neovaleric acid $(CH_3)_3CCO_2H$-(PiVOH), an isomer of valeric acid known as pivaloyl chloride (PvCl) in the presence of pyridine is effectively used to protect alcohols and amines. Treatment of pivaloyl compounds with LDA has been successfully achieved by Domingo Sanchez et al to liberate amine. Acetylation of hydroxy and amine functional groups can be generally conducted using acetyl chloride in the presence of a base such as triethyl amine or diisopropylethylamine. Acetyl group can be removed in the presence of a base like KOH, NaOH in

EtOH/H_2O. The Steglich esterification has become popular by shortening the reaction times, improving the yields, wherein the process is conducted in the presence of DCC, and DMAP. DCC activates the carboxylic acids and DMAP enhances the reactivity.

Examples:

1. $$CH_3CH_2OH \xrightarrow[PhCO_2H]{H^+} PhCOOCH_2CH_3 + H_20$$

2. $$CH_3CH_2CH_2CH_2OH \xrightarrow{AcOH} CH_3CH_2CH_2CH_2OCOCH_3$$

3. 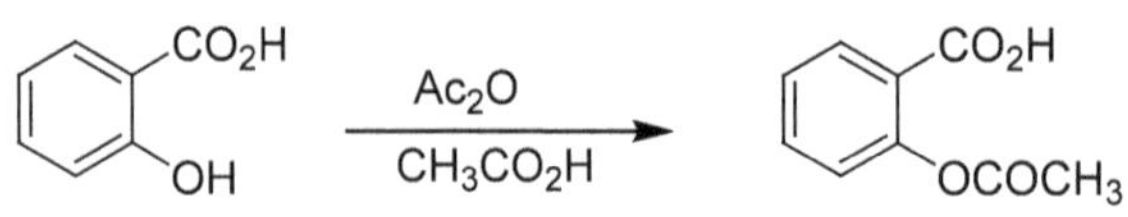

Salicylic acid Aspirin

4. 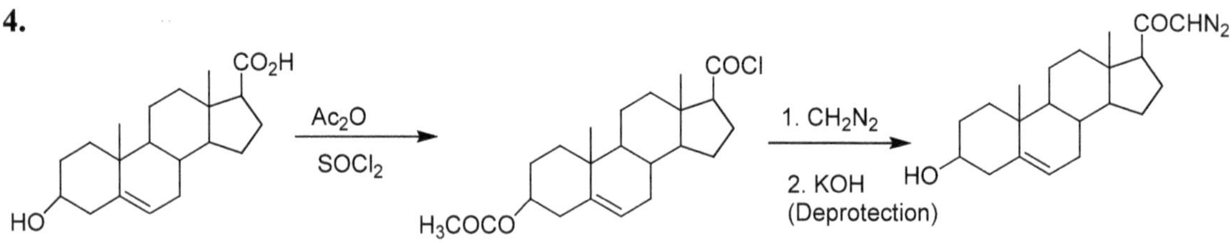

From the synthesis of deoxy corticosterone

5. 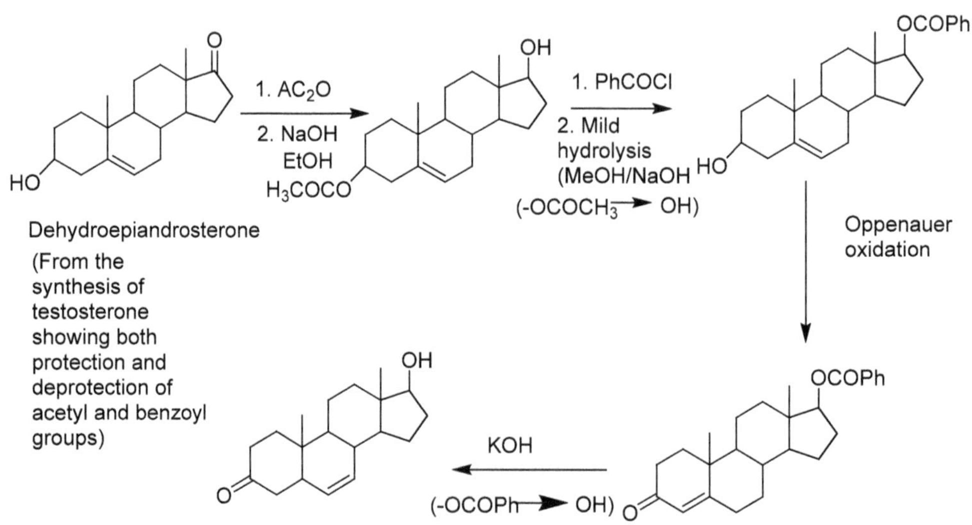

Testosterone

6. 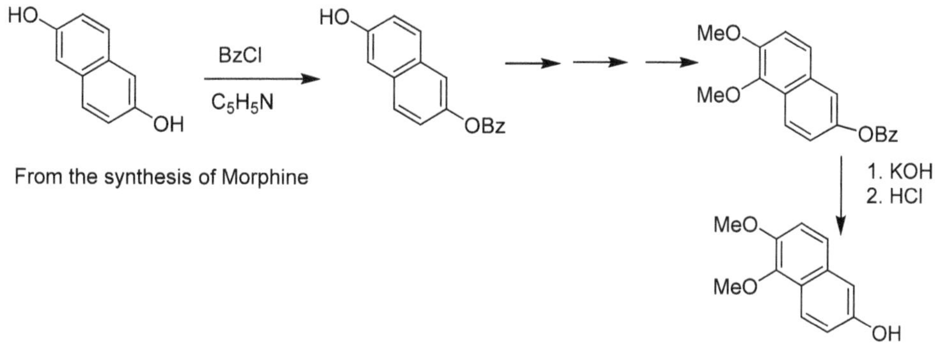

From the synthesis of Morphine

7. 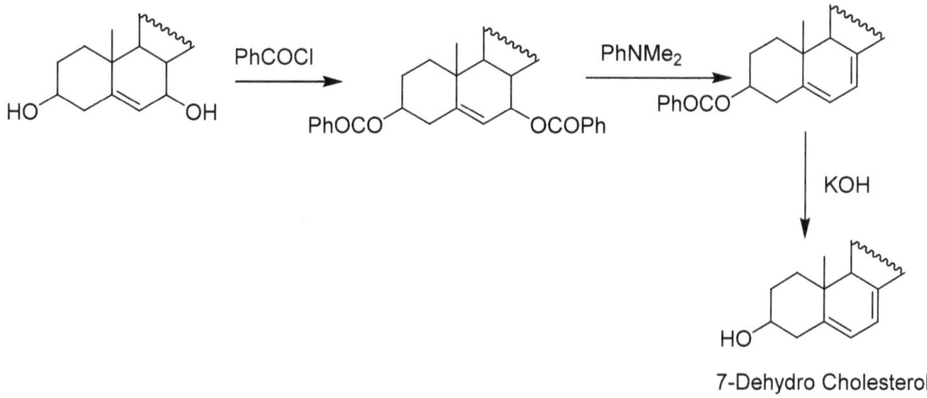

8. 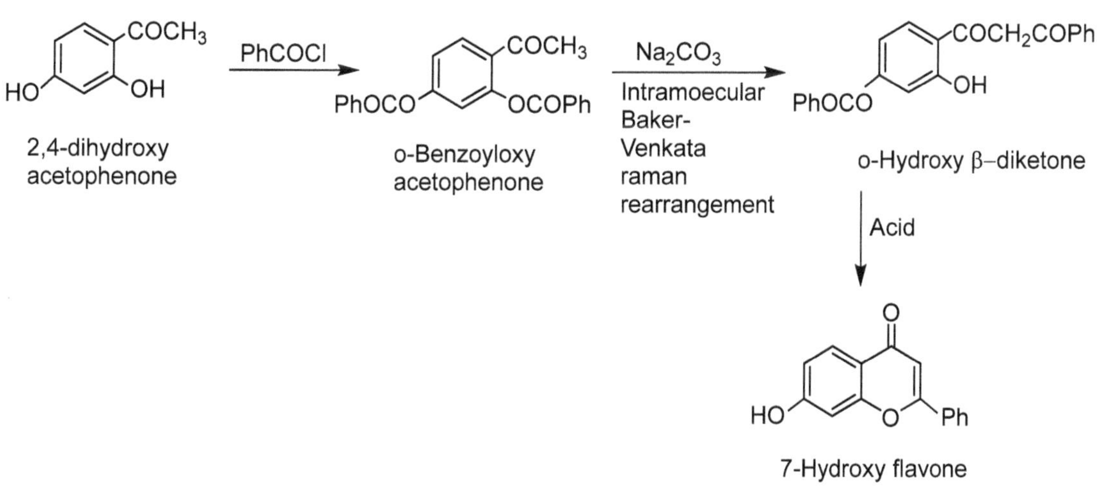

9. 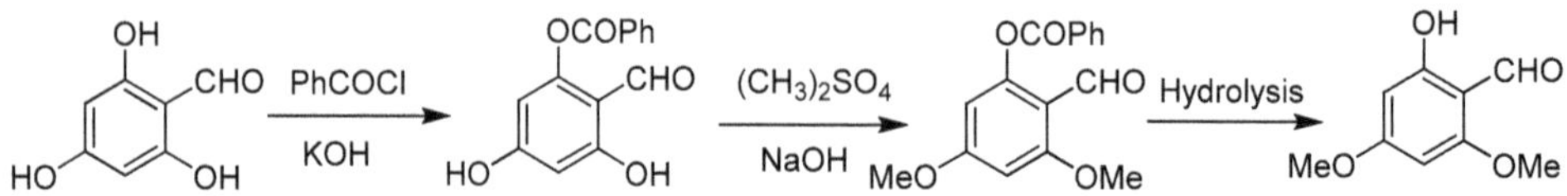

2-Hydroxy-4,6-dimethoxy benzaldehyde

10. 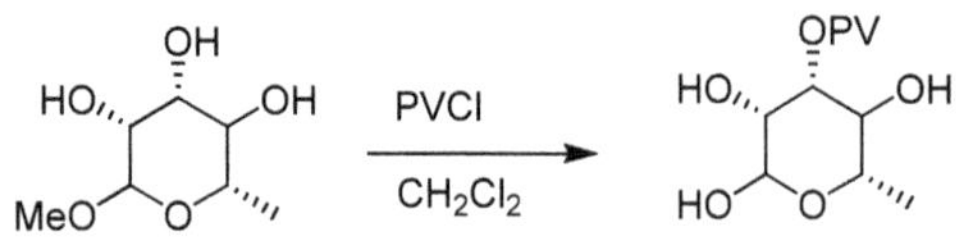

11. $$PhOH + PhCOCl \xrightarrow{NaOH} PhOCOPh$$

12. 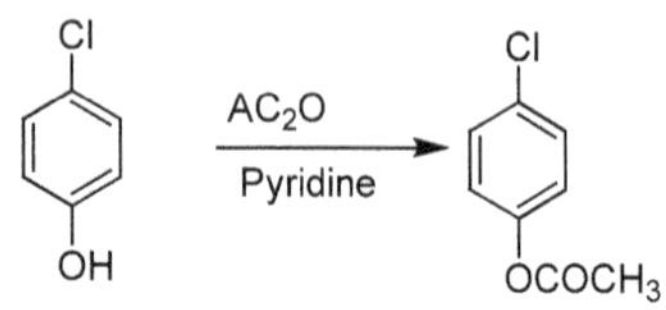

Methyl ethers can be prepared using diazomethane in the presence of HBF_4 or silica, or with methyl iodide in the presence of sodium hydroxide. Various reagents are available to deblock ethers like trimethylsilyl iodide. Alcohols can also be converted to methoxymethyl ethers (MOM) using chloromethyl methyl ether in the presence of a strong base like sodium hydroxide. Primary, secondary, and tertiary hydroxyls can be protected using this technique. These can be deprotected using $ZnBr_2$, $AlBr_3$, PhSe, Ph_2P, EtSH etc. Selective protection of alcohols is also possible by converting them into 2–methoxyethoxymethyl ether (MEM) by reacting with $CH_3OCH_2CH_2OCH_2Cl$ (MEMCl) in the presence of DIPEA or sodium hydroxide. These can be deprotected with several reagents like TiC14, $ZnBr_2$, Cerium(III) chloride, Me_2BBr_2 etc., MOM or MEM ethers are reportedly hydrolysed to their respective alcohols with 10% CBr_4 in iprOH. Methoxy ethoxy methyl ethers can be converted to alcohols using trimethylsilyl chloride also.

The utilization of ethoxyethyl (EE) or methoxypropyl (MOP) protecting groups, even though not quite common plays an important role in the carbohydrate chemistry. Both attachment and removal of these can be carried out under mild conditions. These are stable under basic conditions. These can be removed under acidic conditions.

1. $$ROH + R'\text{—}Lg \longrightarrow ROR'$$ Lg: Leaving group , R= Alkyl;Aryl

2. $$ROMOM \xrightarrow[CH_2Cl_2]{ZnBr_2} ROH$$

3. 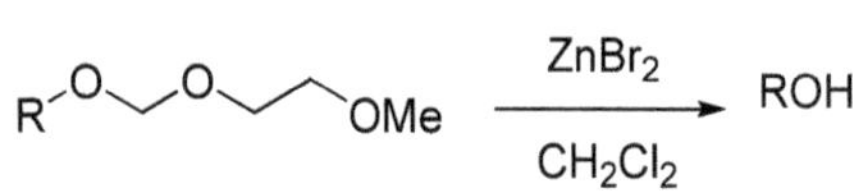

4. $$ROMEM \xrightarrow[CH_3CN,\ Heat]{CeCl_3.7H_2O} ROH$$

5. $$ROCH_2OCH_2CH_2OMe \xrightarrow[(Br_4, iprOH)]{10\ mol\%} ROH$$

Examples:

1. 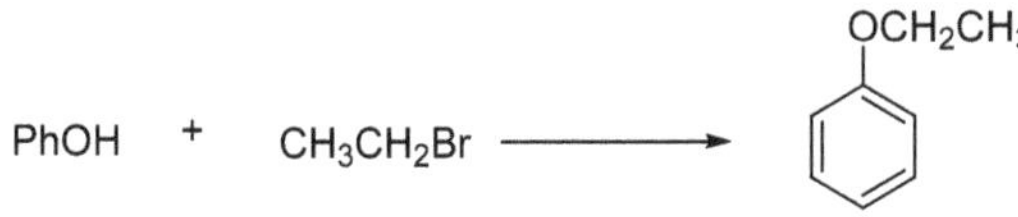

(Williamson synthesis)

2. 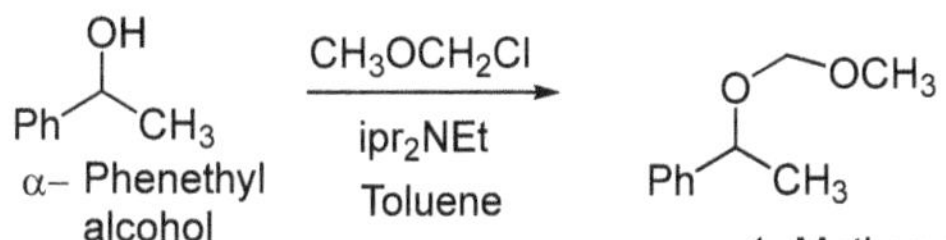

1- Methoxy-methoxy-1-phenethyl ethane

3. 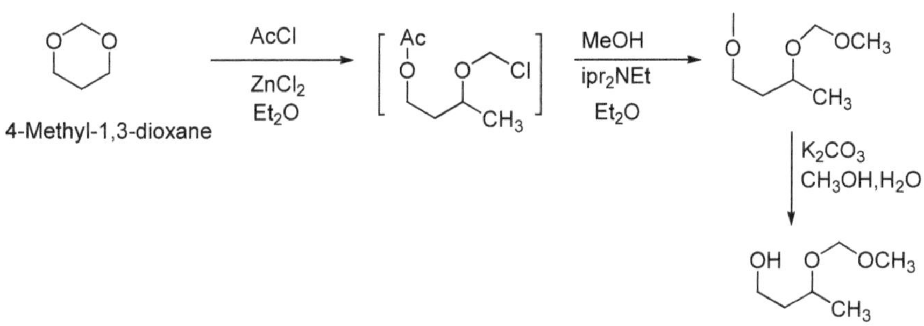

3-(Methoxy methoxy)1-butanol

4. 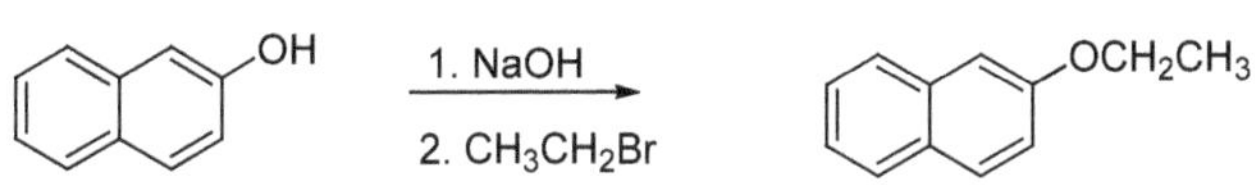

2- Ethoxy naphthalene
(Nerolin)

5. 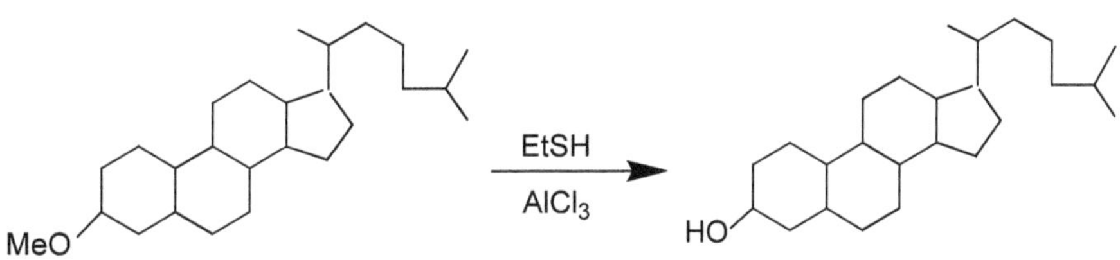

Methylthiomethyl ethers (MTM) can also be obtained from primary secondary or tertiary alcohols by reacting them with dimethyl sulfoxide in acetic acid and acetic anhydride mixture. The reaction follows Pummerer rearrangement. MTM etherification is more useful in the case of tertiary alcohols. These can be cleaved selectively employing neutral compounds like silver nitrate/THF, H_2O or mercuric chloride/CH_3CN, H_2O or MgI_2/Ac_2OorCH_3I/$NaHCO_3$, CH_3COCH_3, H_2O. These can be prepared using MTM chloride by Williamson synthesis.

MTM ethers can be easily prepared under mild conditions using chloromethyl methyl sulphide. Both alkoxy methyl ethers (MOM) and methoxy ethoxy methyl ethers (MEM) are stable to basic and mild acidic conditions.

$$ROH \xrightarrow[\text{NaH,THF}]{\text{ClCH}_2\text{SMe}} ROCH_2SMe$$

$$ROCH_2SMe \xrightarrow[\text{AgNO3,THF, 2,6-Lutidine}]{} ROH$$

E. J. Corey and co-workers first explored the use of methyl thiomethyl ether group in the preparation of antibiotics like erythronolide etc. MTM ethers are stable in acidic conditions but the presence of sulphur group is prone to oxidation by peracids, Cr(VI) or NBS etc.,

1. $$ROCH_2SMe \xrightarrow[\text{CH}_3\text{CN,H}_2\text{O}]{\text{HgCl}_2} ROH$$

2. $$ROH + ClCH_2SMe \xrightarrow[\text{Et}_3\text{N,C}_6\text{H}_6]{\text{AgNO}_3} ROCH_2SMe$$

3. 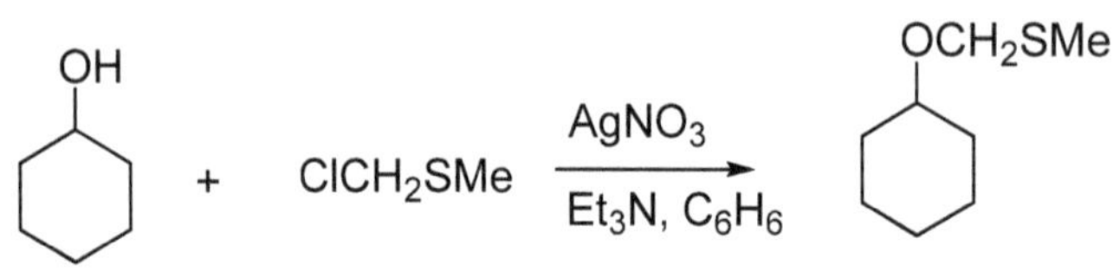

4. 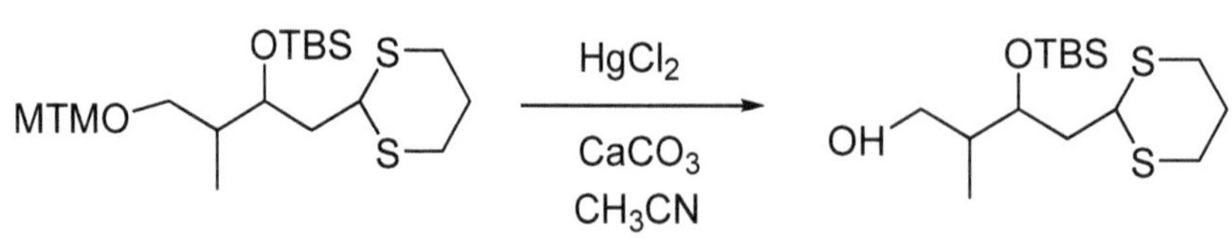

Tetrahydropyranyl group is frequently employed as a common protecting group for alcohols generating tetrahydro pyranyl ethers. The group is useful for both alcohol and phenol protection. THP ethers are stable to bases. These are also stable to hydrides organometallics and other alkylating agents. The THP group can be easily attached and removed under conditions that will not harm other functionalities. Alcohols can be regenerated by acid catalyzed hydrolysis using p-toluene sulphonic acid in water or acetic acid or pyridine p-toluene sulphonate (PPTS) in ethanol or amberlist-15 in methanol.

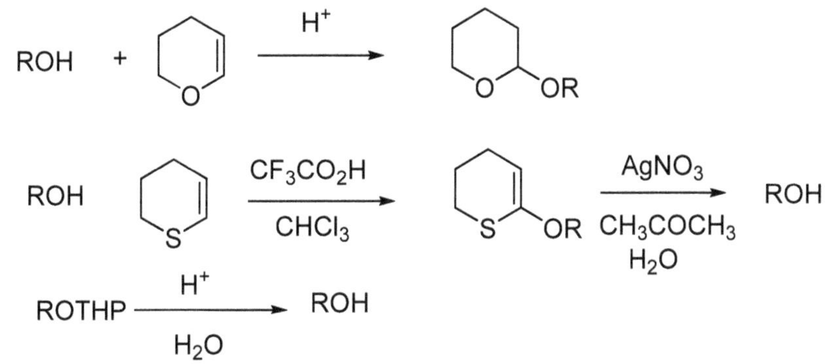

These can also be removed under wide range of oxidizing conditions using CrO_3/AcOH or O_3 or NBS or NIS or $(CH_3)_3SiI/CH_2Cl_2$ etc., The advantages for the group is ease of formation, cost effectiveness, relative stability and also facile removal.

Benzyl ether formation offers versatile method of protection of alcohols. These can be prepared under basic conditions using benzyl bromide, or benzyl iodide, in the presence of sodium hydride in dimethylformamide or in the presence of sodium hydride and tetrabutylammonium iodide in THF. Benzyl bromide reacts with alcohols in the presence of silver triflate generating benzyl ethers under neutral conditions. Benzyl ethers can also be produced by the reaction of benzyl trichloroacetimidate /triflicacid or phenyl diazomethane / tetrafluoroboric acid under acidic conditions. These can be effectively removed to restore alcohols employing classical hydrogenolysis (H2/Pd/C). Alternatively, catalytic transfer hydrogenolysis using HCO2NH4/Pd/C works efficiently. Birch reduction conditions using Na/NH3or treatment with anhydrous FeC13 also liberate alcohols. These can also be removed under wide range of oxidizing conditions using CrO3/AcOH or 03 or NBS or NIS or (CH3)3SiI/CH2C12 etc.,

Examples:

1. $ROH \xrightarrow[KOH]{PhCH_2Br} ROCH_2Ph$

2. $ROH \xrightarrow[BrCH_2CHCH_2]{KOH} ROCH_2CH{=}CH_2$

3. $PhCH_2OH \xrightarrow[KOH]{PhCH_2Br} PhCH_2OCH_2Ph$

4. $CH_3(CH_2)_8CH_2OH \xrightarrow[KOH]{PhCH_2Br} CH_3(CH_2)_8CH_2OCH_2Ph$

5. 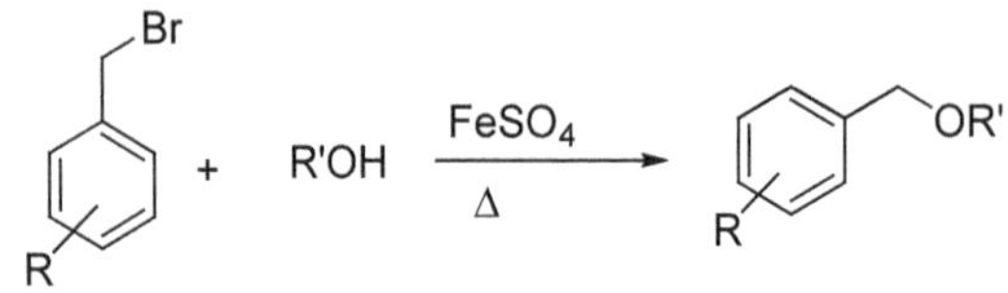

R= H; NO_2; Br; OMe
R'= Me; Et; Br; C_6H_{11}; $PhCH_2$

P.H.Seeberger etal **(Seeberger, P.H., et al., Org. Lett., 2021.,23,514-18.)** described facile visible light mediated oxidative debenzylation using 2,3 -dichloro 5,6-dicyano 1,4-benzoquinone (DDQ) as a catalytic photo oxidant in the presence of tertiary butyl nitrite (TBN) as a co-catalyst. The research group proved that benzyl ethers can be cleaved even in the presence of other functionalities like azides, alkenes, and alkynes. Benzyl ethers are stable over a broad range of reaction conditions and so are ideal protecting groups particularly in the carbohydrate chemistry. Their cleavage required harsh reaction procedures like oxidation with Ozone or DDQ or BC13. Apart from benzyl ethers, halobenzyl ethers and allyl ethers are also commonly employed to protect alcohols or phenols in the synthetic sequences.

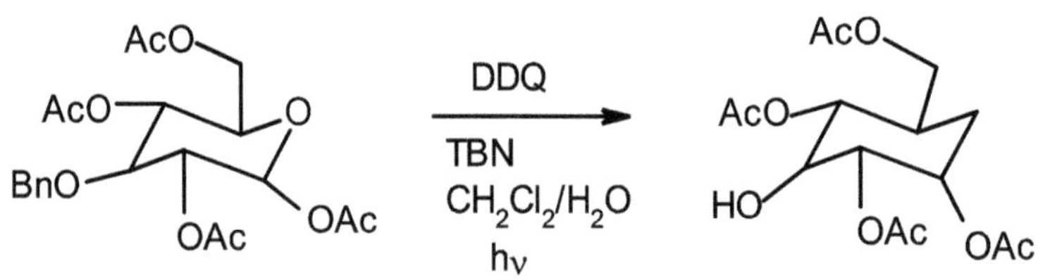

Allyl ethers can be prepared from the corresponding alcohols using several allyl compounds like allyl bromide, allyl carbonate, allyl ethyl carbonate etc.,

$$PhCH_2OH \xrightarrow[\text{KOH, PTC}]{BrCH_2CH{=}CH_2} PhCH_2OCH_2CH{=}CH_2$$

p.Methoxy benzyl group (PMB) can be introduced as a protecting group in the presence of strong bases like KOH, or NaOH or Buli or NaH with p.Methoxy benzyl halide. DDQ, NBS, TFA, CAN, or Br2 are often used to reproduce alcohols. These are more readily cleaved than unsubstituted benzyl ethers by oxidative methods.

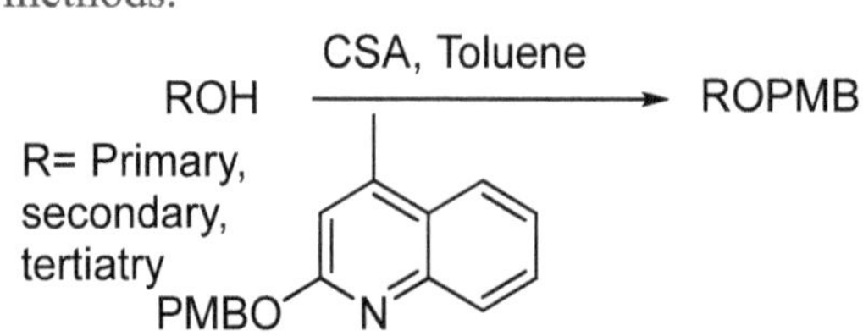

Examples:

1.

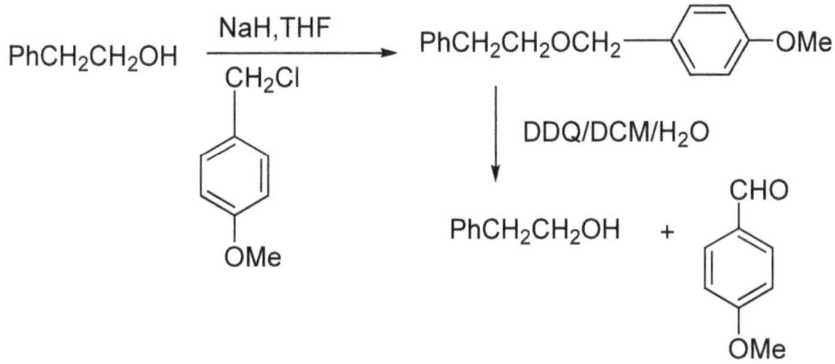

2.

$$CH_3(CH_2)_8CH_2OPMB \xrightarrow[\text{1,3-dimethoxy benzene, } CH_2Cl_2]{\text{TfOH}} CH_3(CH_2)_8CH_2OH$$

3.

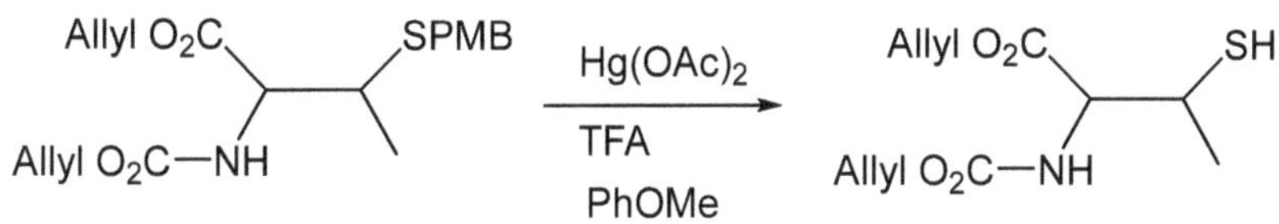

4.

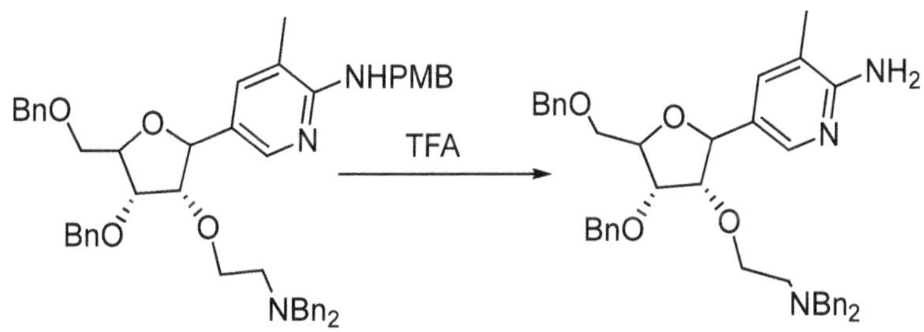

The triphenyl methyl group (trityl group) is an important protecting group used in organic synthesis. It can be introduced using trityl chloride in the presence of a base such as TEA, Pyridine, or 2,4,6-collidine, or 4-dimethoxy amino pyridine etc.

$$ROH \xrightarrow{\text{TrCl}} RO{-}C(Ph)_3$$

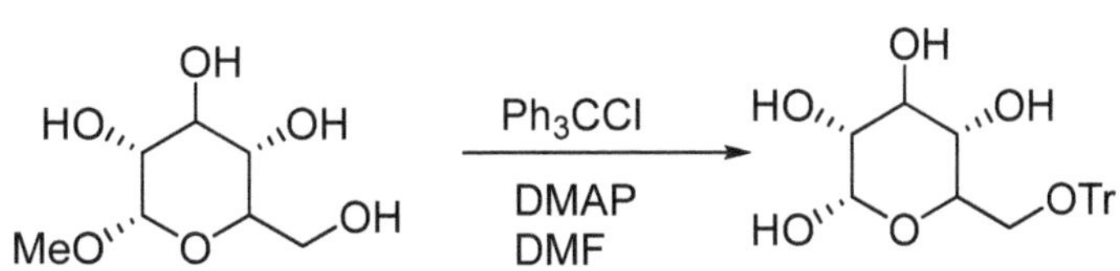

Trityl chloride reacts selectively and converts alcohols to ethers. Trityl chloride is used in the manufacture of many active pharmaceutical ingredients. The removal of trityl group can be affected using Lewis acids or mineral acids. These are stable to neutral and basic conditions. Solvents like CH2C12, CH3CN, THF or CHC13 can be used. Reports indicate that tritylation can be achieved using trityl alcohol also. Trityl group can be employed as a protecting group for both alcohols and amines. The technique is widely used in carbohydrate and nucleo side chemistry.

Both allyl chloride and trityl chloride are used as protecting groups in the complex synthesis of 6-O-alkylcelluloses.

Examples:

1. $CH_3CH_2—(OCPh_3)—(CH_2)_4CH_2OCPh_3 \xrightarrow[PH_3CBF_4,\ DCM]{} CH_3CO(CH_2)_4CH_2OH$

2.

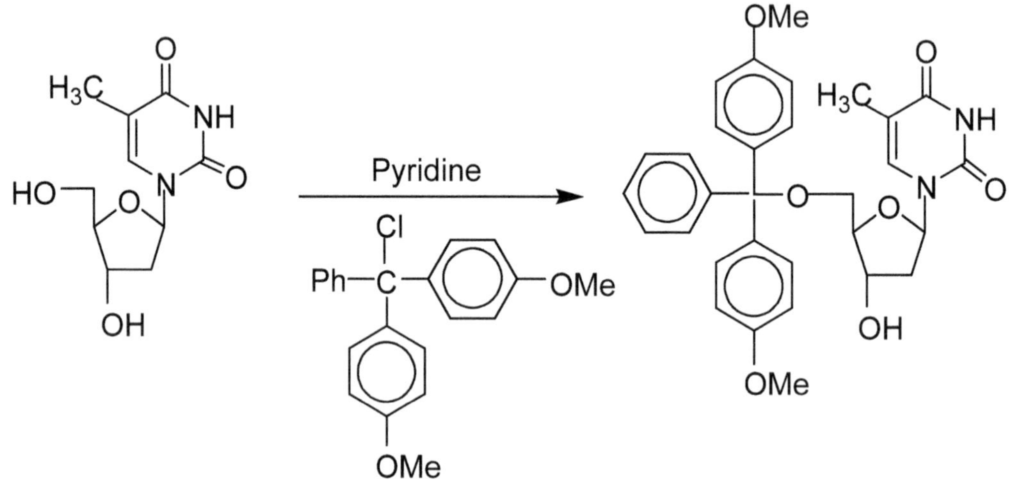

Silylation is the introduction of substituted silyl groups to replace active hydrogen from a molecule and is the most commonly used method in the synthetic organic chemistry. The process is used to block the hydroxy, amine, thiol and carboxy functionalities. Tri-methyl silyl halide, tri-ethyl silyl halide, tri-isopropyl chlorosilane, trialkyl silyl azides, trialkyl silyl triflates, allyl trimethyl silane and N, N-bis trimethyl silyl urea (BSU) are some of the generally used as reagents. Trimethyl isopropyl silyl (TIPS), or tertiary butyl dimethyl silyl (TB or TBDMS) or tertiary butyl diphenyl silyl (TBDPS) or hexamethyl disilazane (HMDS) groups are also employed for attaching robust substituents. These are stable in basic conditions but can be removed under mild acidic conditions or by using fluoride compounds, such as CsF, KF, HF/DCM, SiF4/DCM, Bu4NF, NH4F, HF/Pyridine, Et3N.3HF., etc., The Silicon protecting groups are most frequently employed in modern synthetic organic chemistry.

The steric and electronic properties of the silyl protecting agents can be fine- tuned by varying the substituents attached to silicon. This allows them to be employed in a wide range of reactions. As a leaving group this feature is very important in the selection of protection process. Electron withdrawing groups on silicon increases susceptibility toward basic hydrolysis. At the same time, they decease sensitivity to acid stability toward acid increases as- TMS < TES < TBDMS < TIPS < TBDPS. Stability to base increases in the following order- TMS < TES < TBDMS-TBDPS < TIPS. Migratory aptitude of silicon groups from one hydroxyl to another is an important feature of these groups. The TBDMS migrates frequently. The migration is solvent dependent and proceeds faster in protic solvents. This intramolecular migration occurs both in basic and acidic conditions. Sterically less hindered alcohols undergo silylation easily.

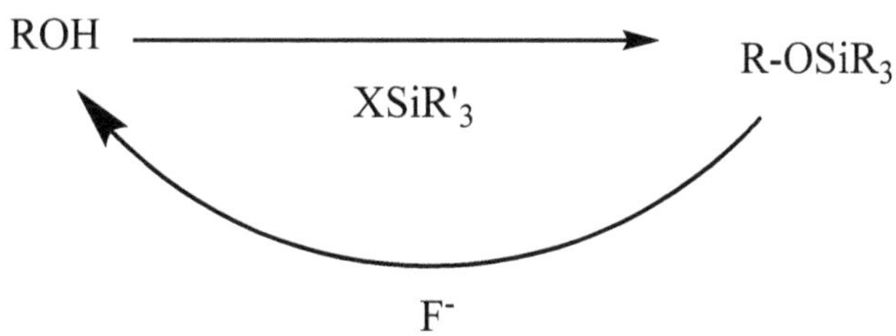

Examples:

1. 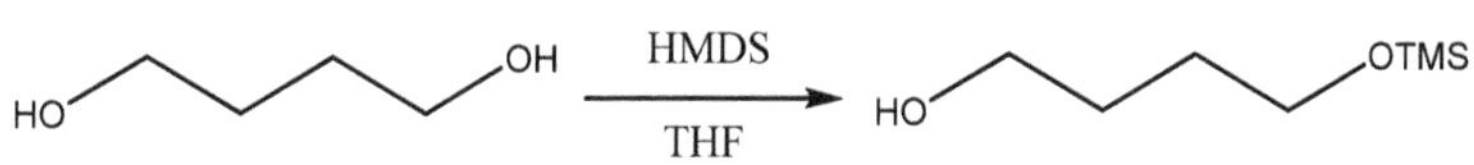

2. 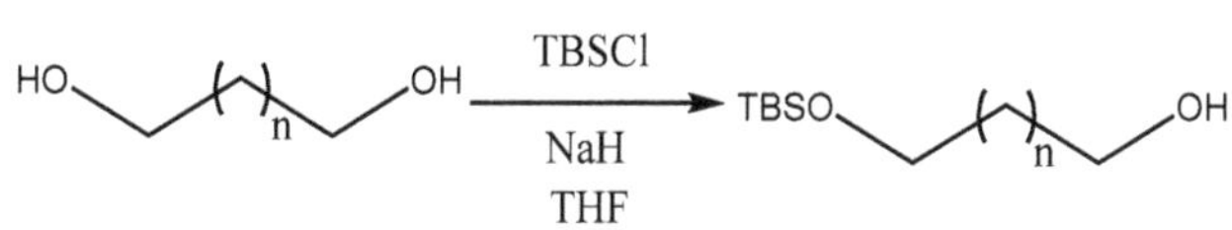

3. 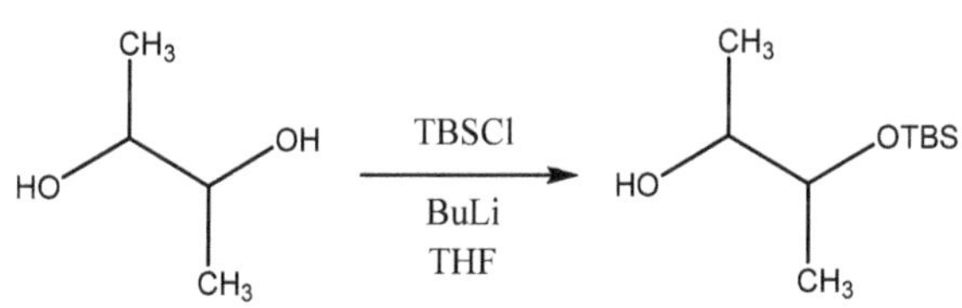

4. 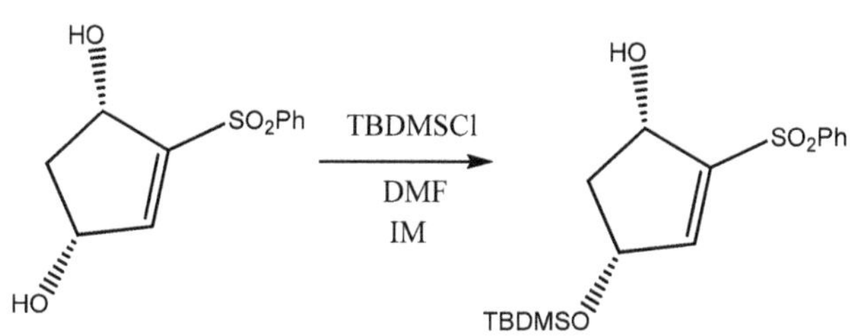

5.

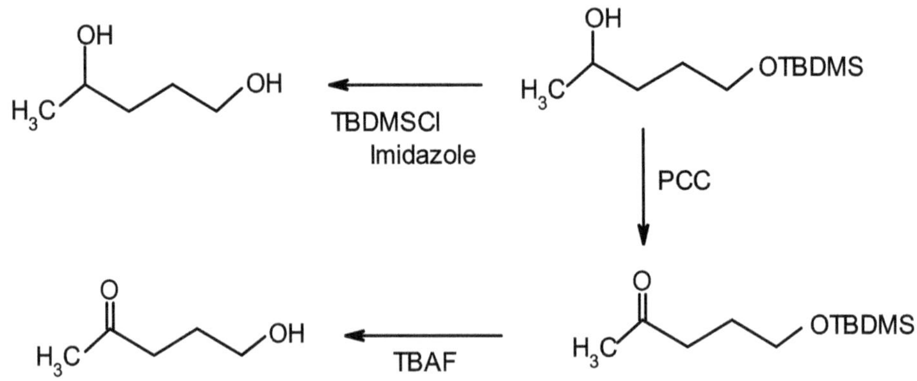

Acetonide is another common protecting group used for 1,2- 1,3- diols, obtained by the reaction with Acetone. Acetals or Ketals can be easily removed by the hydrolysis using dilute aqueous acids. During the preparation of acetonides of triols generally 1,2- derivative is preferred over 1,3-derivative, depending on the structure. The method is frequently employed in carbohydrate and steroid chemistry. An example is the application employed in the synthesis of taxol by Nicolaou. Some of the acetamides are corticosteroid topical applicants used in the dermatological applications. Ex. Fluclorolone acetonide, Fluocinolone acetonide and Triamcinolone acetonide.

Apart from acetonides, benzylidene acetals are also in practice in glycol- chemistry for example hydroxyl groups of aldonolactones react with benzaldehyde to generate benzylidene derivatives. Some research reports indicate that benzylidene acetals can be removed using triethyl silane/Pd/C in methanol. The six-membered rings are hydrolyzed faster than the five-membered rings. 4-Methoxybenzylidene acetal undergoes hydrolysis faster than simple benzylidene acetal.

Examples:

1.

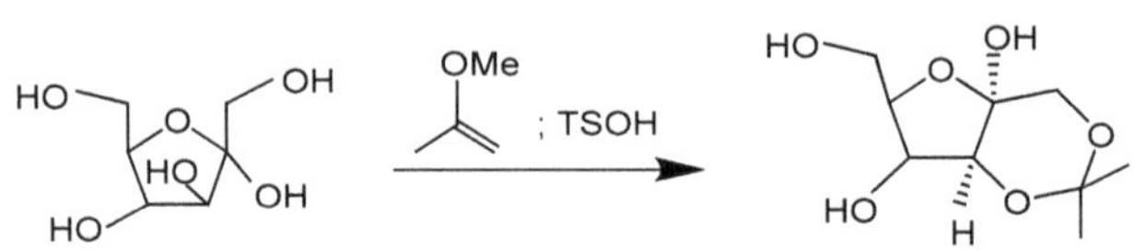

2.

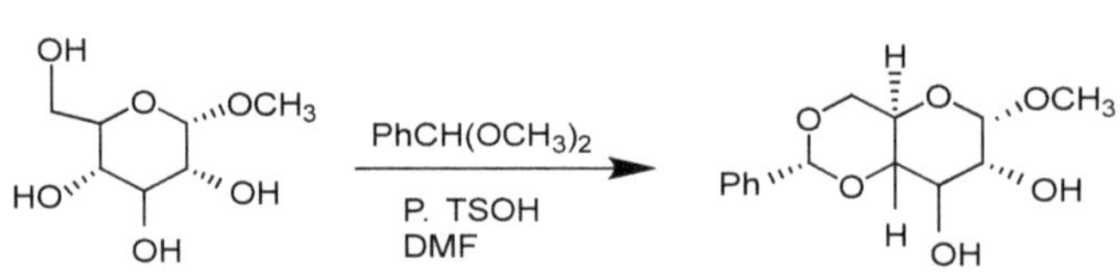

Methyl-α-D-glucopyranoside

3.

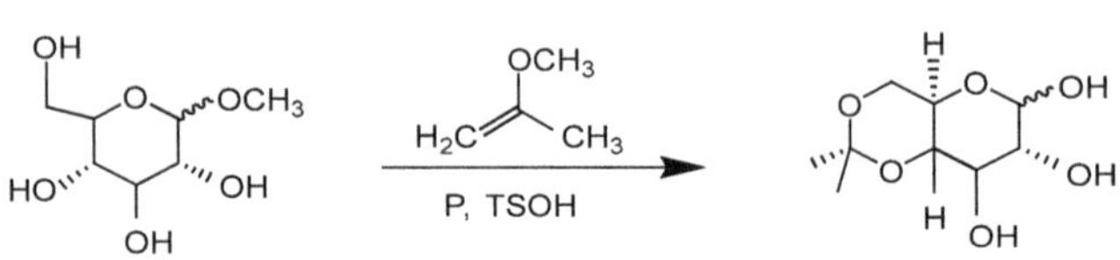

D-glucose

4.

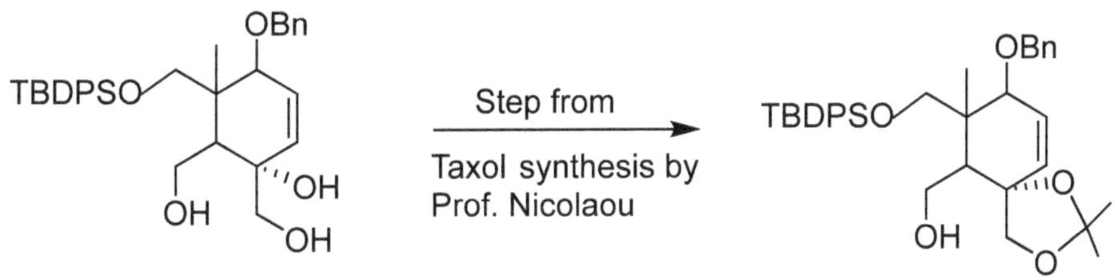

5.

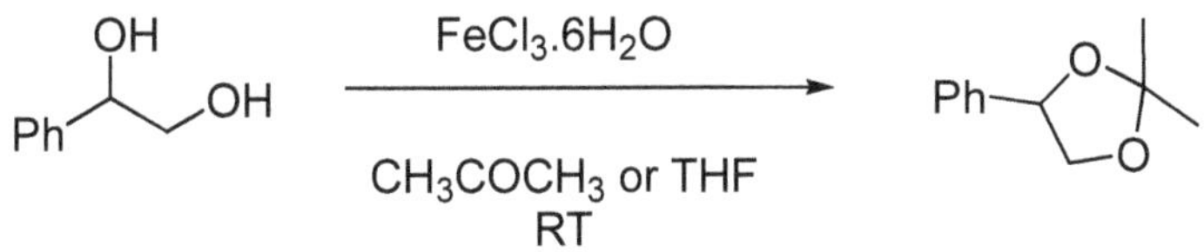

Cyclic carbonates or carbonate esters which play an important role in carbohydrate chemistry are obtained by the reaction of diols with phosgene, thiophosgene or chloroformates in the presence of base. These can be hydrolysed in the presence of strong bases like KOH etc., The carbonate esters can also be prepared from epoxide on reaction with CO2. Carbonyl diimidazole is a more user-friendly reagent than phosgene.

Carboxyl group Protection

Esters:

Generally, the carboxylic acids whether aliphatic, or aromatic, substituted or unsubstituted display similar functional properties related to the carboxyl group. During the course of a synthetic sequence, these are protected either to mask the acidic proton from interference in base-catalyzed reactions or to shield the carbonyl group from nucleophilic addition reactions. A large number of protective groups are developed which can be removed under a variety of conditions. Esterification, amidation and conversion to hydrazides are significant. Hydrolysis is an important method of deprotection, normally using hydroxide in an organic aqueous medium such as MeOH/H2O. Nucleophilic displacement of the carboxylate is another way. Lipase, esterase, and alkaline protease are known to cleave methyl and benzyl esters.

An ester can be prepared from an acid chloride or anhydride and an alcohol in the presence of a base like triethylamine or pyridine in a suitable solvent. In the case of sterically hindered alcohols, the reaction is accelerated by the addition of dimethylaminopyridine (DMAP). Initially, the acid is converted to acid chloride by reacting with SOC12, POC13 under reflux conditions. The reaction of oxalyl chloride with the carboxylic acid in the presence of a catalytic amount of DMF in CH2C12 at ambient temperatures also generate acid chloride. Sc (OTf)3 as a cocatalyst enhances the esterification process in the case of tertiary alcohols. Many substituted methy, ethyl, alkylphenyl and benzyl esters are in practice. Tertiary butyl esters are less susceptible to nucleophilic attack than methyl ester. Aliphatic acids are esterified even in the presence of aromatic acids by using NaHSO4.SiO2. Fe3+ –K10 montmorillonite clay can be also used to esterify aliphatic acids.

Examples:

1. $PhCO_2H + CH_3OH \xrightarrow{H^+} PhCOOCH_3 + H_2O$

2. $CH_3CO_2H + PhCH_2OH \xrightarrow{H^+} PhCOOCH_2Ph + H_2O$

3. $PhCO_2H + PCl_5 \xrightarrow{100^0C} PhCOCl + POCl_3 + HCl$

4. $3CH_3CO_2H + PCl_3 \xrightarrow{50^0C} 3CH_3COCl + H_3PO_3$

5. $n\text{-}C_{17}H_{35}CO_2H + SOCl_2 \xrightarrow{Heat} n\text{-}C_{17}H_{35}SOCl + SO_2 + HCl$

6. 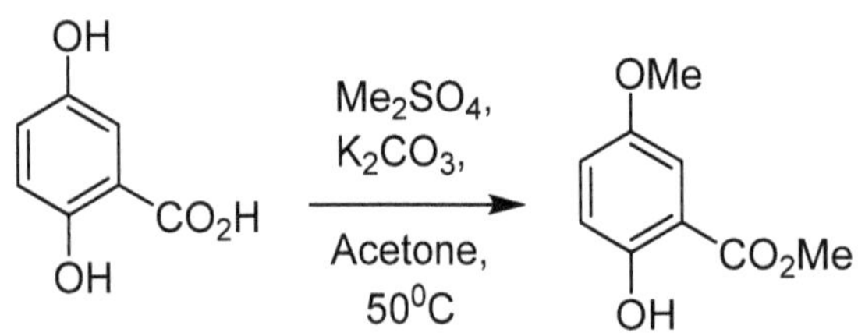

7. $(CH_3)_3CCO_2H \xrightarrow[2.\ EtOH]{1.\ SOCl_2} (CH_3)_3CCO_2Et$

Trimethyl acetic acid → Ethyl trimethyl acetate

8. $CH_3CO_2H + PhCH_2OH \xrightarrow{H^+} CH_3CO_2CH_2Ph$

Acetic acid + Benzyl alcohol → Benzyl acetate

9. 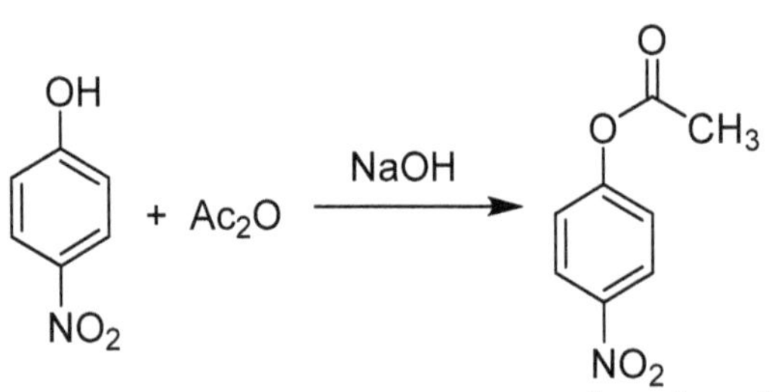

p-nitro phenyl acetate

10. $PhCO_2H + (CH_3)_2CHCH_2OH \xrightarrow{H^+} PhCOOCH_2CH(CH_3)_2$

Benzoic acid Isobutyl alcohol Isobutyl benzoate

11. 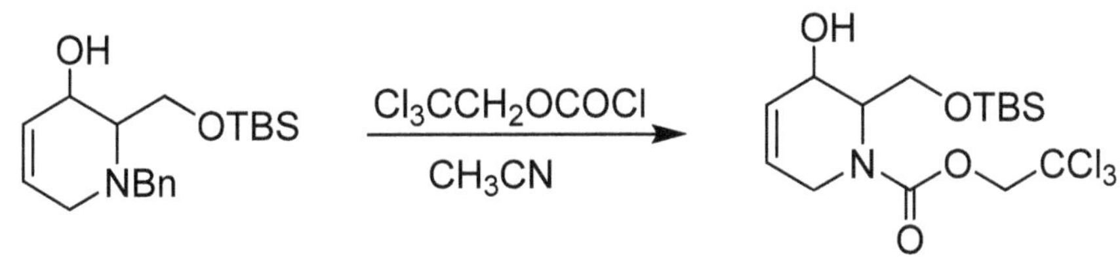

Boric acid or N-alkyl-4-boronopyridinium chloride act as best catalysts when α-hydroxy acids are used.

Benzyl esters can be prepared using many classical methods and by many new methods. These are relatively acid stable. (RCO2CH2C6H5, RCO2Bn) These can be cleaved by hydrogenolysis or electrolytic reduction.

Acetol esters are prepared by DCC coupling from acid and acetol (hydroxy acetone). These can be removed with TBAF/THF. These are stable to hydrogenolysis and useful in peptide synthesis.

Silylation of acids to silyl esters is also a potential protection protocol. Preparation of trimethylsilyl esters (TMS) – RCOOSi (CH3)3, triethylsilyl esters (TES)- RCOOSi (C2H5)3, t-Butyldimethylsilyl esters (TBDMS)- RCOOSi(CH3)2C(CH3)3 , t-butyldiphenylsilyl esters (TBDPS) - t-(CH3)3C(C6H5)2Si–O2CR, i-propyldimethylsilyl esters -RCOOSi(CH3)2CH(CH3)2, and triisopropylsilyl esters (TIPS) - (i-Pr)3Si–O2CR, are some of the important esterifications. The esters are prepared generally from concerned carboxylic acid and a silyl halide. These are stable to nonaqueous reaction conditions. These can be cleaved under mild acidic or basic hydrolytic environment.

More active thiol esters are used to activate carboxyl groups both for lactonization and for peptide bond formation. These increase the acidity of the hydrogens α to the carbonyl group. Use of AgNO3 or Hg(O2CCF3)2 is known for cleavage.

Amides and hydrazides

Amides and hydrazides are prepared from an -ester or an acid chloride and an amine or hydrazine. These can also be prepared directly from the acid. Several activating agents are employed for the conversion of carboxylic acids to amides, especially in peptide chemistry. These are stable to mild alkaline hydrolysis under which esters are not stable. NBS/H2O, 60% HClO4, POCl3, HCl/HOAc, or HBr/HOAc are some reagents that cleave hydrazides. Carbodiimide and HOBt are usually employed to access the hydrazide of amino acids. In peptide chemistry, phenylhydrazides are prepared from amino acid esters and phenylhydrazine. Cu (OAc)2, or FeCl3/1 N HCl, are generally used to cleave phenylhydrazides. The N, N′ -diisopropylhydrazide used to protect penicillin derivatives is cleaved oxidatively employing Pb (OAc)4/Pyr, Aq. NBS/THF–Pyr, CrO3/HOAc, or NaIO4/H2O–THF, H2SO4.

Amine group protection

A large variety of protective groups have been developed for the amino group, including carbamates (>NCO2R), used in peptide and protein syntheses, as well as amides (>NCOR), used particularly in the syntheses of alkaloids and the nitrogen bases of nucleotides. Apart from the above, N-alkylation, N-arylation N-sulfenylation and N-sulfonylation are also popular methods. Moreover, N-metal, N-silicon, N-phosphorous derivatizations are also in practice. Amides can be formed from the acid chloride. Activated esters readily react with amines.

Carbamates

Carbamates are prepared with the help of a wide variety of reagents including the chloroformate. N-Alkyl carbamates can be cleaved by acid-catalyzed hydrolysis and N-alkylamides are deprotected under acidic or basic hydrolysis at reflux conditions. Primary and secondary amines are known to readily react with CO2, and these adducts can be alkylated to form a variety of carbamate derivatives. Methyl chloroformate (CH3OCOCl) is the most common reagent employed for the preparation of methyl carbamate. TEA and pyridine are the frequently used bases. Many substituted methyl (H3COC(O)NR2), ethyl (H3CH2COC(O)NR2) and benzyl carbamates apart from t-Butyl, Vinyl, Allyl, and Propargyl carbamates are some others in use. t-Butyl, 2-(biphenylyl) isopropyl, benzyl (Cbz), 9-fluorenylmethyl (Fmoc–NR2), isonicotinyl, 1-adamantyl, trimethylsilylethyl and allyl carbamates are readily cleaved respectively by acidic hydrolysis, by dilute acetic acid, by catalytic hydrogenolysis, by β-elimination with base, by reduction with zinc in acetic acid, by trifluoroacetic acid, by fluoride, and by Pd-catalyzed isomerization or by nucleophilic addition to the π-allylpalladium complex. The azidomethyl carbamate (Azoc–NR2 - N3CH2OCONR2) prepared by azide displacement on the chloromethyl carbamate is cleaved easily with trimethylphosphine or triphenylphosphine. Cl3CCH2OCOCl reacts with amines in Pyridine or aq. NaOH to form 2,2,2-Trichloroethyl Carbamate (Troc–NR2) -Cl3CCH2OC(O)NR2, which can be cleaved by electrolysis or by Zn/THF/H2O. 2-Phenylethyl Carbamate- R2NCO2CH2CH2Ph can be prepared from the chloroformate, and can be cleaved with H2/Pd–C.

t-Butyl Carbamate (BOC Group) - (CH3)3COC(O)NR2 is the most commonly and extensively used in peptide and heterocyclic synthesis for amine protection. It can be introduced easily by mixing (BOC)2O and the amine in THF with gentle heating or in the presence of aq.NaOH or using TEA/MeOH or TEA/DMF. BOC derivative was also obtained using (BOC)2O in β-cyclodextrin/ H2O at rt. BOC derivative was also prepared from (BOC)2O/EtOH or MeOH/ NaHCO3, under ultrasound conditions. BOC derivative was also developed from (BOC)2O/ sulfamic acid at rt under ultrasound/ neat conditions. It is inert to many nucleophilic reagents and is not easily hydrolyzed under basic conditions. It can be cleaved with strong acids generating t-BuOH or isobutylene and CO2 as by-products. HCl/ EtOAc, or 50% TFA/ CH2Cl2 or AcCl/ MeOH, or TMSCl/ MeOH, or Me3SiCl/ PhOH/ CH2Cl2 or TsOH/ THF/ CH2Cl2 or HNO3/ CH2Cl2 or aq.H3PO4/ THF/ CH3CN are some of the reported conditions for deprotection of BOC group.

Allyl Carbamate (Alloc–NR2 or AOC–NR2) - CH2^CHCH2OC(O)NR2 is prepared with CH2^CHCH2OCOCl in Pyridine or (CH2^CHCH2OCO)2O in dioxane. Common method for cleavage is based on Pd (0) in the presence of a nucleophile.

Benzyl Carbamate (Cbz–NR2 or Z–NR2) - PhCH2OC(O)NR2, another widely applied group can be formed by the reaction of amine with PhCH2OCOCl in the presence of aq. Na2CO3 or NaOH/ THF or DIPEA/ CH3CN/ Sc (OTf)3. The benzylation was also performed in β-cyclodextrin/ water at rt. I2 /MeOH, or SSA, ionic liquid can also help in getting benzylation product. It can be readily cleaved by using TBAF/ THF, or BF3/Et2O/ CH3SCH3, or Trifluoroacetic anhydride/ pyridine or BBr3/ CH2Cl2, or BBr3 / trifluoroacetic acid, or TMSBr/ PhSMe/ TFA or BCl3/ CH2Cl2 or by catalytic hydrogenolysis with using H2/Pd–C, NH3 or PdCl2, MeOH, H2 or Pd(OAc)2/ H2 or Pd–C or Pd black/ hydrogen donor or by photolysis or electrolysis. The above mentioned are only some of the reported reaction conditions.

Amides

Amides are generally prepared from the acid chloride or the anhydride. A large number of coupling agents and methodologies were developed for amide formation. These are generally stable to acidic or basic hydrolysis but can be cleaved by heating in strongly acidic or basic solutions. Moreover, the deprotection is facilitated in the presence of a neighboring hydroxyl group which can participate in the hydrolysis. Hydrolytic stability increases from formyl to acetyl to benzoyl. Among the haloacetyl derivatives the lability increases with the number of halide atom substitution: acetyl < dichloroacetyl <trichloroacetyl< trifluoroacetyl. Formamide- R2NCHO, Acetamide- R2NAc, Chloroacetamide- R2NCOCH2Cl, Trichloroacetamide- R2NCOCCl3, Trifluoroacetamide (TFA)- R2NCOCF3, Phenylacetamide-R2NCOCH2C6H5, Benzamide- R2NCOC6H5 and N-Phthalimide are some of the commonly used amide derivatives.

Methylamines are generally prepared by reacting the amine with a methylating agent such as MeI or dimethyl sulfate and can be cleaved photochemically. The reaction of allyl chloride or bromide or iodide with amines in the presence of Cu (0), Cu (ClO4)26H2O, or activated silica gel or K2CO3, or CsOHH2O, 4 Å MS, or LiOHH2O, 4 Å MS, or KF–Celite, provides N-Allylamines-(CH2^CHCH2NR2). Use of Pd (Ph3P)4, or Pd/C, or Rh (CO)H(PPh3)3, or Cl2(Cy3P)2Ru^CHPh (Grubbs' carbene) are some of the reported methods for the deprotection of allyl amines.

N-Benzylamine (R2N–Bn) - R2NCH2Ph can be prepared from amines using BnCl, or BnBr, or BnOH, or PhCHN2, or dibenzyl carbonate, or polymer-supported benzylating agents. The group can be cleaved by hydrogenolysis using Pd (OH)2/ H2, or H2/Pd–C or Na/ NH3, or Li, (CH2NH2)2, TEA, which are some of the reported protocols.

Benzyl or other alkyl groups, can be modified to various carbamates by a variation of the von Braun reaction

Allyl chloroformate is reported to convert benzyl amine to an Alloc carbamate. Some reagents like CAN, RuO4, MCPBA, or BBr3, or NIS or o-iodoxybenzoic acid (IBX) are reported to cleave benzyl group.

Amino Acids

Amino acids are difunctional moieties containing both acidic carboxyl group and basic amino functionality. These are building blocks for peptides and proteins. Except glycine the alfa carbons of amino acids are chiral. Naturally occurring alfa amino acids are L-amino acids. Peptide synthesis dealing with many amino acids is a difficult task as many different amide bonds are to be formed in a specific sequence. To overcome the problem, protection and deprotection of both the functional groups is important. Many different protecting groups are developed for both amino and carboxyl groups. In practice, some are widely implemented. Carboxyl groups are protected generally as methyl or benzyl esters, which can be easily introduced and removed under standard conditions.

Example: Leucine

Amino groups are commonly protected as tertiary butyloxy carbonyl amide (BOC) or fluorenyl methyl oxy carbonyl amide (FMOC) derivatives.

Example: Alanine

To make a dipeptide five steps are important. Protection and deprotection of both carboxyl and amino functionalities and coupling of both protected amino acids using reagent like DCC. The sequence is repeated whenever an amino acid is to be added to the sequence.

BOC-Ala+Leu-OCH3----→BOC-Ala-Leu-OCH3----→Ala-Leu-OCH3----→Ala-Leu

1st step-DCC, 2nd step-CF3CO2H, 3rd step-NaOH/H2O

-CO_2H protection

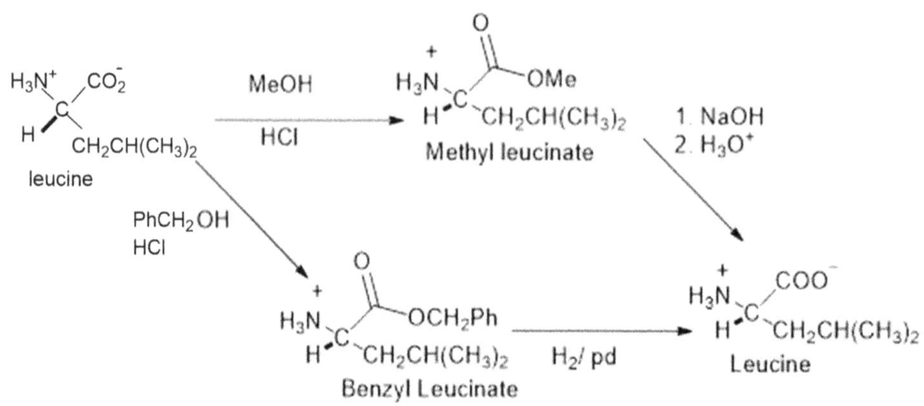

-NH_2- protection

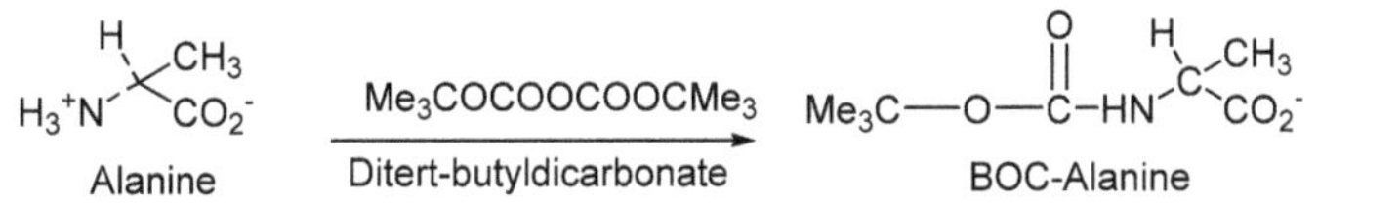

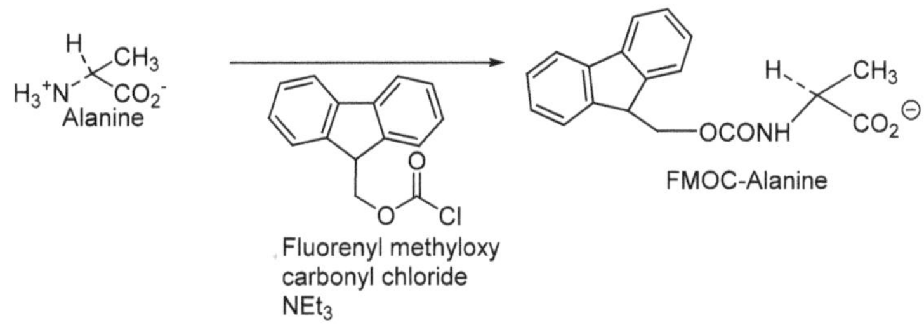

Peptide synthesis:

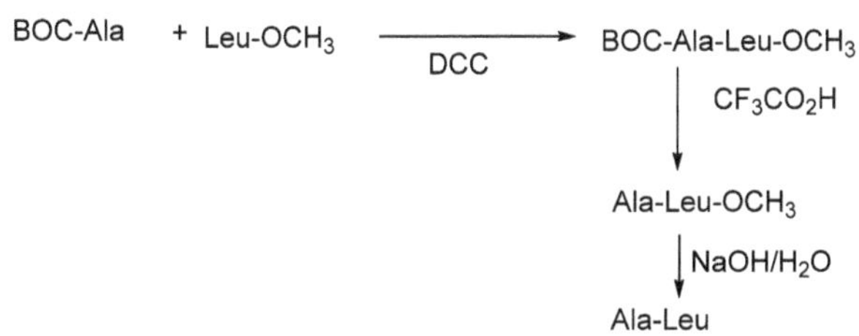

TsCl, introduced by Fischer and carbobenzoxy (CbO) chloride introduced by Bergmann are two more interesting protecting groups for amino group. Carbobenzoxy group can be removed by reduction with Pd/H2. But when amino acid contains sulphur catalytic reduction cannot be used as sulphur poisons the catalyst. In that case, Na/NH3 or phosphonium iodide can be used. The group can also be cleaved with HBr/AcOH or nitromethane. 4- Nitro or 4- bromo benzoxy chlorides are also used as protecting groups. Dimedone was also introduced as protecting group for amino group. It can be removed by bromination. Amino group can also be protected by tritylation which can later be removed with AcOH. Sheehan et al in 1949 adopted Gabriels phthalimide synthesis to protect amino group during peptide synthesis.

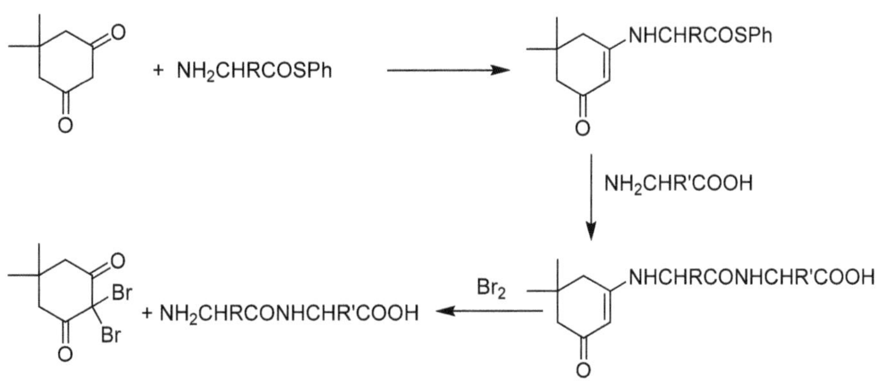

CHAPTER 4

Heterocyclic Chemistry and Synthesis of Representative Drugs

1. Bernthsen Acridine Synthesis

The reaction of diarylamine with a carboxylic acid (or acid anhydride) in the presence of zinc chloride at 200-270 °C for 24 hours forming 9-substituted acridine was reported by Bernthsen in 1884. A major improvement of the Bernthsen synthesis was reported in 1961 by Popp using polyphosphoric acid (PPA) as both the solvent and acid, which shortened the reaction time to 15 minutes. o – Substituted aryl diphenylamine is supposed to be an intermediate. Acridines are privileged structures in medicinal chemistry and exhibit wide variety of diverse properties. Example: Mepacrine (antimalarial) bucricaine (anaesthetic) Aminacrine, Euflavine (antibacterial).

General reaction

Bernthsen's method

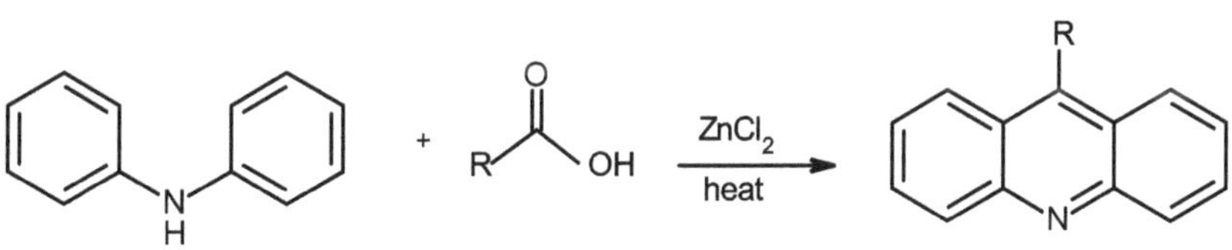

Mechanism:

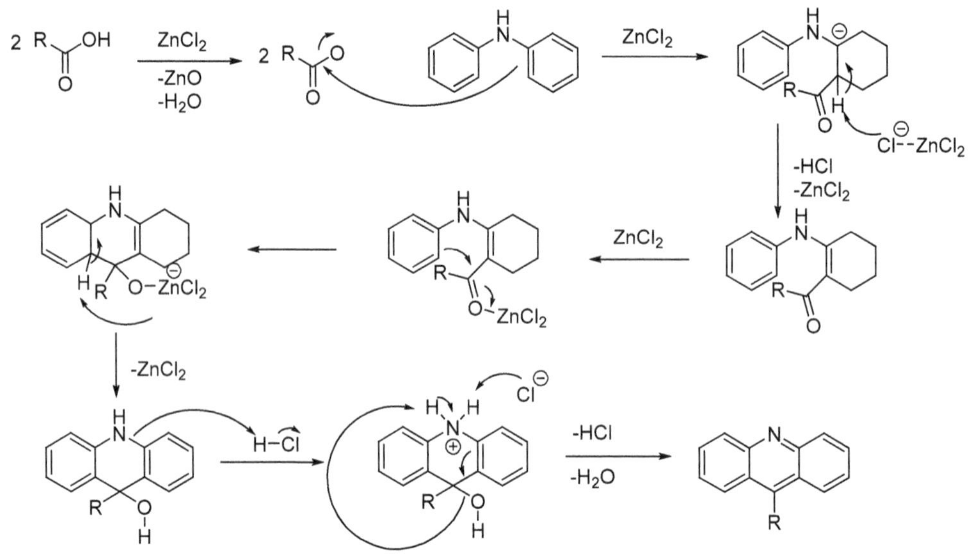

Applications and examples:

1. Preparation of 9-Phenyl acridine

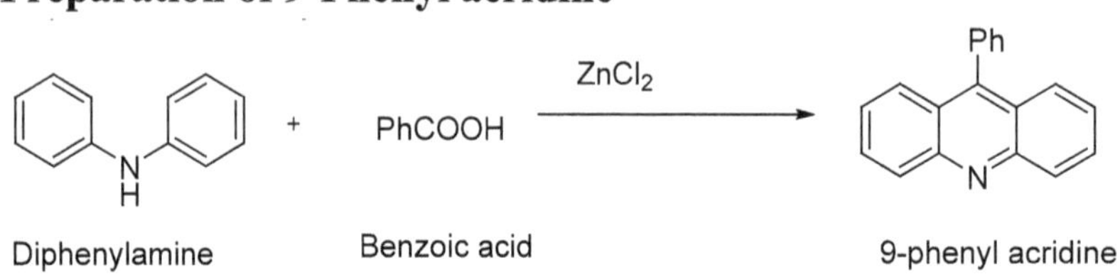

2. Preparation of 1-amino acridine

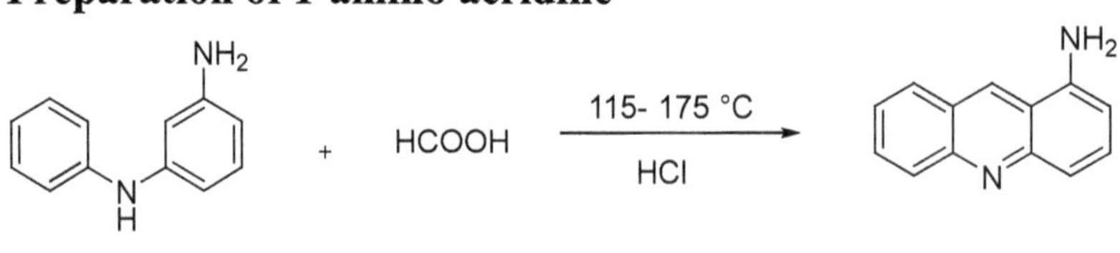

3. Preparation of 9-Chloroacridine

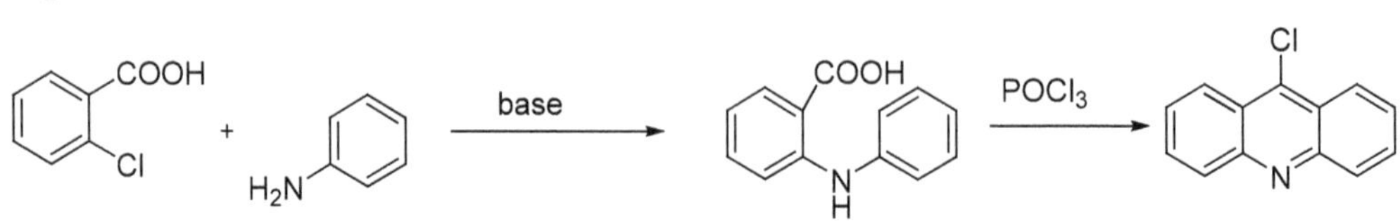

4. Synthesis of 9- substituted acridines under microwave conditions[31]:

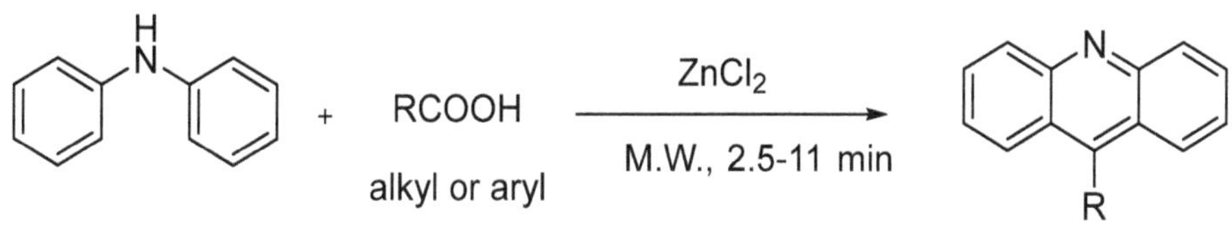

2. Combes quinoline synthesis

Quinoline is an important heterocyclic scaffold that serves as a building block for many pharmacologically active compounds and appear in common antimalarial drugs, fungicides, antibiotics, dyes, and flavoring agents. The quinoline derivatives exhibit cardiovascular, anticancer, and anti-inflammatory activities. There are several synthetic methods to prepare quinoline derivatives. The Combes quinoline synthesis is one among them.

In 1888 Edmond Combes reported the condensation of unsubstituted anilines with β-diketones to form 2,4-disubstituted quinolines in the presence of an acid via ring closure of the intermediate Schiff base.

General reaction:

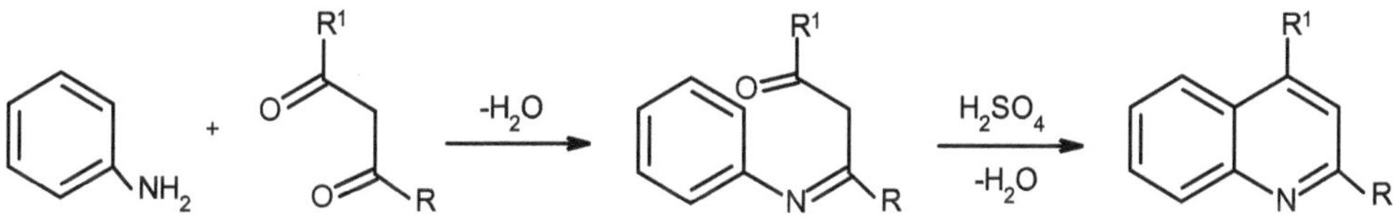

Mechanism:

The reaction is initiated by the protonation of the oxygen on the carbonyl in the β-diketone, which then undergoes a nucleophilic addition reaction with the aniline followed by an intramolecular proton transfer by an E2 mechanism with the loss of water molecule. Deprotonation at the nitrogen atom generates a Schiff base, which forms an enamine on tautomerization. This in acidic medium (con.H2SO4) gets protonated followed by annulation, proton transfer onto N-atom, protonation of OH-group and dehydration forms quinoline molecule. The annulations are the rate-determining step. Both steric and electronic effects influence the regioselective formation of the products. Concentrated sulphuric acid, con. HCl, acetic acid, chloroacetic acid, lactic acid, p-toluene sulphonic acid, HF, polyphoshoric acid, and PPE are some of the acidic reagents used for the reaction.

Mechanism:

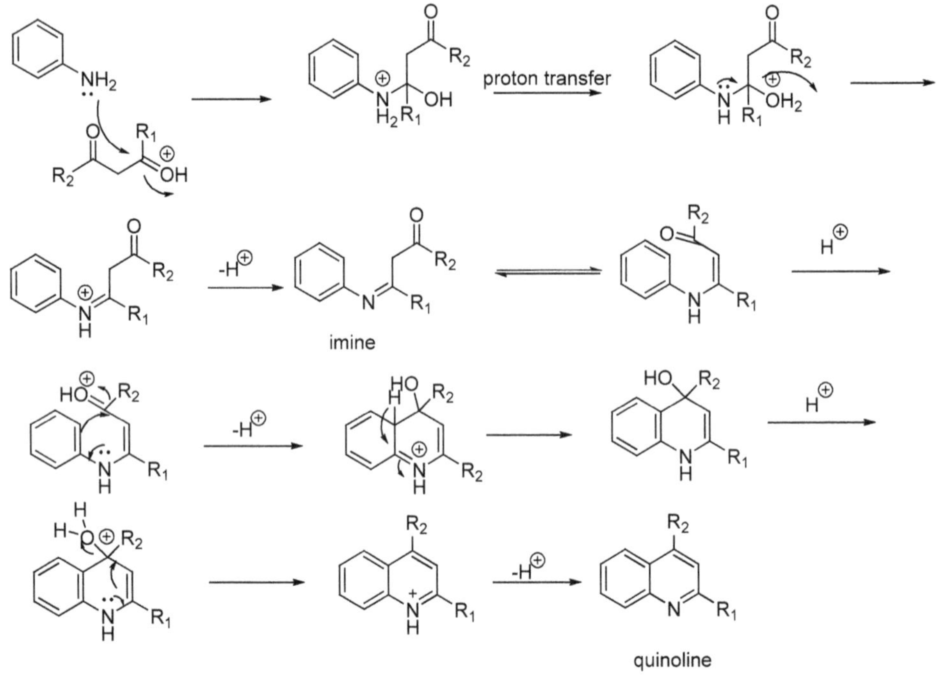

Applications and examples:

1. Combes Quinoline Synthesis:
Applications and exmaples:

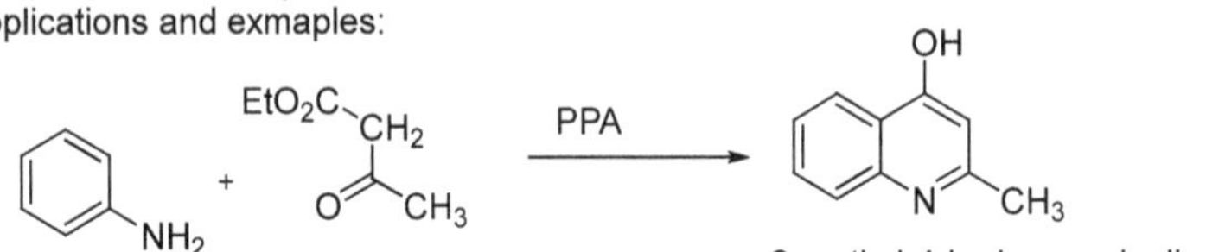

2-methyl-4-hydroxy quinoline

2.

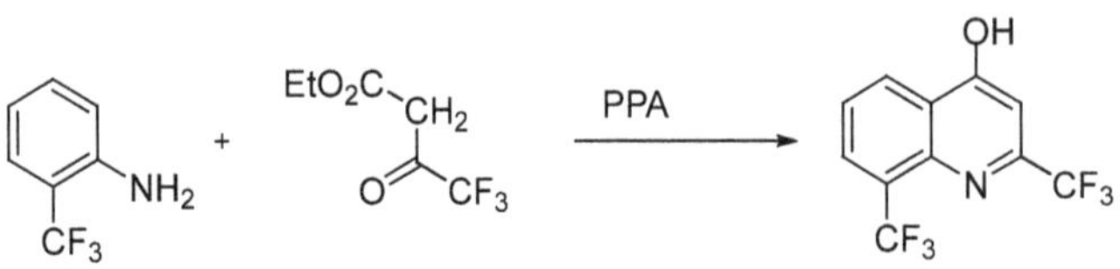

2,8 (ditrifluoromethyl) 4-hydroxy quinoline

3.

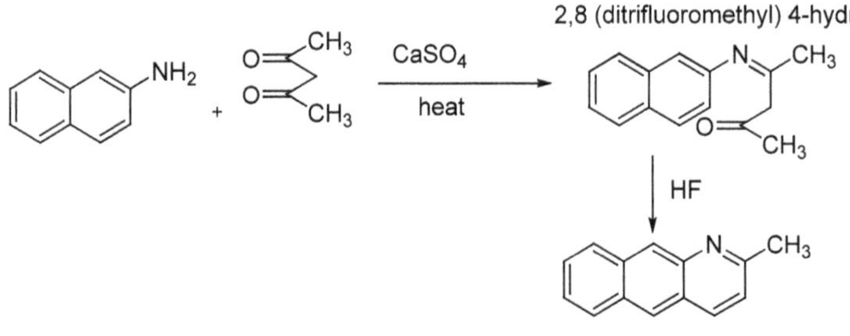

3. Debus–Radziszewski imidazole synthesis

In medicinal chemistry and pharmacology, Imidazole and its derivatives occupy a potential position. These exhibit various biological activities such as antimicrobial, anti-inflammatory, analgesic, antitubercular, antidepressant, anticancer activity, antiviral, and anti-leishmanial activities.

This is a widely applied, multicomponent, two-stage reaction involving the condensation of a dicarbonyl, an aldehyde, and ammonia, leading to the formation of imidazoles. This reaction is named after Heinrich Debus and Bronisław Leonard Radziszewski. The dicarbonyl component is commonly glyoxal, but can also include various substituted 1,2-diketones and ketoaldehydes. In the first step, the dicarbonyl and ammonia condense to give a diimine. The condensation of diimine with the aldehyde is the second step.

Ammonium carbonate, or aq. ammonia can also be used in place of ammonium acetate. If aryl amines are used 1,2,4,5-tetrasubstituted imidazoles will be formed. This reaction was first reported by Debus in 1858, then developed by Radziszewski in early 1882, and further modified by Weidenhagen in 1935.

General reaction:

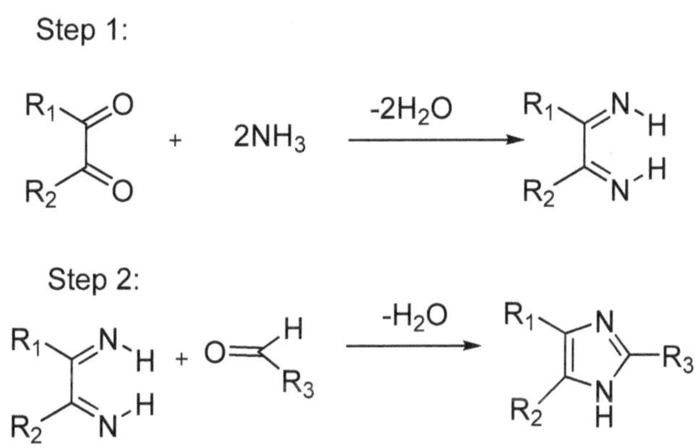

N-Substituted imidazoles can be obtained by a modification of the above method by using 1 equivalent of amine in place of ammonia.

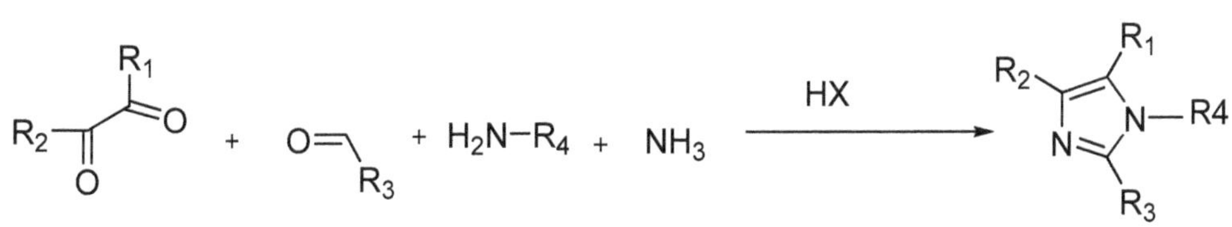

Mechanism:

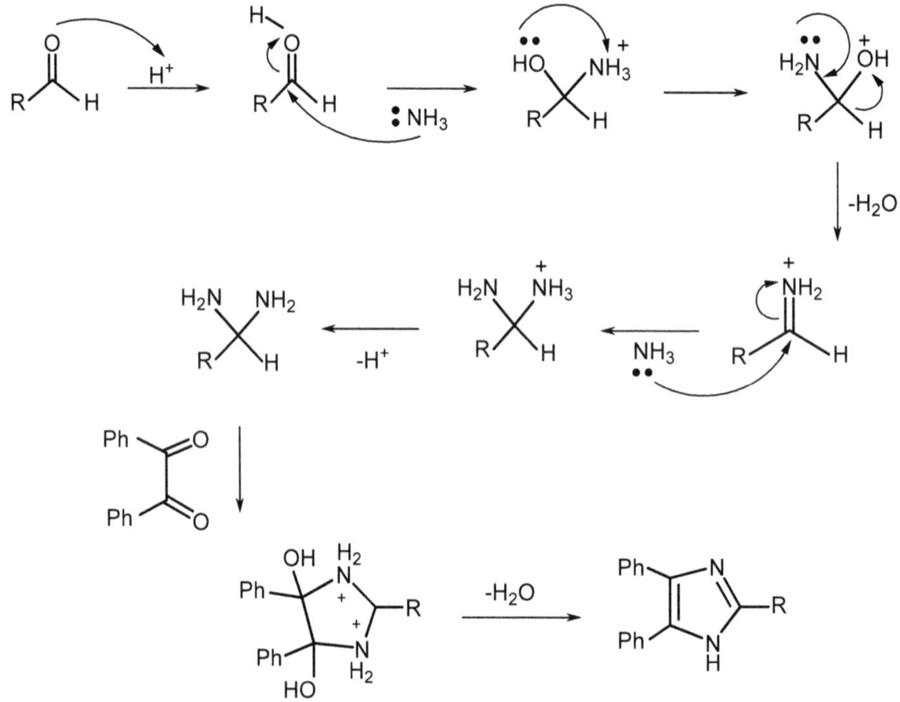

Applications and examples:

Debus-Radziszewski imidazole synthesis

Application and examples

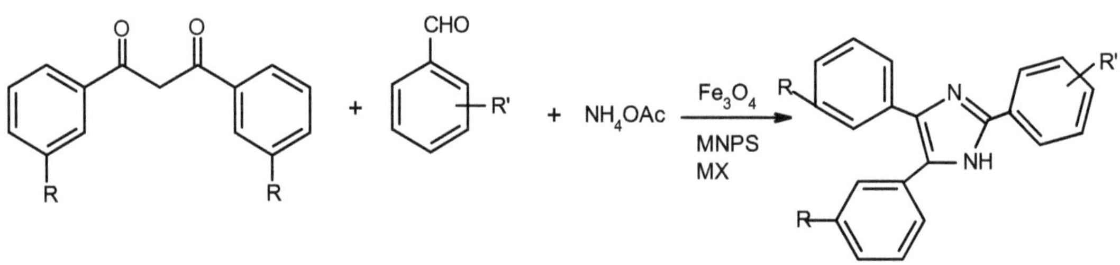

1. Microwave assisted synthesis of trisubstituted imidazoles

A one-pot microwave-assisted 2,4,5- trisubstituted imidazoles using a freshly prepared Schiff's base nickel catalyst (Ni-C) complex, under microwaves was reported[32].

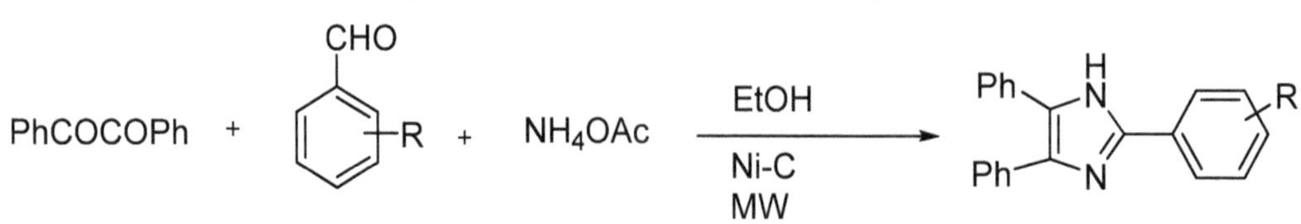

2. Preparation of 2,4,5- trisubstituted Imidazoles using lactic acid

2,4,5-Trisubstituted imidazoles were efficiently prepared by reacting aromatic aldehyde, benzil and ammonium acetate in the presence of biodegradable lactic acid at 160 °C[33].

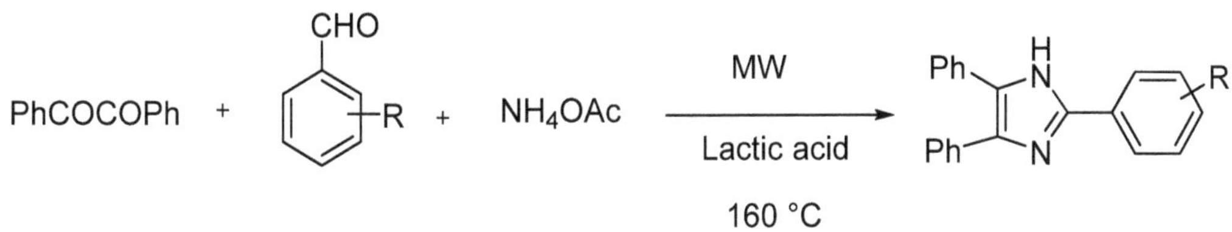

3. Synthesis of 2,4,5-triarylimidazoles using $KMnO_4$ and $CuSO_4$

A one-pot three-component condensation of bis-aryl α-hydroxyketones, aromatic aldehydes and ammonium acetate in the presence of KMnO4/CuSO4 as catalyst under mild reaction conditions was developed[34].

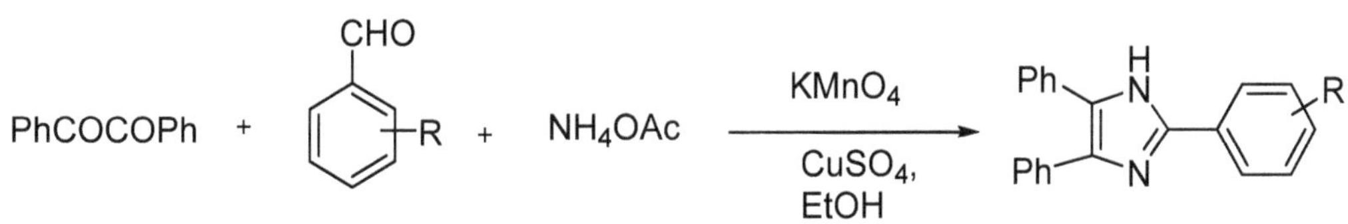

4. Synthesis of 2,4,5-trisubstituted and 1,2,4,5-tetrasubstituted imidazoles using DABCO

These are prepared by the condensation of benzaldehyde, ammonium acetate, and benzil in the presence of DABCO (1,4- diazabicyclo [2.2.2]octane) as catalyst using t-butanol as solvent at 60–65°C[35].

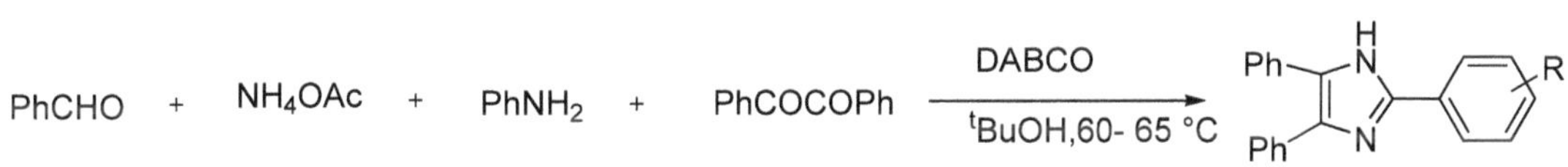

5. Preparation of Metronidazole

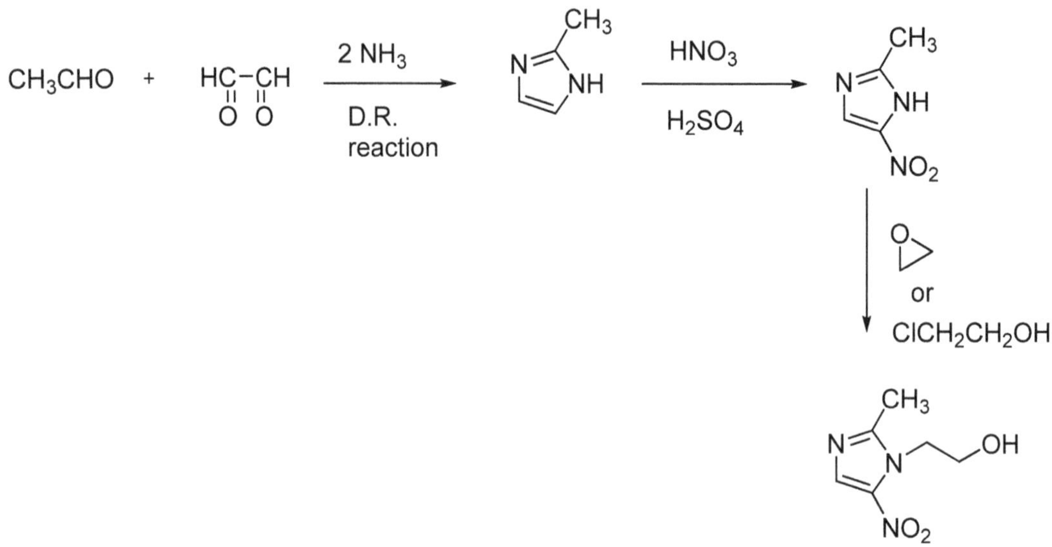

Metronidazole

6. Preparation of 1,2,4,5- tetrasubstituted imidazoles

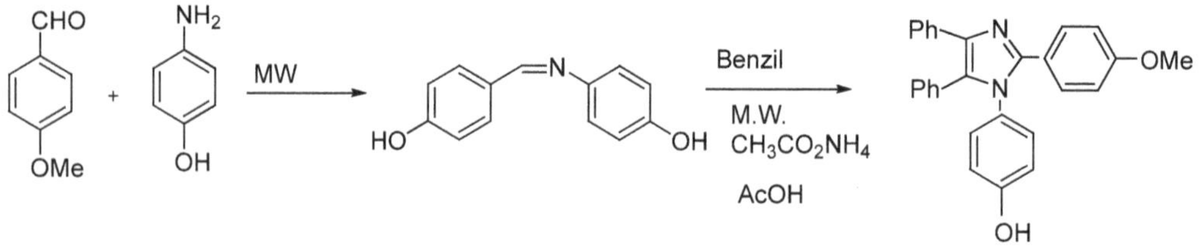

4. Knorr pyrazole synthesis

In Knorr pyrazole synthesis hydrazine or substituted hydrazines like phenylhydrazine or cyanoethylhydrazine and hydrazides, or semicarbazides or aminoguanidines are reacted with 1,3-dicarbonyl compounds like acetyl acetone, pyruvic aldehyde, acetoacetic ester, or β-ketonitrile. In the presence of acid medium, an imine is formed, later the other nitrogen of the hydrazine derivative also attacks the other carbonyl group which has also been protonated by the acid and results in second imine group. On deprotonation this diimine regenerates the acid catalyst and produces the pyrazole compound. There can be two different regioisomer pyrazole products depending on which carbonyl group is attacked first. This is the major limitation of the process. The best example is the Synthesis of antipyrine.

General reaction:

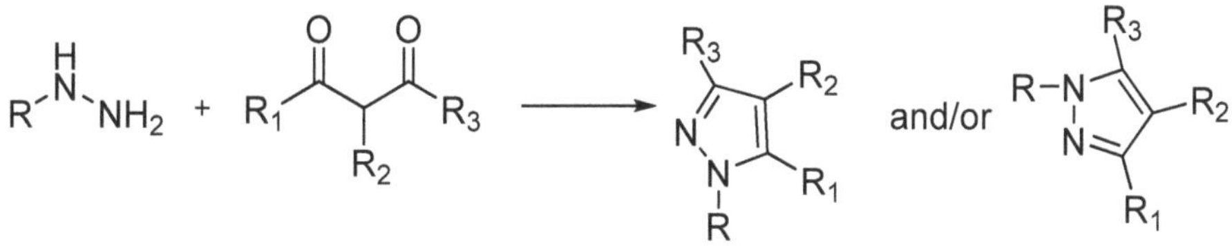

Mechanism:

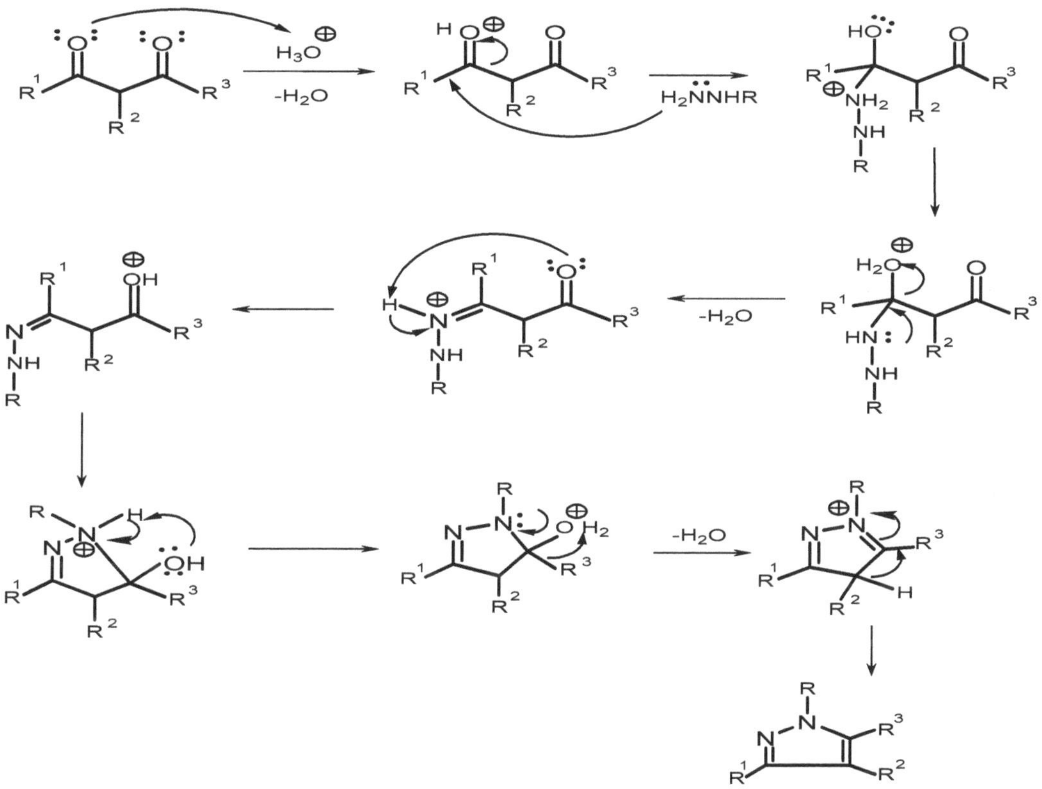

Applications and examples

1. Synthesis of Antipyrine

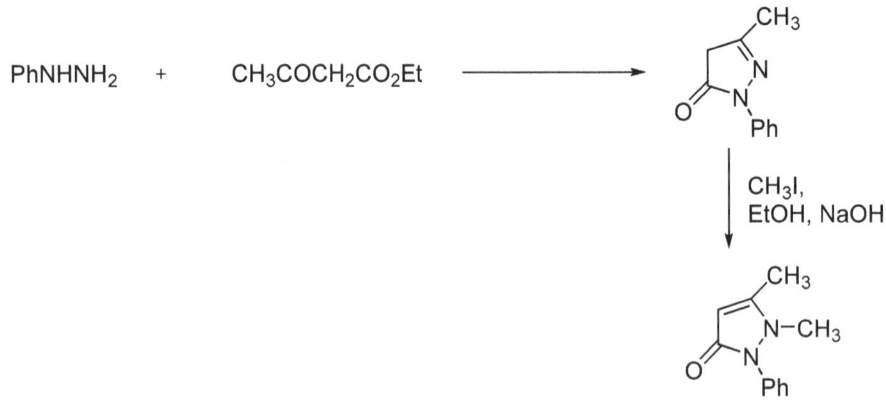

2. Preparation of 3(3,5-dimethyl pyrazole-4-yl)-pentane 2,4-dione

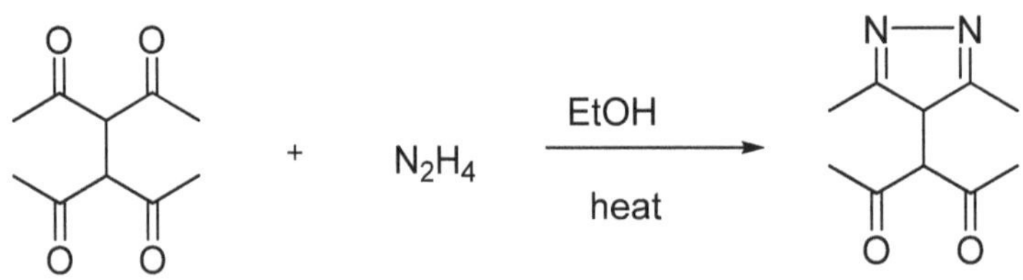

3(3,5-dimethyl pyrazol-4'-yl) pentane-2,4-dione

5. Pinner pyrimidine reaction

The synthesis of pyrimidines is a very active area of research, due to the wide applicability of such compounds in pharmaceutical or coordination chemistry. Grimaux in 1879 reported the preparation of barbituric acid from urea and malonic acid in the presence of phosphorus oxychloride. Pyrimidine derivatives widely occur in nature as well as in synthetic compounds. Pyrimidine structure is present in several biologically active compounds such as nucleotides, cytosine, thymine and uracil, thiamine (Vitamin B1) and alloxan as well as in barbiturates. Many sulfa drugs like sulfamerazine, trimethoprim, and anti-HIV drug Zidovudine also contain pyrimidine nucleus. The pyrimidine compounds have great potential in medicinal chemistry due to the diverse pharmacological activities exhibited such as antibacterial, antiplasmodial, anticancer, antineoplastic, anti-inflammatory, antiviral, and antimalarial activities.

Pinner pyrimidine reaction is a strong acid -promoted condensation between a β-ketoester or β-diketone and non-N-substituted amidine affording pyrimidine derivatives. In 1885 Pinner observed that amidines react with acetoacetic esters forming 2,6-dimethyl-4-hydroxyl- pyrimidines. As original Pinner reaction had problems such as low yields and harsh reaction conditions various approaches including cycloaddition reactions, MCRs and tandem synthesis have come up with efficient methodologies. Large number of synthetic methods are reported for the preparation of pyrimidine compounds. Primarily these can be prepared by the cyclization of β-dicarbonyl compounds with N–C–N compounds. Reactions of β-dicarbonyl compounds with amidines provide 2-substituted pyrimidines, with urea give 2-pyrimidinones, and guanidines produce 2-aminopyrimidines. Some of the examples are discussed here.

General Reaction:

Mechanism:

Pinner pyrimidine reaction

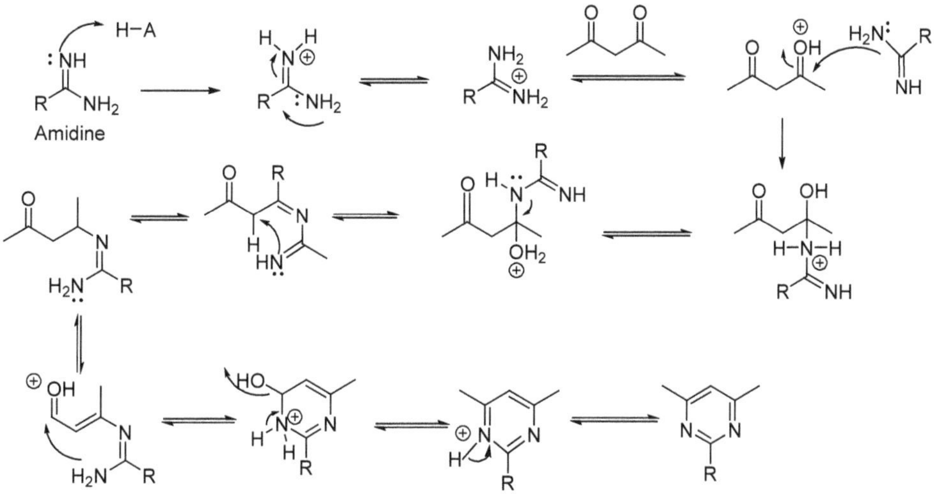

Drugs with pyrimidine nucleus:

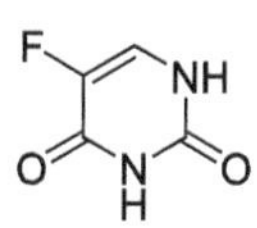

5-Fluoro uracil
(anti-cancer)

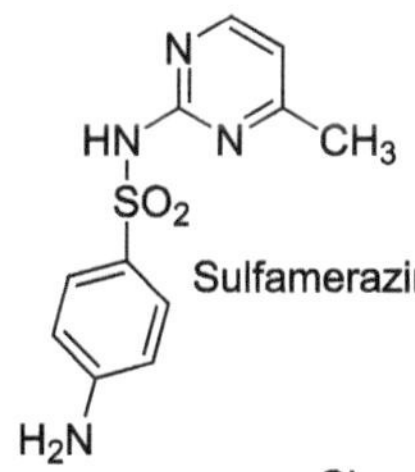

Sulfamerazine

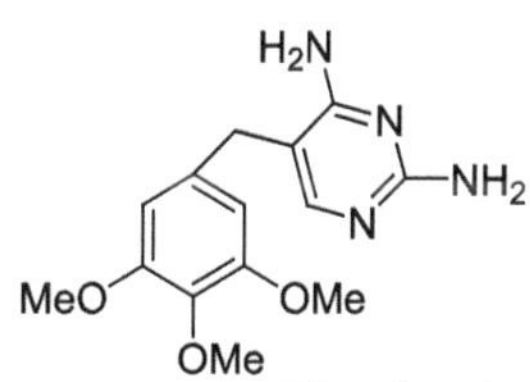

Trimethoprim

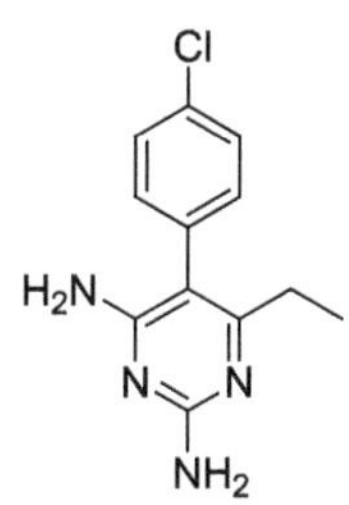

Pyrimethamine
(antimalarial)

Applications and examples:

General Reaction:

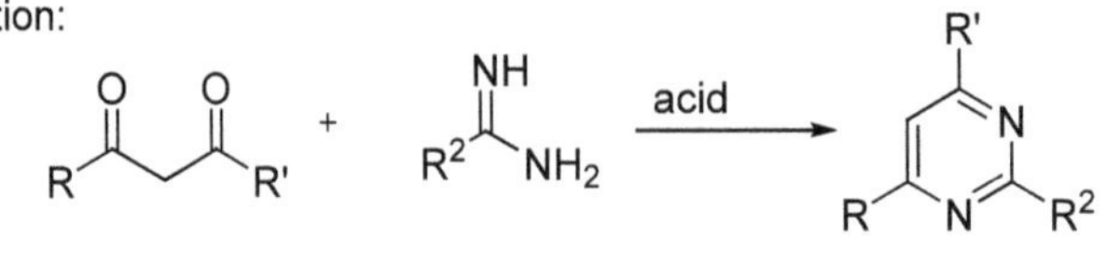

1,3 dicarbonyl compounds

Applications and examples:

1.

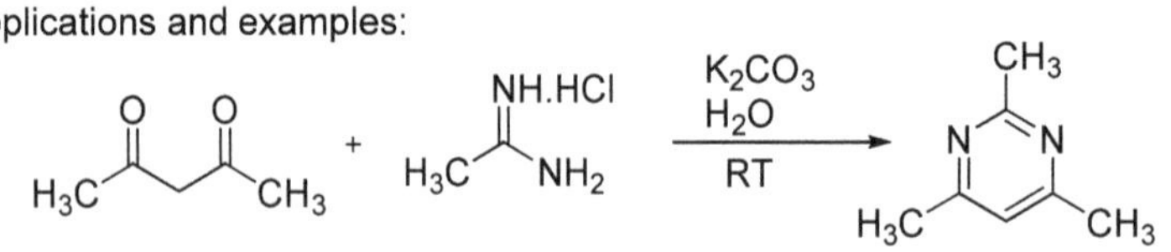

2,4,6- trimethyl pyrimidine

2.

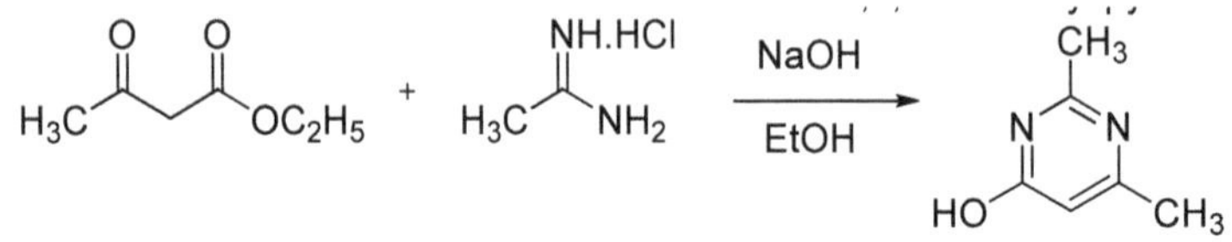

2,6- dimethyl 4-hydroxy pyrimidine

3.

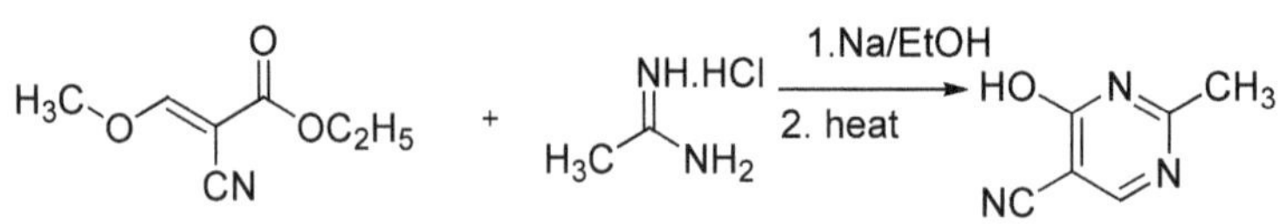

2-methyl 6-hydroxy 5-cyano pyrimidine

4. $CH_3COCH_2CH_2ONa$

Sodium formyl acetone

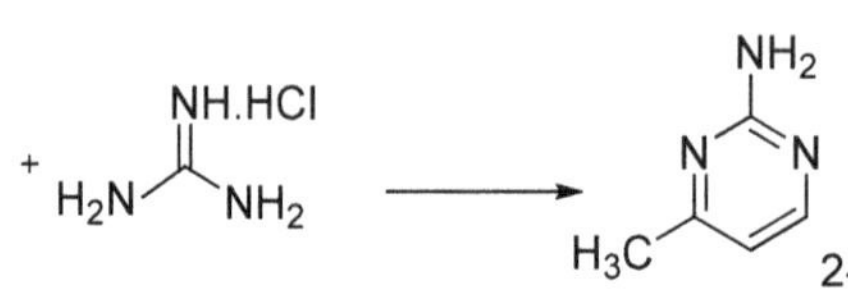

2-amino-4-methyl pyrimidine

5. Synthesis of Trimethoprim

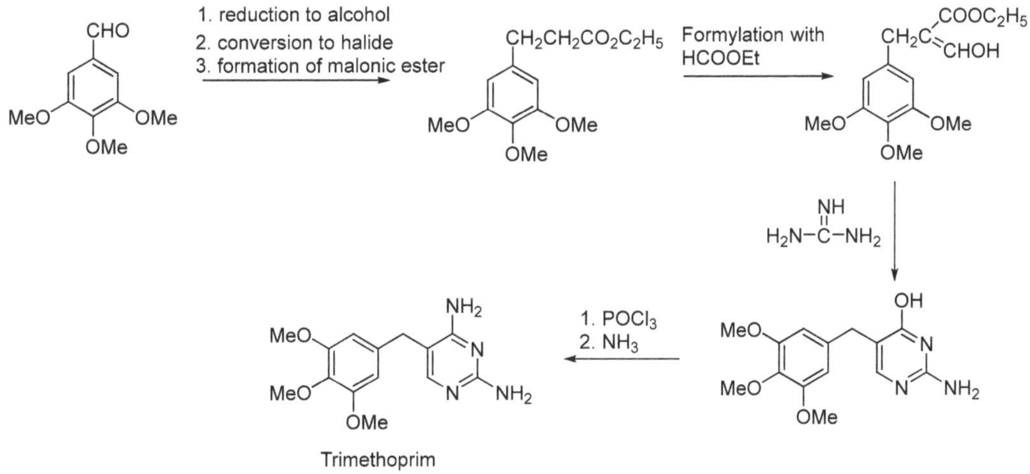

6. Smiles rearrangement

The Smiles rearrangement is an intramolecular nucleophilic aromatic substitution (SNAr reaction), named after British chemist Samuel Smiles. Original reaction was reported in 1894 by Henriques for naphthol sulfones. Smiles worked extensively in 1930s. The reaction involves breaking of a C–X single bond and forming a new C–X or C–C bond though ipso substitution. It has wide scope, in terms of nucleophile, leaving group, and ring-size of the transition state. It is a powerful tool for arene functionalization working under simple and economic reaction conditions.

General reaction

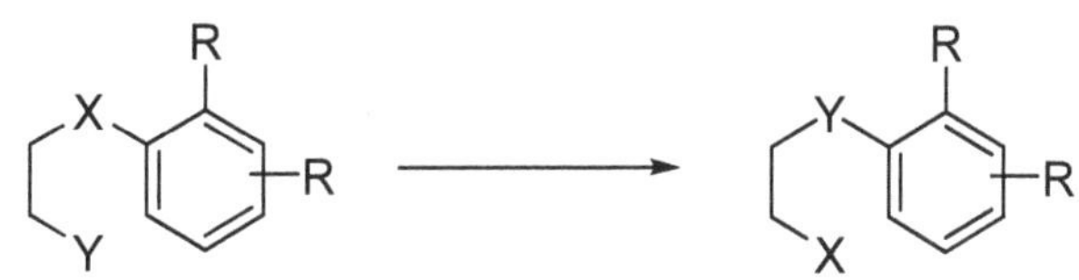

X in the arene compound can be a sulfone, a sulfide, an ether or any substituent capable of dislodging from the arene carrying a negative charge. Y can be an alcohol, amine, or thiol that can act as a strong nucleophile. The arene requires activation by an electron-withdrawing group preferably in the ortho position. Strongly electron-withdrawing nitro or p-sulfonyl or 2-pyridyl groups were primarily used to activate the migrating aromatic ring. The Truce–Smiles rearrangement is a modification in which the incoming nucleophile is sufficiently strong and the arene does not require activation. Ex: The conversion of an aryl sulfone into a sulfonic acid by the action of n-butyl lithium. Many reviews appeared on this reaction. Many variations and improvements were reported in literature.

Applications and examples:

1.

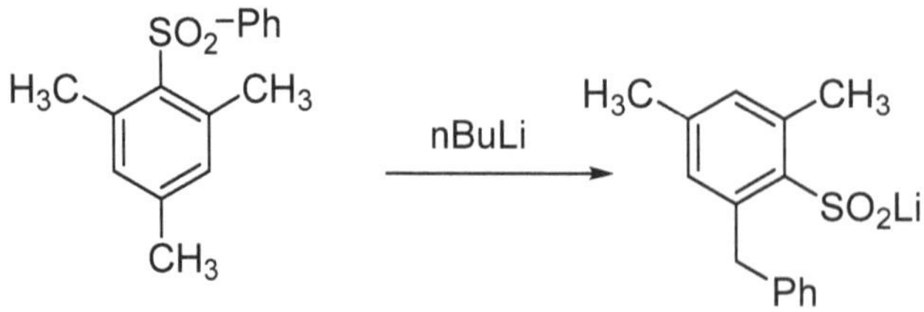

Truce–Smiles rearrangement

2. Alkyl nitroarylethers with a pendant primary or secondary amino group undergo a facile Smiles rearrangement on treatment with KOH/DMSO/H_2O to give the corresponding *N*-alkylnitroaniline[36].

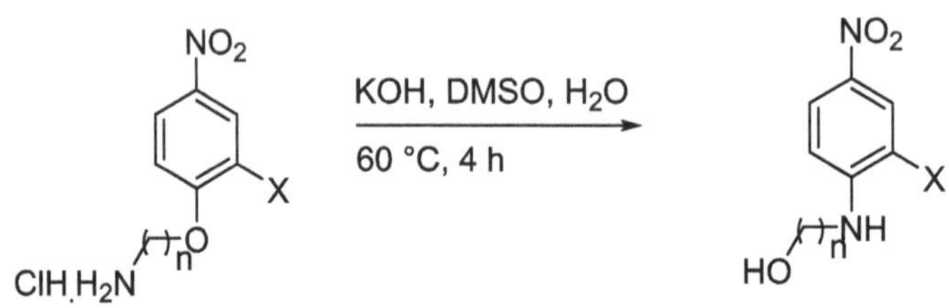

X= F, NO_2
n= 1, 2

3. **Clayden rearrangement:** An unprecedented intramolecular aryl migration was reported by Clayden and co-workers. This developed into a rich area of chemistry for lithiated ureas, carbamates, and thiocarbamates. This is also related to Smiles rearrangement[37].

4. **Vinylogous Truce–Smiles rearrangement:** A series of three nitrostyrene substrates successfully produced rearranged stilbene products[38].

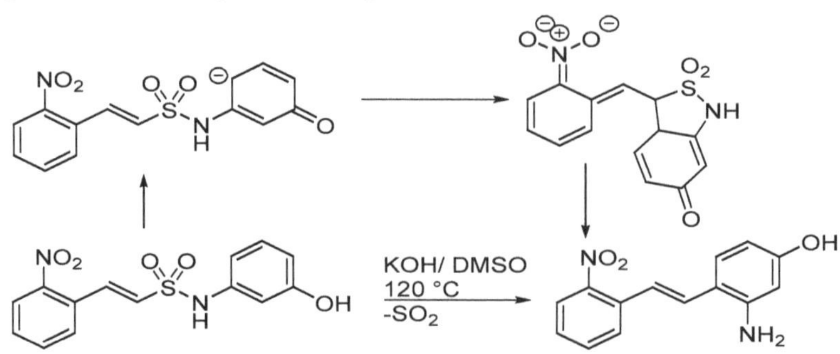

5.

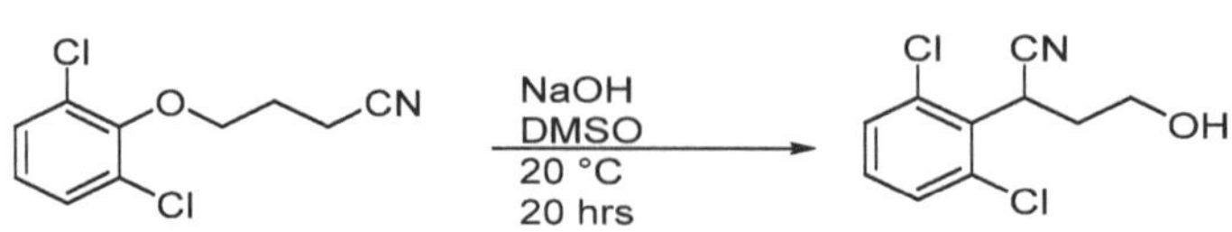

6. Synthesis of diclofenac sodium

The industrial six-step continuous flow method for the synthesis of diclofenac sodium was reported via cascade esterification and Smile rearrangement strategy. This employs 2,6-dichloro-N-diphenylaniline as a key intermediate, and involves the Smiles rearrangement of phenoxyacetamide. This involves removal of a C_2 unit as waste in the form of 2-hydroxyacetic acid sodium salt. A new C_2 group is again introduced using corrosive and toxic chloroacetyl chloride. In this traditional batch process causes waste and reduces efficiency, leading to laborious operations. To improve the processes new continuous-flow synthetic routes to diclofenac sodium are being invented[39].

(Six-step continuous flow synthesis of diclofenac Sodium via cascade etherification/Smile rearrangement strategy: Tackling the issues of batch processing)

7. Traube purine synthesis

Purine is a water soluble, widely occurring, nitrogen containing heterocyclic aromatic compound consisting two ring fused system with pyrimidine and imidazole. It is present in high in animal products like meat, meat extracts, internal organs such as liver, brain, and kidneys. It is also present in fish, seafood, and poultry. Some legumes, spinach, cauliflower, spirulina, mushrooms, and algae also contain purine compounds. These play significant role in DNA and RNA as bases adenine and guanine. These are also potential constituents in many biomolecules like ATP, GTP, cyclic AMP, NADH, and coenzyme A.

Some of the important molecules having purine nucleus are caffeine, uric acid, theophylline, theobromine, xanthine, hypoxanthine and isoguanine.

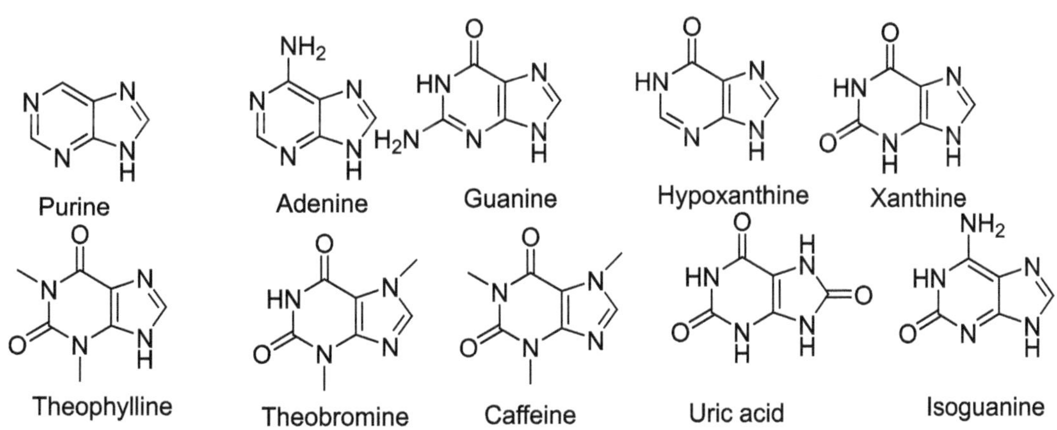

Purine synthesis by Emil Fischer.

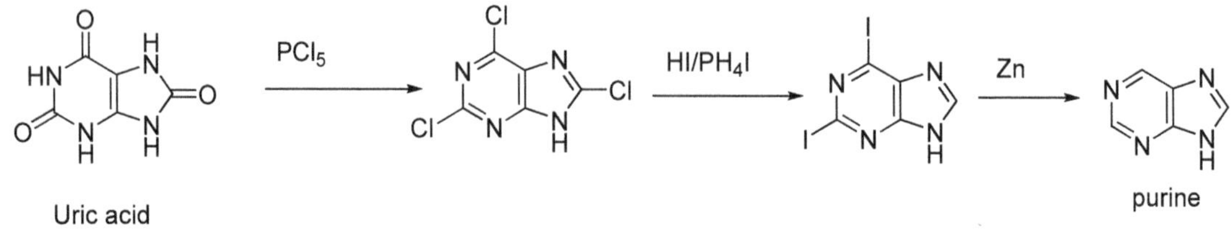

In 1898, Emil Fischer synthesized purine for the first time starting from uric acid by chlorination with PCl_5 to give 2,6,8-trichloropurine, followed by iodination to 2,6-diiodopurine with HI, PH4I and reduction with zinc dust. Earlier in 1776, Carl Wilhelm Scheele isolated uric acid from kidney stones.

Wilhelm Traube, in 1900 reported the important reaction now termed as -The Traube purine synthesis starting from formic acid and 4,5-diaminoprimidine compounds. This general method is widely used to make different purine derivatives and is also the basis of various commercial methodologies aiming to generate purines synthetically.

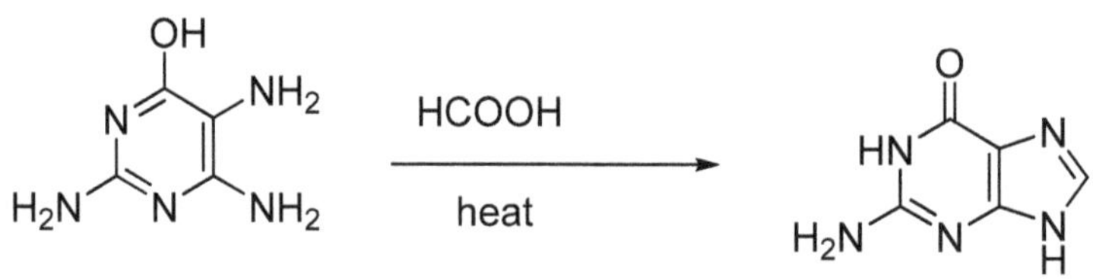

Mechanism:

Applications and examples:

1. Synthesis of 8-Hydroxy purine

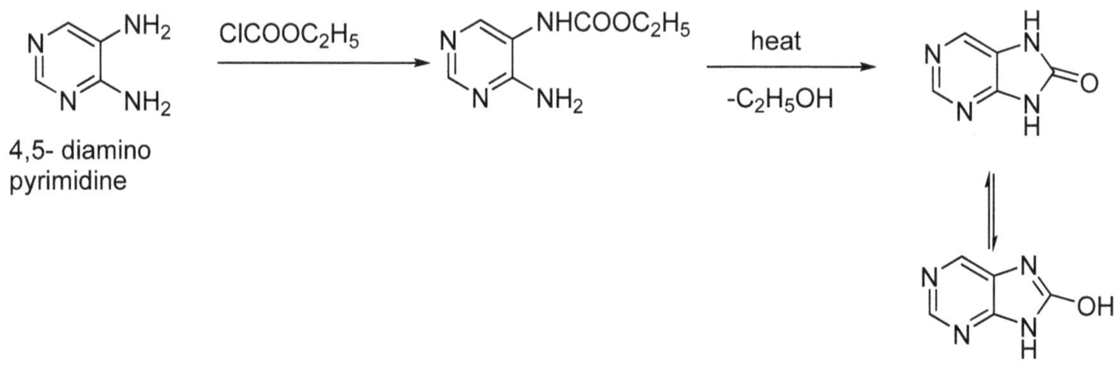

2. Synthesis of hypoxanthine

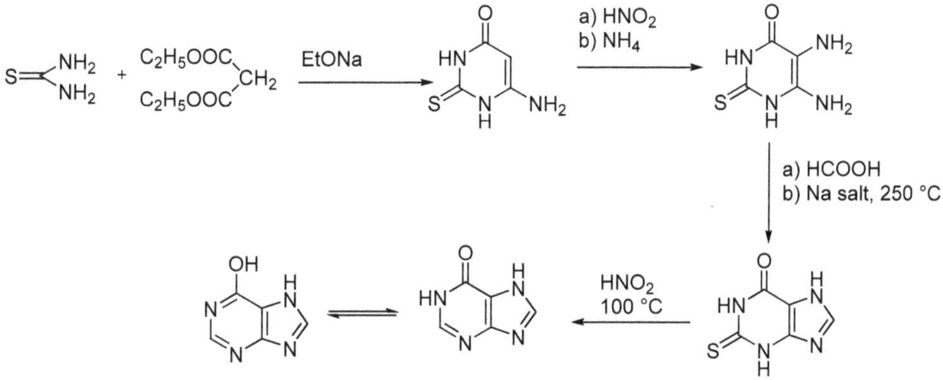

3. Synthesis of xanthine

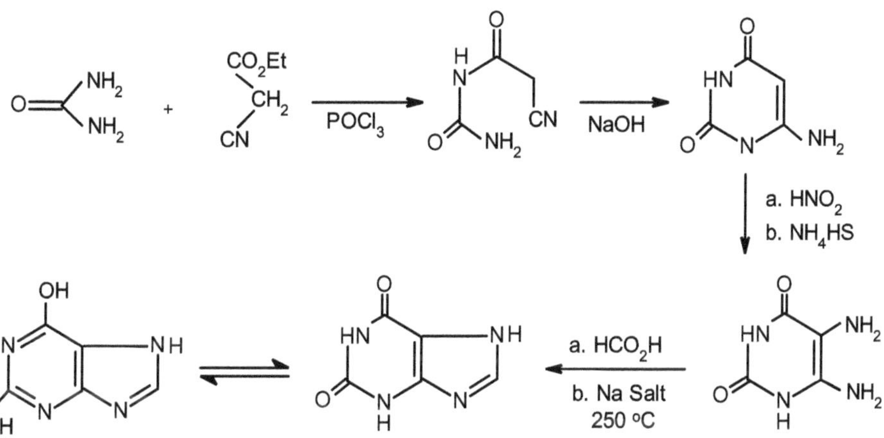

4. Synthesis of guanine

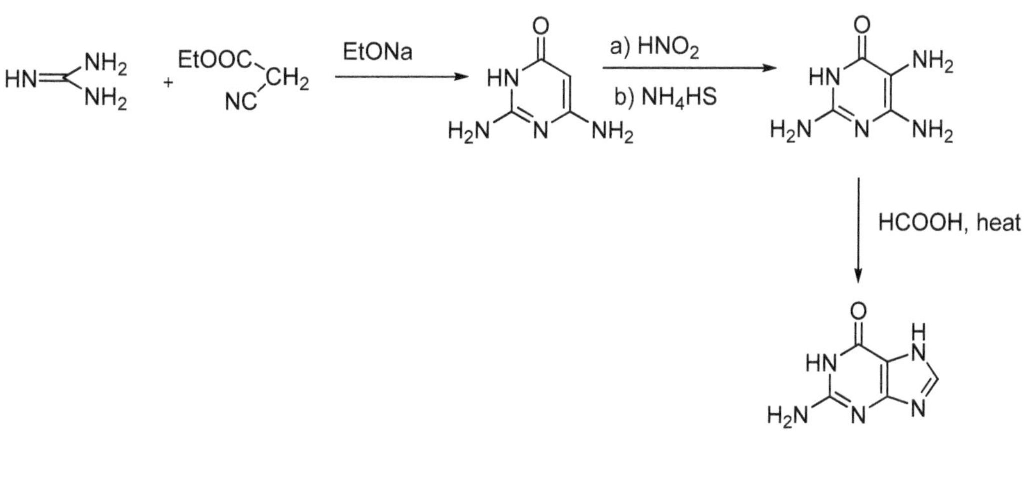

5. Synthesis of Caffeine

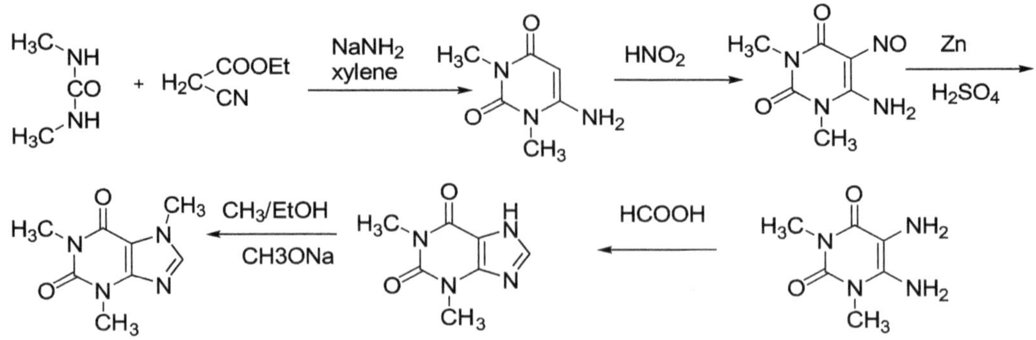

6. Synthesis of theophylline

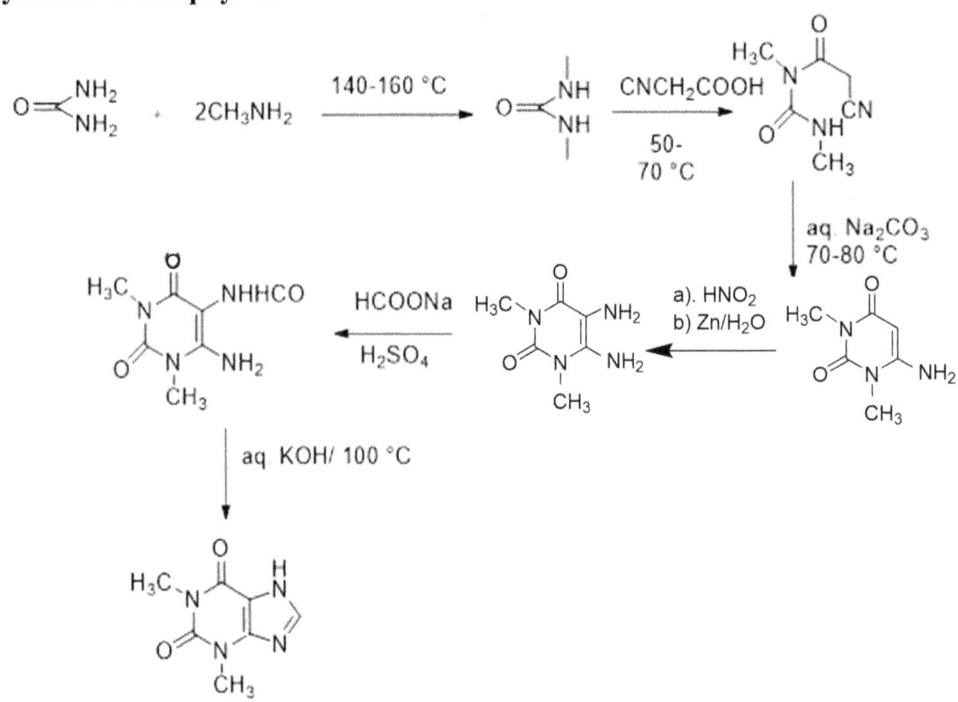

Synthesis of Representative Drugs

1. Alprazolam
2. Amsacrine
3. Antipyrine
4. Celecoxib
5. Chloroquine
6. Chlorpromazine
7. Hydroxychloroquine
8. Ketoconazole
9. Mercaptopurine
10. Metamizole sodium

11. Metronidazole
12. Miconazole
13. Prochlorperazine
14. Promazine
15. Quinacrine
16. Quinine
17. Sulfamerazine
18. Terconazole
19. Theophylline
20. Thioguanine
21. Triamterene
22. Trimethoprim

1. Alprazolam

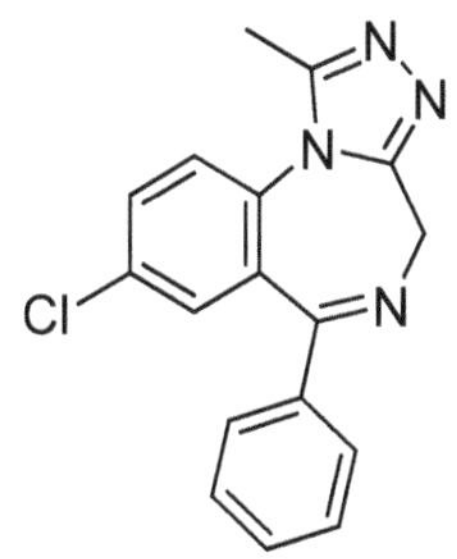

8-Chloro-1-methyl-6-phenyl-4*H*- [1,2,4] triazolo[4,3-a] [1,4] benzodiazepine

a) Molecular formula: $C_{17}H_{13}ClN_4$

b) 308.77

c) It was invented by Dr. Jackson Hester at the Upjohn Company and patented in 1971 and approved for medical use in 1981. Alprazolam is a schedule IV-controlled substance and is a common drug of abuse. In 2020, it was the most commonly prescribed medication. It is also a chemical analog of triazolam_which differs by the absence of a chlorine atom in the o-position of the 6-phenyl ring.

d) Uses: It is a fast-acting potent tranquilizer of medium duration. It is used as a medication in the management of anxiety disorders, panic of general category.

e) Side effects: Amnesia, ataxia, drowsiness, dizziness, vertigo, hallucinations, rashes, and fatigue. Benzodiazepines have general physical dependence, abuse, addiction, and withdrawal symptoms.

f) Mechanism of action: It exhibits antidepressant, muscle relaxant, anticonvulsant and antianxiety properties. It is a positive allosteric modulator of the gamma amino butyric acid (GABA) type A receptor. Effects of GABA are enhanced and inhibits neurons in the brain. Therapeutically, it is similar to other benzodiazepines and is a high potency triazolobenzodiazepine. It is similar to tricyclic antidepressants. It causes marked suppression of the hypothalamic-pitutory-adrenal axis.

g) Metabolism: It gets metabolized to less active 4-hydroxyalprazolam and more active alpha hydroxyalprazolam in liver by cytochrome P4503A1 and P4503A4. Half-life is 12hours. The metabolites are excreted in urine. It gets absorbed very well. It binds to proteins in serum.

h) Synthesis: 2,6-Dichloro-4-phenylquinoline, reacts with hydrazine giving 6-chloro-2-hydrazino-4-phenylquinoline, which on boiling with triethyl orthoacetate in xylene leads to the heterocyclization into a triazole derivative. This on oxidative cleavage with sodium periodate and ruthenium dioxide in H_2O/CH_3COCH_3 gives 2-[4-(3′-methyl-1,2,4-triazolo)]-5-chlorobenzophenone. On oxymethylation using HCHO followed by the substitution of the OH-group with PBr_3, gives 2-[4-(3′-methyl-5′-bromomethyl-1,2,4-triazolo)]-5-chlorobenzophenone. Br group is replaced by an amino group using ammonia followed by intermolecular heterocyclization gives alprazolam[40].

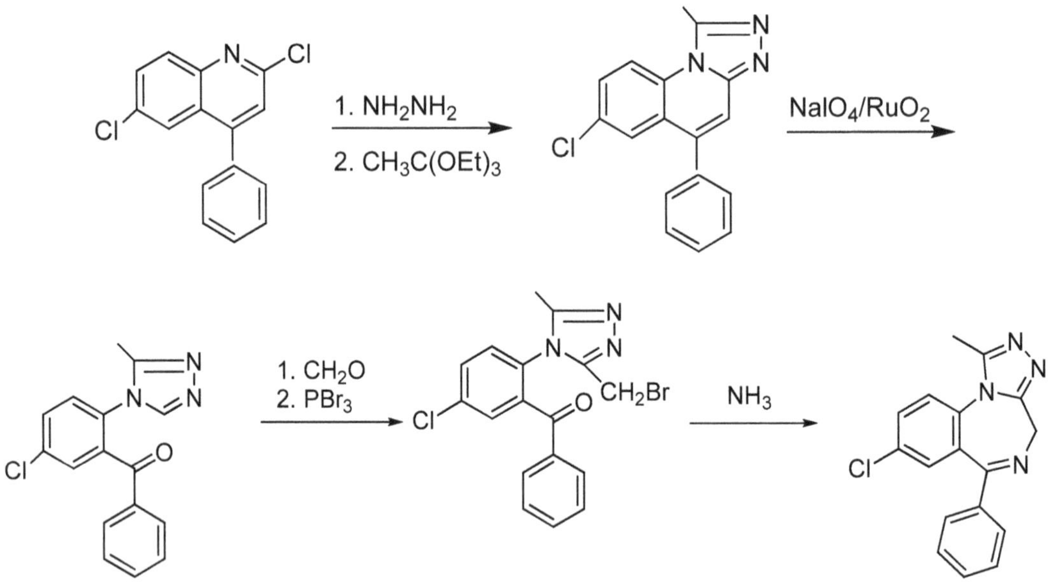

2. Amsacrine

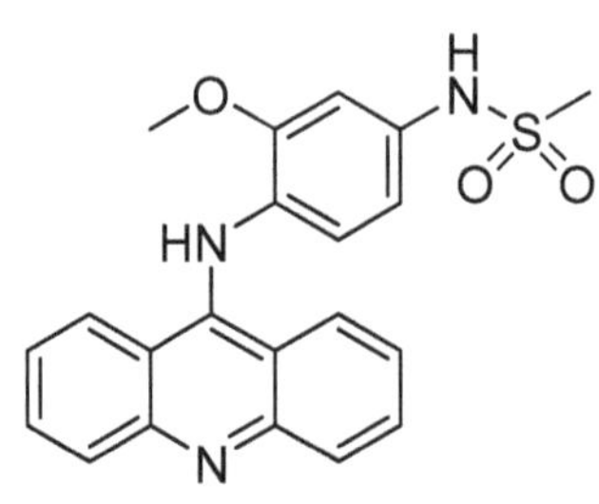

a) Molecular formula: C21H19N3O3S

b) Mol. wt. 393.46

c) Amsacrine, an anticancer drug was first synthesised in 1970 by Professor Cain and colleagues. It underwent clinical trials in 1978 under the US National Cancer Institute, exhibited excellent activity against acute lymphoblastic leukaemia.

d) Uses: This acridine based cytotoxic antineoplastic agent is used for treating acute lymphoblastic leukaemia and malignant lymphomas.

e) Side effects: Cough, fever, chills, sores, ulcers, white spots, bloody urine and stools, accumulation of pus.

f) Mechanism of action: It inhibits topoisomerase isomerase II. It binds to DNA through intercalation and external binding, there by altering the DNA structure inhibiting DNA replication and transcription. It reduces the number of RBC in the blood. It induces DNA double-strand breaks and arrests S/G2 phase of the cell cycle leading to cell death.

g) Metabolism: This poorly absorbed drug is extremely and primarily metabolized in the liver. It is excreted in the bile and urine. Half life is 8 to 9 hours. It undergoes oxidative metabolism. It gets converted to 5, and 6-glutathione conjugates. Other metabolites are N-methanesulfonyl-N4-(9-acridinyl)-3-methoxy-2,5-cyclohexadiene-1,4-diimine and 3-methoxy-4-(9-acridinylamino-2,5-cyclohexadiene-1-one.

h) Synthesis: Amsacrine, 4-(9-acridinylamino)-3-methoxyphenyl-*N*-methansulfonamide, is prepared by the sulfonation of 4-nitro-*m*-anisidine with methanesulfonyl chloride, to form sulfonyl amide, followed by the reduction of the nitro group to an amino group with Fe/HCl, affording 4-amino-3-methoxyphenyl-*N*-methansulfonamide. Reacting this with 9-chloroacridine generates amsacrine[41].

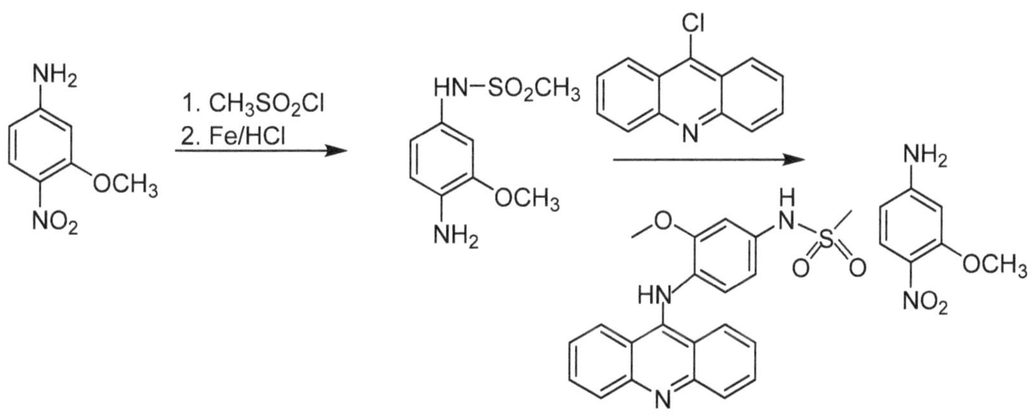

3. Antipyrine

1,2-Dihydro-1,5-dimethyl-2-phenyl-3*H*-pyrazol-3-one

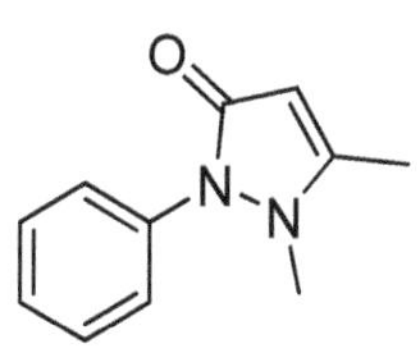

a) Molecular formula: $C_{11}H_{12}N_2O$

b) Mol. wt: 188.230

c) It was first synthesized by Ludwig Knorr and later patented by Knorr in 1883. Antipyrine is also known as phenazone, or phenazon. It is known as the "the 'mother' of all modern antipyretic analgesics.

d) Uses: It is an earliest widely used analgesic, antipyretic and anti-inflammatory drug and can be categorized as nonsteroidal anti-inflammatory drug (NSAID). It is slowly replaced by phenacetin, aspirin, paracetamol and followed by other NSAIDs such as ibuprofen.

e) Side effects: Allergy, nausea, hepatotoxicity and agranulocytosis.

f) Mechanism of action: Antipyrine acts primarily in the CNS, increasing the pain threshold by inhibiting both isoforms of cyclooxygenase, COX-1, COX-2, and COX-3 enzymes involved in prostaglandin (PG) synthesis. It acts by blocking the synthesis of prostaglandins by inhibiting cyclooxygenase, which converts arachidonic acid to cyclic endoperoxides, precursors of prostaglandins.

g) Metabolism: 3-Hydroxymethyl antipyrine, 4-hydroxy antipyrine and norantipyrineare known metabolites.

h) Synthesis: 1. Phenazone is prepared by the condensation of phenylhydrazine and ethyl acetoacetate under basic conditions and methylation of the resulting intermediate compound 1-phenyl-3-methylpyrazolone with dimethyl sulfate or methyl iodide.

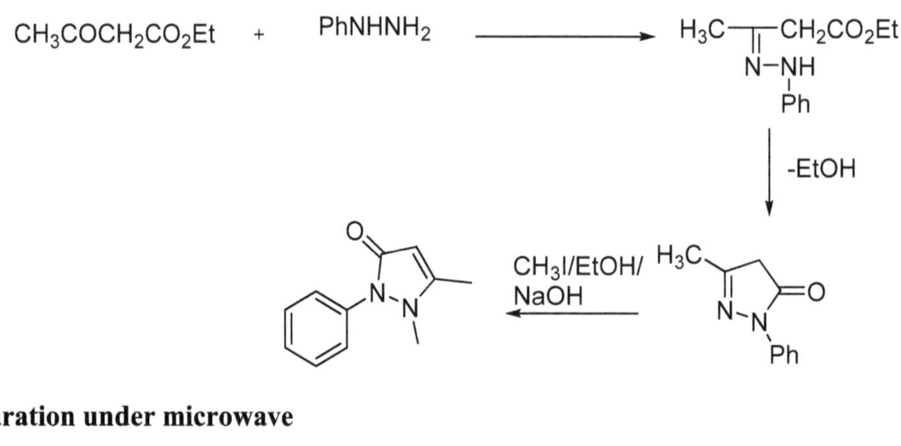

2. Preparation under microwave

The mixture of ethyl acetoacetate and phenylhydrazine was refluxed for 15 min in microwave oven to obtain phenazone[42].

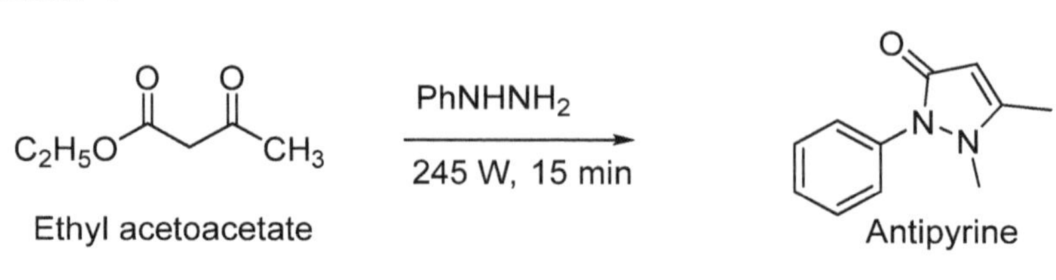

4. Celecoxib

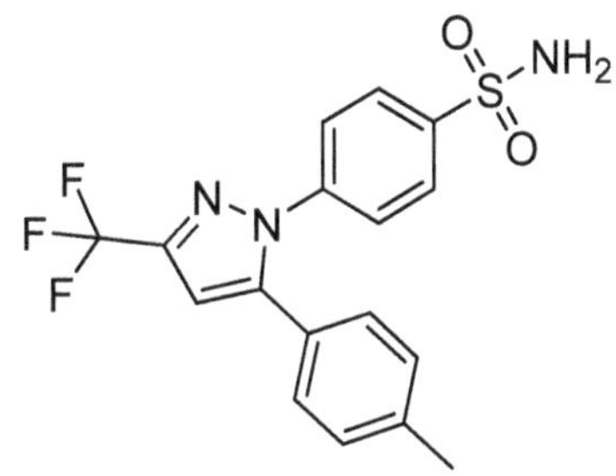

4-[5-(4-Methylphenyl)-3-(trifluoromethyl) pyrazol-1-yl] benzenesulfonamide

a) Molecular Formula: C17H14F3N3O2S

b) Mol. wt: 381.37

c) It was first patented in 1993 and was in medical use since 1999. In 2020, it was one of the most commonly prescribed medication. Along with other COX-2 inhibitors such as Valdecoxib etc., celecoxib was discovered by Monsanto, Searle division team led by John Talley.

d) Uses: It is a COX-2 inhibitor and nonsteroidal anti-inflammatory drug (NSAID). It is widely used to treat the pain and inflammation in osteoarthritis, rheumatoid arthritis, ankylosing spondylitis, painful menstruation, and acute pain in adults. It has analgesic and antipyretic properties also. It is used as an adjunct to surgeries.

e) Side effects: Nausea, diarrhea, GI bleeding, ulcers, heart attacks, kidney failures and anaphylaxis.

f) Mechanism of action: It exerts anti-inflammatory and analgesic activities by blocking the synthesis of different inflammatory prostanoids. It acts as a selective noncompetitive inhibitor of cyclooxygenase -2 (COX-2) enzyme, expressed in inflammed tissues. Inhibition of COX-2 reduces the synthesis of mediators like PGE-2, Prostacyclin (PG-12), PGD-2, PGF-2 and thromboxane (TXA-2), leading to reduction of pains well as inflammation and providing relief.

g) Metabolism: It is rapidly absorbed and reaches peak serum concentration in approximately 3 h.It is extensively metabolized in the liver. It is metabolized primarily through methyl hydroxylation to form hydroxycelecoxib, largely catalyzed by CYP2C9. Hydroxycelecoxib is oxidized further to carboxycelecoxib by the action of cytosolic alcohol dehydrogenases ADH1 and ADH2, followed by conjugation with glucuronic acid by the action of UDP glucuronosyltransferases generating the 1-*O*-glucuronide. The metabolites are not pharmacologically active. It is eliminated by hepatic metabolism and excreted through faeces and urine. Half-life is 11hours.

h) Synthesis: 1. The synthesis starts with the reaction of 4-methylacetophenone with *N*-(trifluoroacetyl)imidazole in the presence of sodium *bis*(trimethylsilyl)amide forming 4,4,4-trifluoro-1-(p-tolyl) butane-1,3-dione. This condenses with 4-sulfamoylphenylhydrazine generating celecoxib[43].

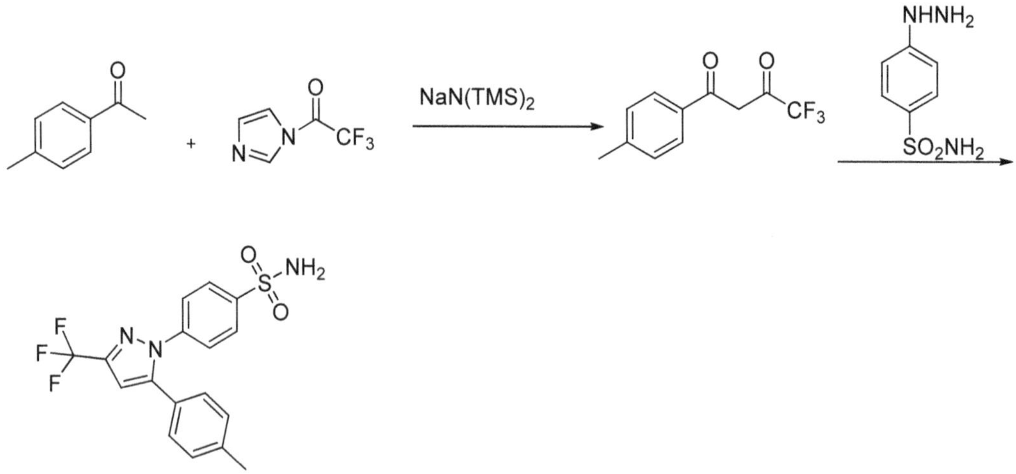

2. Other method[44]

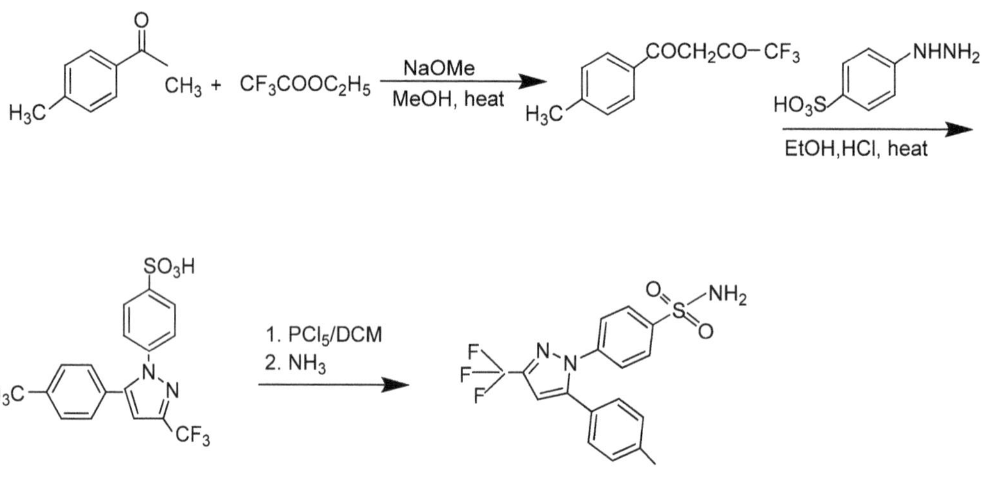

5. Chloroquine

(*RS*)-*N*′-(7-chloroquinolin-4-yl)-*N*, *N*-diethyl-pentane-1,4-diamine

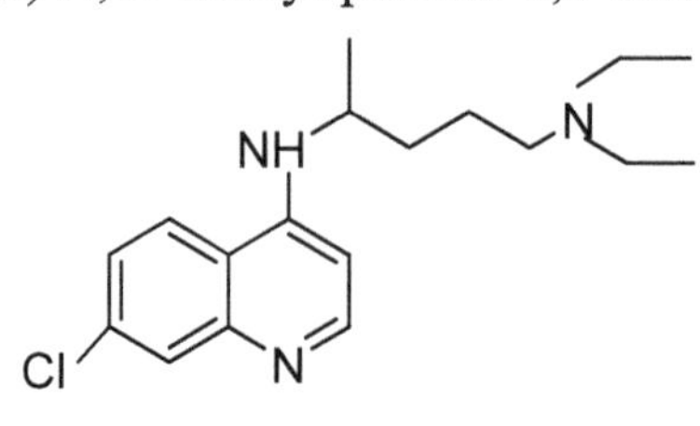

a) Molecular formula: $C_{18}H_{26}ClN_3$

b) Mol. wt: 319.88

c) The indigenous people of Peru used the extract of the bark of the *Cinchona* tree (Cinchona officinalis) to fight chills and fever. It was later introduced in Europe where they used it against malaria also. In 1820, quinine an antimalarial drug was isolated from the extract. In 1934, Hans Andersag and co-researchers at the Bayer laboratories, discovered chloroquine, a structural analogue with similar type of action. This was initially named as Resochin. It was introduced into clinical use in 1947 for the prophylactic treatment of malaria. It is on the WHO's List of Essential Medicines.

d) Uses: It is primarily and extensively used to prevent and treat malaria from *Plasmodium vivax*, *P. ovale*, and *P. malaria*. Chloroquine is not useful for malaria caused by *Plasmodium falciparum*. Rheumatoid arthritis, amebiasis, and lupus erythematosus, are also treated with this. It has antiviral effects against some viruses.

e) Side effects: Nausea, vomiting, blurred vision, abdominal cramps, headache, diarrhea, pale lips/nails/skin, muscle weakness, swelling legs/ankles, shortness of breath, easy bruising/bleeding, hearing and mental problems.

f) Mechanism of action: It inhibits the action of heme polymerase in malarial trophozoites, preventing the conversion of heme to hemozoin. Accumulation of toxic metabolic wastes such as heme kills the parasite. Chloroquine diffuses through cell membranes and into endosomes, lysosomes, and Golgi vesicles; where it increases pH. The raised pH in endosomes prevents viruses from utilizing their activity. Inhibition of DNA replication, DNA and RNA biosynthesis, and protein synthesis are the main features of Chloroquine. It produces rapid degradation of ribosomes.

g) Metabolism: It is a weak base and a half-life of around 20-60 days. It has good bioavailability. Metabolized in liver. N-desethylchloroquine, N-bidesethylchloroquine and 7-chloro-4-amino quinoline are the metabolites. It is eliminated through urine.

h) Synthesis[44]: The first synthesis of chloroquine was disclosed in a patent filed by IG Farben in 1937. Chloroquine, 7-chloro-4-(4-diethylamino-1-methylbutylamino)-quinoline, is prepared by reacting 4,7-dichloroquinoline with 4-diethylamino-1-methylbutylamine at 180 °C.

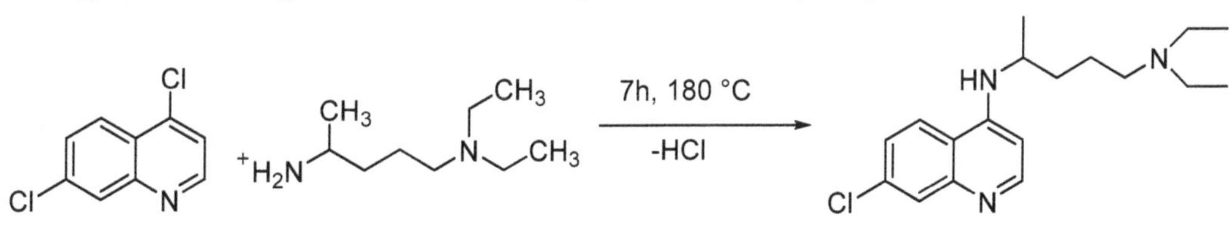

Part A

Synthesis of 4,7-dichloroquinoline.

Method 1: 3-Chloroaniline is reacted with ethoxymethylenmalonic ester to make (3-choroanilino)-methylenemalonic ester, it undergoes high-temperature heterocyclization to form the ethyl ester of 7-chloro-4-hydroxyquinolin-3-carboxylic acid. On hydrolysis with sodium hydroxide, it produces 7-chloro-4-hydroxyquinolin-3-decarboxylic acid. On heating at 250–270 °C it is decarboxylated, giving 7-chloro-4-hydroxyquinoline. Treatment with $POCl_3$ it forms 4,7-dichloroquinoline.

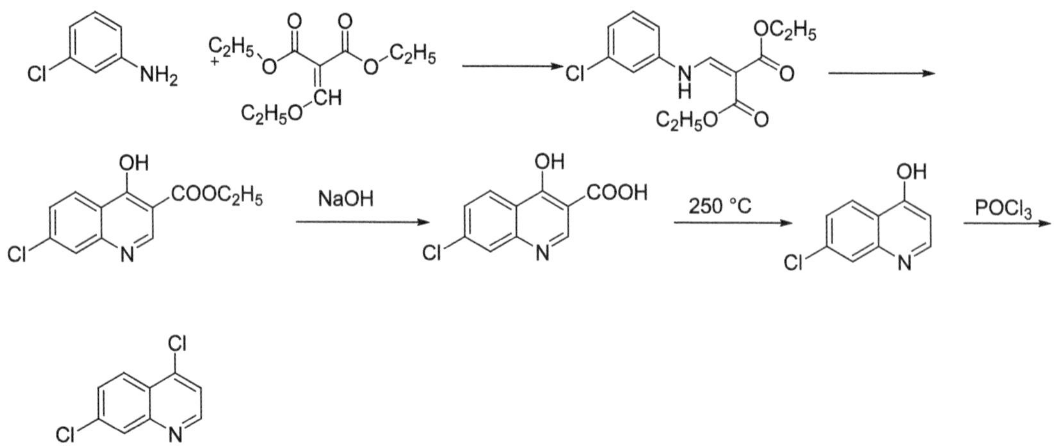

Method 2: In another method 3-chloroaniline is reacted with the ethyl ester of formylacetic acid to produce the enamine. On heating this directly cyclizes to 7-chloro-4-hydroxyquinoline. On treatment with phosphorus oxychloride forms 4,7-dichloroquinoline.

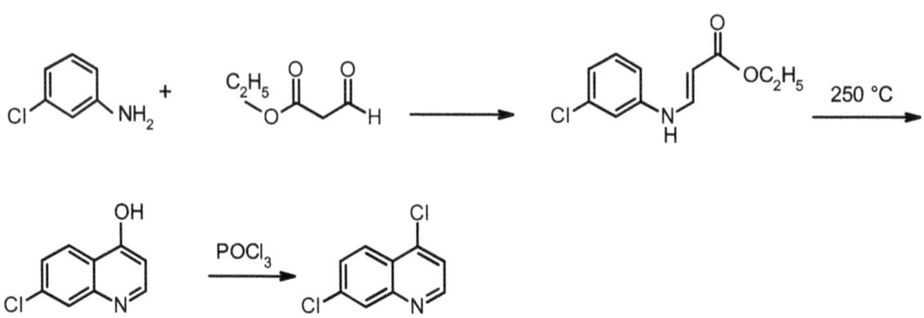

Part B

Synthesis of 4-diethylamino-1-methylbutylamine

Method 1: Acetoacetic ester is alkylated with 2-diethylaminoethyl chloride to give 2-diethylaminoethylacetoacetic acid ester, which undergoes acidic hydrolysis with HCl and further decarboxylation forms 1-diethylamino-4-pentanone. This on reductive amination with H_2/NH_3 /Raney nickel produces 4-diethylamino-1-methylbutylamine.

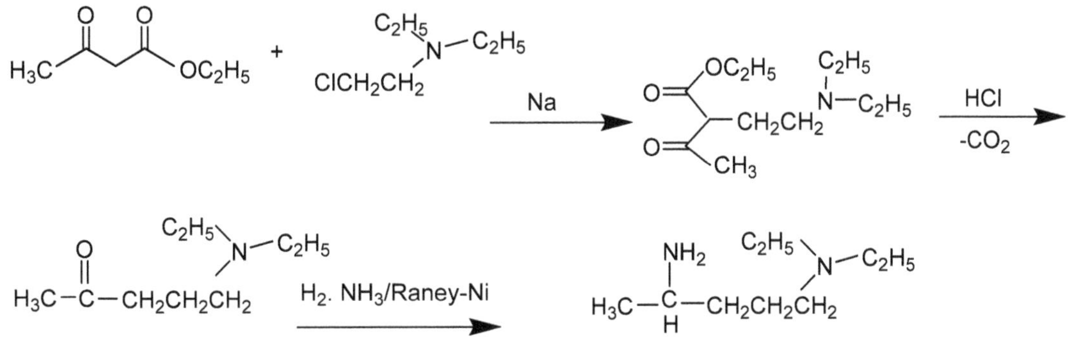

Method 2: 3-Acetylbutyrolactone, formed by the reaction between ethylacetoacetate and ethylenoxide undergoes hydrolysis followed by decarboxylation to give 1-bromo-4-pentanone. This on reaction with diethylamine forms 1-diethylamino-4-pentanone, which on reductive amination with H_2/NH_3/ Raney nickel produces 4-diethyl-1-methylbutylamine.

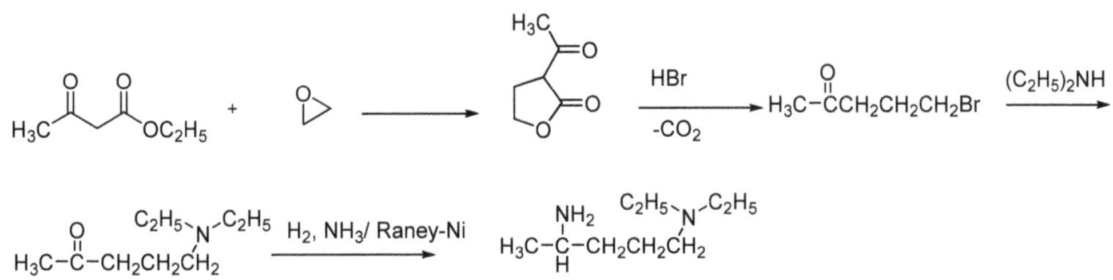

6. Chlorpromazine

2-Chloro-10-(3-dimethylaminopropyl) phenothiazine

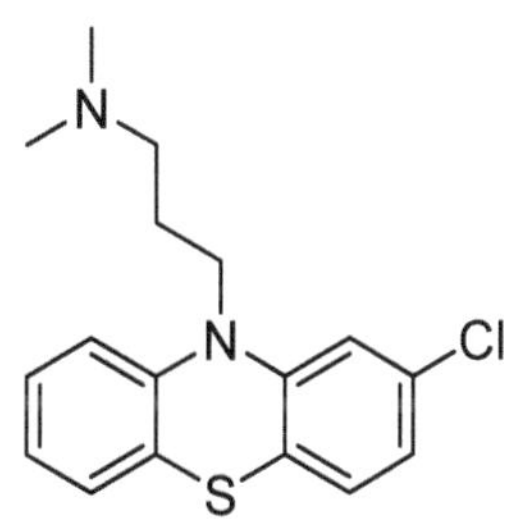

a) Molecular formula: $C_{17}H_{19}ClN_2S$

b) Mol. wt: 318.86

c) In 1947, the French pharmaceutical company Laboratoires Rhône-Poulenc synthesized promethazine, a phenothiazine derivative, which has more pronounced sedative and antihistaminic effects than earlier drugs. While searching for compounds with better properties, in 1950, Paul Charpentier produced a series of compounds that included, chlorpromazine. In 1955, it was approved in the United States for the treatment of emesis (vomiting). The popularity of the drug came down from the late 1960s as a number of other similar antipsychotics were developed, leading to the discovery of a class of antidepressants.

d) Uses: It belongs to antipsychotic phenothiazine class of compounds. It is used to treat psychotic disorders like schizophrenia, bipolar disorders, nausea, vomiting, hiccup, severes migraine. It has wide spectrum of anthelmintic effect. This works as antagonist of several insect mono amine receptors. It is also prescribed to manage severe anxiety, psychotic aggression, amphetamine induced psychosis.

e) Side effects: Sedation, parkinsonism, low hypotension, dizziness and movement disorders.

f) Mechanism of action: It works as an antagonist on different presynaptic and postsynaptic receptors-dopamine D1, D2, D3, D4), serotonin receptors (5HT2, 5HT6, 5HT7), histamine (H1) and muscarinic acetyl choline (M1, M2) receptors, as well as alpha 1 alpha 2 adrenergic receptors.

g) Metabolism: It is mainly metabolized in liver (cytochrome P450) and also kidney as well as GI tract. It is excreted in urine, bile, and faeces. Half-life 23 and 37 hrs. It is highly lipid soluble and 98% bound to plasma proteins and is extensively distributed in the body. The major routes of metabolism include hydroxylation, demethylation, deamination, N-oxidation, sulfoxidation, and conjugation. About 10 to 12 major metabolites have been identified for chlorpromazine. N-dedimethylchlorpromazine, 7-hydroxychlorpromazine, chlorpromazine-N-oxide, 3-hydroxychlorpromazine, chlorpromazine sulfoxide are the main metabolites.

h) Synthesis: It is prepared by the alkylation of 2-chlorophenothiazine with 3-dimethylaminopropylchloride[45].

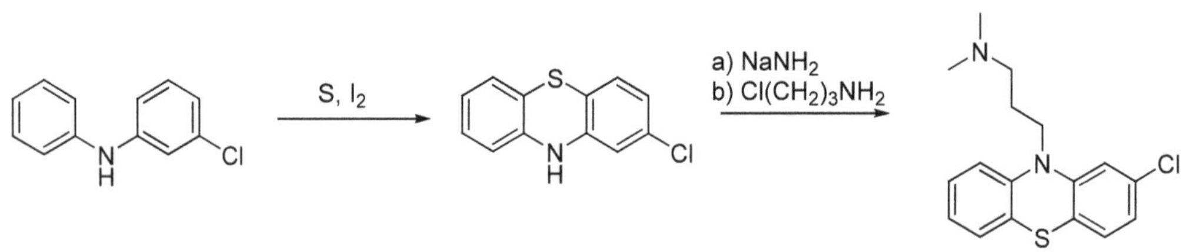

5. Another method[46]

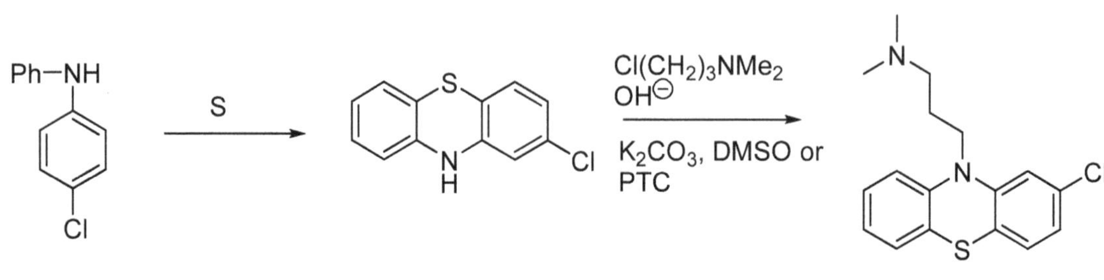

7. Hydroxychloroquine

(RS)-2-[{4-[(7-chloroquinolin-4-yl)amino]pentyl}(ethyl)amino]ethanol

a) Mol.for:$C_{18}H_{26}ClN_3O$

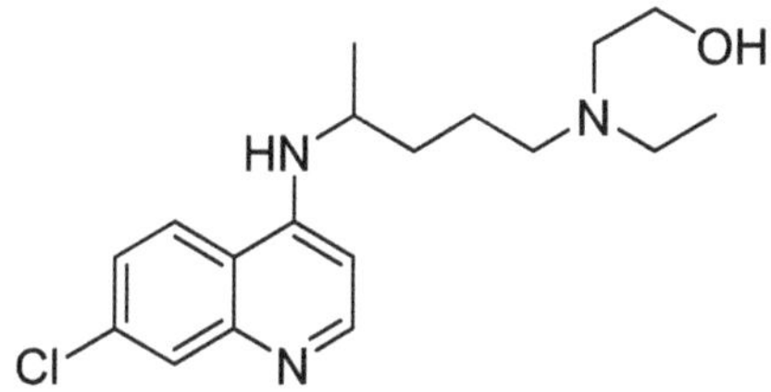

b) Mol. wt**:** 335.88

c) After World War I, alternatives to quinine for treating malaria effectively became significant priority in medical research across the world. In 1934, Chloroquine, a synthetic analogue with the same mechanism of action was discovered, by Hans Andersag and coworkers at the Bayer laboratories. It came into clinical practice in 1947 for the prophylactic use against malaria. Further attempts to discover structural analogues with superior properties led to the discovery of hydroxychloroquine. This was approved for clinical use in 1955. It is on the WHO's List of Essential Medicines. It is the most widely prescribed medicine. It is also studied for an ability to prevent and treat COVID-19

d) Uses: It is used to prevent and treat malaria in the cases sensitive to chloroquine. It is also useful to treat rheumatoid arthritis, and systemic lupus erythematosus.

e) Side effects: Nausea, vomiting, stomach cramps, itching, diarrhea, headache, muscle weakness, allergic reactions, tinnitus, vertigo, retinopathy, and changes in vision.

f) Mechanism of action:It acts by the inhibition of hemozoin biocrystallization, which facilitates the aggregation and accumulation of cytotoxic heme, causing parasitic cell death. In parasites this interferes with the endocytosis and proteolysis of hemoglobin and inhibits the activity of lysosomal enzymes, thereby raising the lysosomal pH.

g) Metabolism: It has good bioavailability. It is metabolized in liver. It is N-dealkylated by CYP3A4 to the active and major metabolite desethylhydroxychloroquine, and the inactive metabolites desethylchloroquine and bidesethylchloroquine. It is excreted renally. It has half-life 537 hours.

h) Synthesis: The first synthesis of hydroxychloroquine was described in a patent filed by Sterling Drug in 1949.

It is prepared by a similar method as that of chloroquine. 1-Chloro-4-pentanone is reacted with 2-ethylaminoethanol to give the corresponding aminoketone, which on reductive amination with H2, NH3/Ra-Ni, produces 4-[ethyl(2-hydroxyethyl) amino]-1-methylbutylamine This on reaction with 4,7-dichlroquinoline affords the hydroxychloroquine.

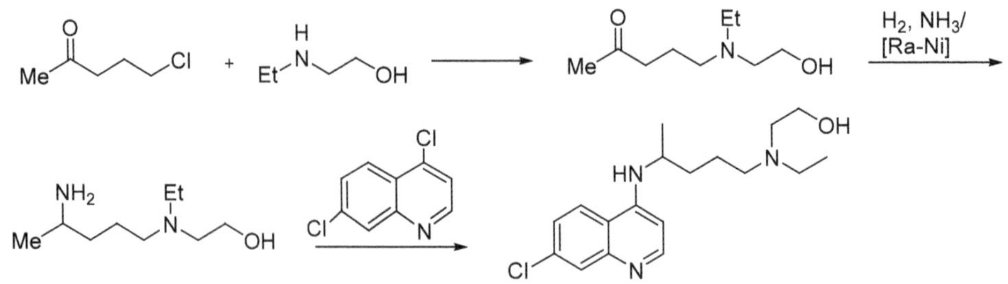

8. Ketoconazole

1-[4-[4-[[2-(2,4-Dichlorophenyl)-2-(imidazol-1-ylmethyl)-1,3-dioxolan-4-yl] methoxy] phenyl] piperazin-1-yl] ethenone.

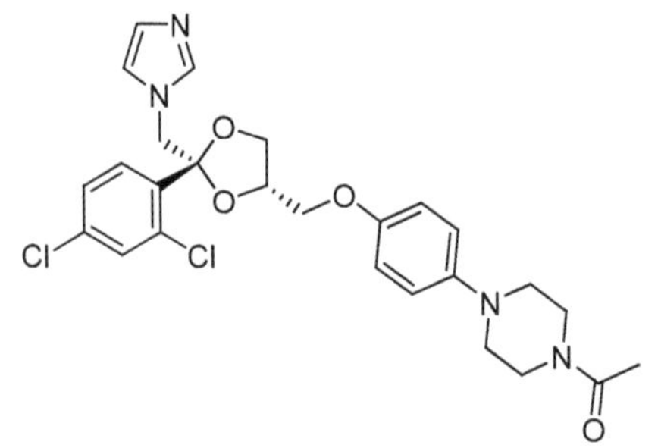

a) Molecular formula: $C_{26}H_{28}Cl_2N_4O_4$

b) Mol. wt: 531.43

c) It was patented in 1977 by Belgian pharmaceutical company Janssen, and was in medical use from 1981. It is most commonly prescribed medication. Janssen pharmaceuticals discovered this in 1976 and patented in 1977. It was the only systemic antifungal medication available for almost a decade. Topical ketoconazole is more widely used and popular as well as safe compared to internal usage.

d) Uses: It was the first broad spectrum antifungal agent with oral activity. It acts as antiandrogen also. It is widely used to treat a number of fungal infections. It is also used in the treatment of Cushing's syndrome. It is mainly used as topical cream and in shampoos for infections of the skin and mucous membranes.

e) Side effects: It causes gastrointestinal, endocrinal toxicity, liver injuries, and hypersensitivity.

f) Mechanism of action: It is an imidazole derivative. It interferes with the fungal synthesis of ergosterol, a constituent of fungal cell membranes and certain enzymes. It works by inhibiting the enzyme cytochrome P450 14-alpha- demethylase (CYP51A1) which participates in sterol biosynthesis. It blocks both testicular and adrenal androgen. Antacids reduce drug absorption well in highly acidic levels. Due to the lipophilic nature, it gets accumulated in fatty tissues.

g) Metabolism: It is extensively metabolized in liver predominantly by oxidation and O-dealkylation. N-Deacetyl ketoconazole is the metabolite.

h) Synthesis: 1. It is synthesized from 2,4-dichlorophenacyl bromide, which on ketalization with glycerol gives cis-2-(2,4-dichlorophenyl)-2-bromoethyl-4-hydroxymethyl-1,3-dioxolane. This on acylation with benzoyl chloride, and then alkylating the resulting compound with imidazole gives the derivative. The benzoyl group is removed by the alkaline hydrolysis. Reacting this with methanesulfonyl chloride forms mesylate. 1-Acetyl-4-(4-hydroxyphenyl) piperazine is reacted with mesylate generating ketoconazole[47].

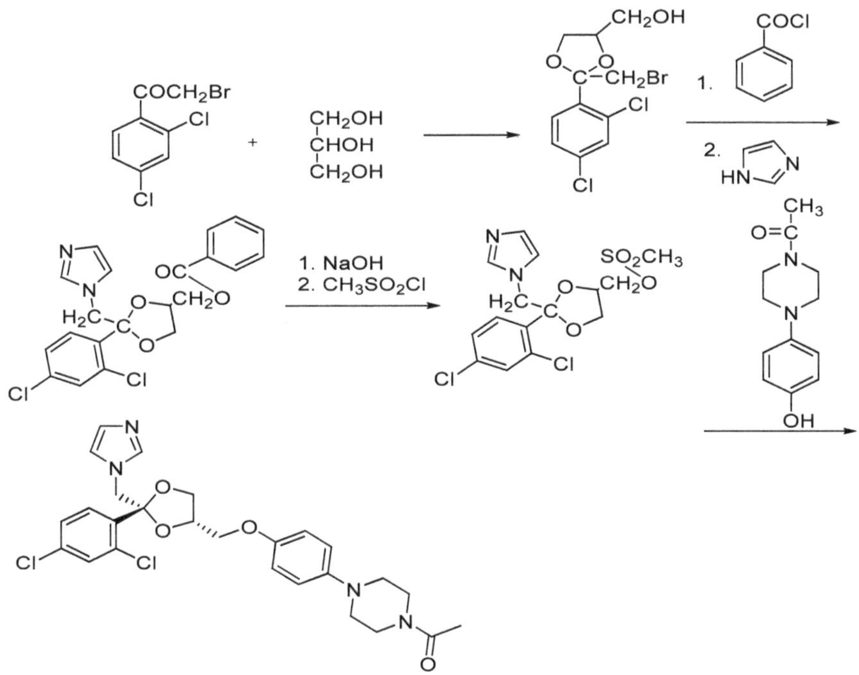

9. Mercaptopurine

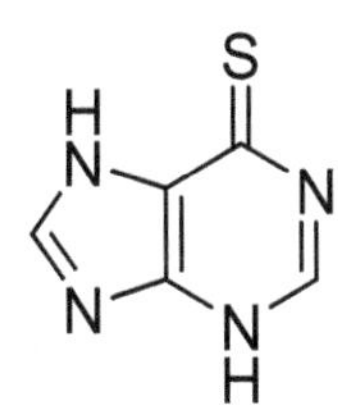

a) Molecular formula: C5H4N4S

b) Mol. Wt.152.18

c) Uses: It is used to treat ulcerative colitis, acute lymphocytic leukemia, and Crohn's disease, it is an antimetabolite and antineoplastic.

d) History: It was discovered by Nobel Prize winners Gertrude B. Elion and George H. Hitchings at Burroughs Welcome, New York, and was approved for medical use in the United States in 1953. It is on the WHO- List of Essential Medicines. It is the most frequently used chemotherapy agent in the management of acute lymphoblastic leukemia and lymphoblastic lymphoma.

e) Side effects: diarrhea, nausea, vomiting, loss of appetite, fatigue, skin rash, darkening of the skin, stomach/abdominal pain, weakness and hair loss, fever, sore throat, bloody urine and stools, swelling and dizziness

f) Mechanism of action: It interferes with normal metabolic processes within cells, typically by combining with enzymes, to disrupt DNA and RNA synthesis (S phase-specific) leading to death of rapidly proliferating cells, especially malignant ones. It also interferes with nucleotide interconversion and glycoprotein synthesis.

g) Metabolism: It has variable absorption, and is widely distributed. It is metabolized in the liver, GI tract and taken up by lymphocytes. It is metabolized in three pathways leading to the formation of thiourea acid, 6-thioguanine nucleotides (6-TGN) and 6-methylmercaptopurine nucleotides (6-MMPN). Half-life is 45 min-2 hours. Excreted in urine.

h) Synthesis:

A) From Hypoxanthine

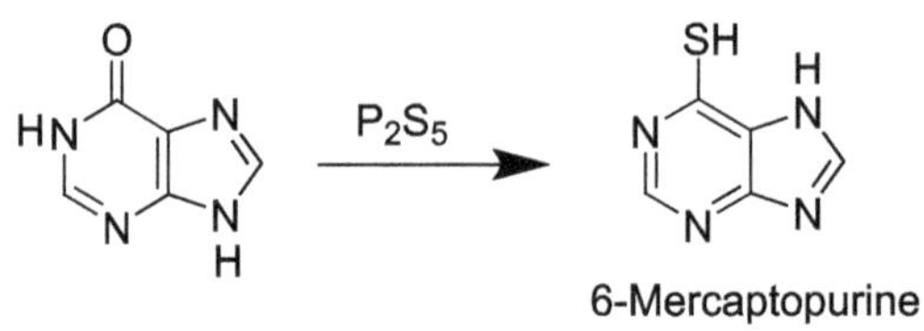

B) From 6-Chloropyrimidine-4,5-diamine

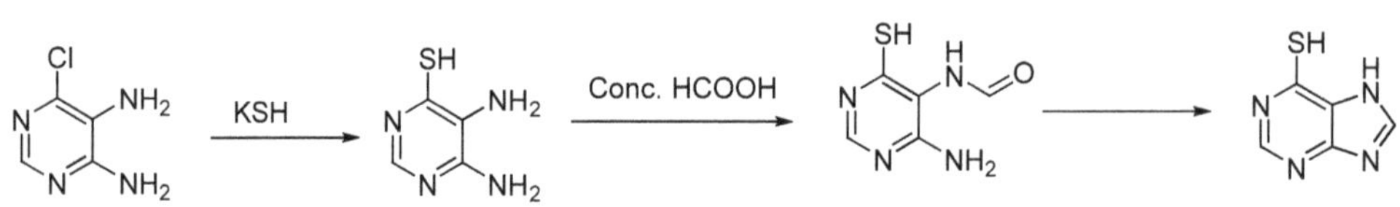

C) From Hypoxanthine

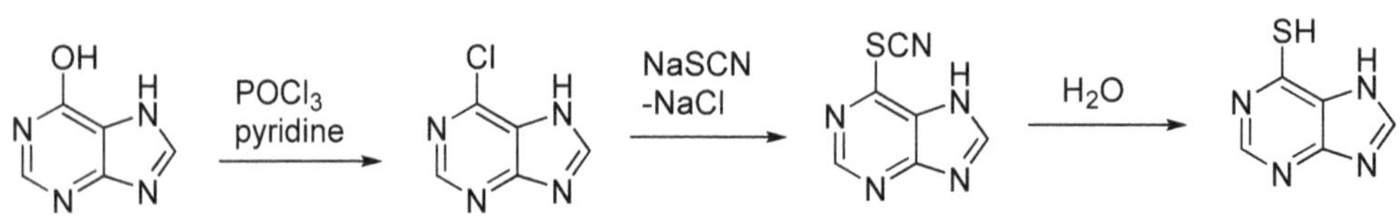

10. Metamizole sodium

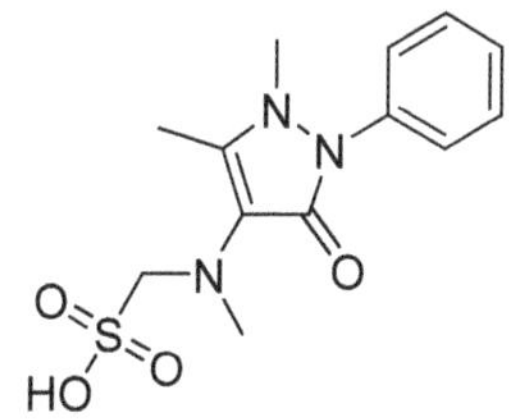

[(2,3-Dihydro-1,5-dimethyl-3-oxo-2-phenyl-1H-pyrazol-4-yl) methyl amino] methanesulfonic acid

a) Molecular formula: C13H17N3O4S

b) Mol. wt: 311.36

c) It is also known as Novalgin, Algocalmin and Dipyrone which belongs to the ampyrone sulfonate family of medicines. It is a pyrazolone derivative that belongs to the group of nonacid nonopioids and is considered a potent analgesic and antipyretic. Knorr, during 1880s while working on quinine derivatives from phenyl hydrazine prepared antipyrine. In 1890s scientists at Teerfarbenfabrik Meister, Lucius & Co invented another derivative- pyramidon which was three times more active than antipyrine.

In 1893, Friedrich Stolz, at Hoechst, reported another derivative of antipyrine- aminopyrine followed by the invention of melubrine (sodium antipyrine aminomethanesulfonate), which was introduced in 1913. Metamizole, a methyl derivative of melubrine, a more soluble prodrug of pyramidon was introduced in 1920s, and was marketed in Germany as Novalgin.

For many years, it was available over-the-counter in most countries, but was withdrawn due to severe adverse effects like agranulocytosis. It is a sulfonic acid and is available as calcium, sodium and magnesium salts. Its sodium salt monohydrate form is a white crystalline powder that is highly soluble in water, but unstable in the presence of light.

d) Uses: Used for relief from pains, fever, and spasms as well as anti-inflammatory agent.

e) Side effects: Blood-related toxicity (blood dyscrasias), bronchospasm, toxic epidermal necrolysis, agranulocytosis, aplastic anaemia, and upper gastrointestinal bleeding.

f) Mechanism of action: It is reported that Its active metabolites, 4-methyl-amino-antipyrine (MAA) and 4-amino-antipyrine (AA), inhibit prostaglandin E2 (PGE_2)-induced hyperalgesia. It has been suggested that the anti-hyperalgesic effect of MAA is mediated by guanosine 3',5'-cyclic monophosphate (cGMP) activation and ATP-sensitive potassium channel opening, while the effects of AA are associated with the activation of cannabinoid receptor type 1 (CB1). It is suggested that metamizole inhibits COX-3 with a higher affinity compared to COX-1 or COX-2.

g) Metabolism: It is quickly absorbed and metabolized by hydrolysis to 4-methyl-amino-antipyrine (MAA) in gastric juice. Its bioavailability is 85-89%. 4-Methyl-amino-antipyrine (MAA). is then metabolized to 4-formyl-amino-antipyrine (FAA) via c-oxidation and 4-amino-antipyrine (AA) via N-demethylation. The N-demethylation of MAA to AA is mainly mediated by CYP3A4, although CYP2B6, CYP2C8 and CYP2C9 may also be involved. AA is acetylated by N-acetyl-transferase to produce 4-acetyl-amino-antipyrine (AAA). Metamizole and its metabolites get eliminated mainly from urine. The half-life of metamizole is 16 minutes. The half-life of 4-methyl-amino-antipyrine (MAA), its active metabolite, ranges from 2.6 to 3.5 hours.

h) Synthesis: 1. It is synthesized from acetoacetic ester and phenylhydrazine. 1-Phenyl-3-methylpyrazolone-5 on methylation with methyl iodide gives 1-phenyl-2,3-dimethylpyrazolone-5 called antipyrine. This on nitrozationwih sodium nitrite under acidic medium, produces 1-phenyl-2,3-dimethyl-4-nitrozopyrazolone-5, which on reduction forms 1-phenyl-2,3-dimethyl-4-aminopyrazolone-5. It is reacted with benzaldehyde, to give 1-phenyl-2,3-dimethyl-4-benzylidenaminopyrazolone-5, which is methylated by dimethylsulfate, giving a quaternary salt. Hydrolysis of the salt gives 1-phenyl-2,3-dimethyl-4-methylaminopyrazolone-5. Treating this with a water solution of a mixture of sodium bisulfite and formaldehyde gives 1-phenyl-2,3-dimethyl-4-methylaminopyrazolone-5-*N*-sodium methanesulfonate- sodium metamizole[48].

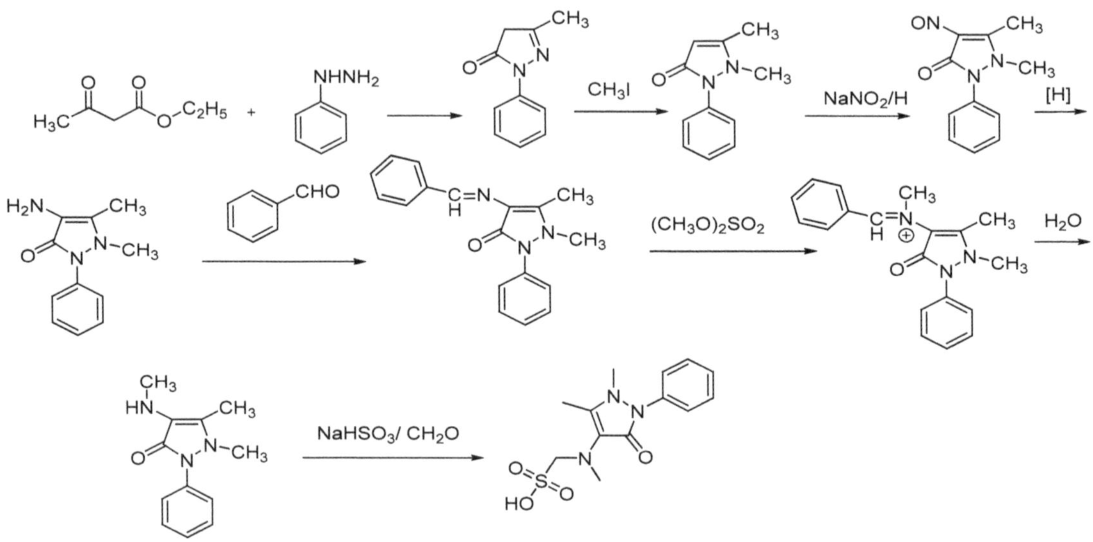

11. Metronidazole

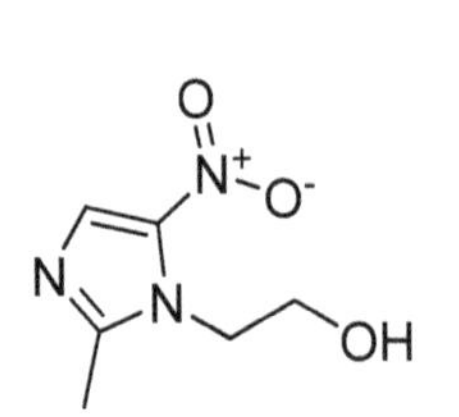

2-(2-Methyl-5-nitro-1H-imidazol-1-yl) ethanol

a) Molecular formula: $C_6H_9N_3O_3$

b) Mol. wt: 171.156

c) The drug was initially developed by Rhône-Poulenc in the 1950s and licensed to G.D. Searle. Metronidazole was started to be used in 1960. It is on the WHO's List of Essential Medicines. It is the most commonly prescribed medication.

d) Uses: It is an antibiotic and antiprotozoal agent. It is used either alone or in combination with other antibiotics to treat endocarditis, and bacterial vaginosis, intra-abdominal infections, fungal wounds, lung abscess, pelvic inflammatory disease. It is effective for trichomoniasis, and amebiasis, dracunculiasis, giardiasis.

e) Side effects: Headache, nausea, a metallic taste, loss of appetite and allergies.

f) Mechanism of action: It works by inhibiting nucleic acid synthesis by forming nitroso radicals, which disrupt the DNA of microbial cells.

g) Metabolism: It is bioavailable via the gut and peak plasma concentrations occur after one to two hours. It is metabolized mainly by oxidation to the main metabolite hydroxymetronidazole and a carboxylic acid derivative, and by glucuronidation. These exhibit antibiotic and antiprotozoal activity *in vitro*. These are excreted via the kidneys and to a lesser extent via the faeces. The half-life is 8 hours.

h) Synthesis: 1. It is prepared by nitrating 2-methylimidazole to make 2-methyl-5-nitroimidazole, which is reacted with ethylenoxide, or 2-chloroethanol to get metronidazole.

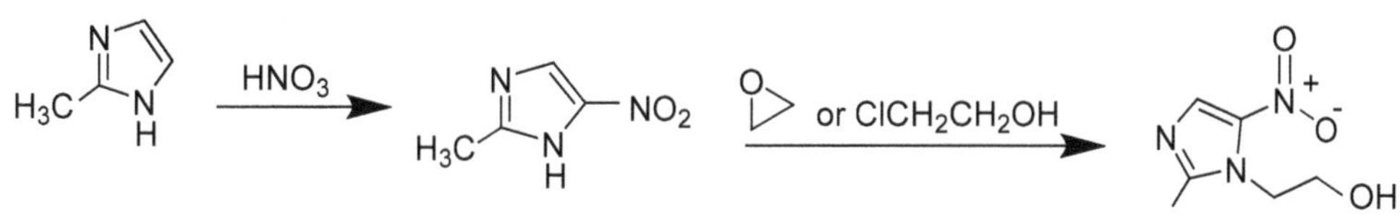

Or

2-Methylimidazole can be prepared via the Debus-Radziszewski imidazole synthesis, or from ethylenediamine and acetic acid, followed by treatment with lime, then Raney nickel. 2-Methylimidazole is nitrated to give 2-methyl-4(5)-nitroimidazole, which is in turn alkylated with ethylene oxide or 2-chloroethanol to give metronidazole[49].

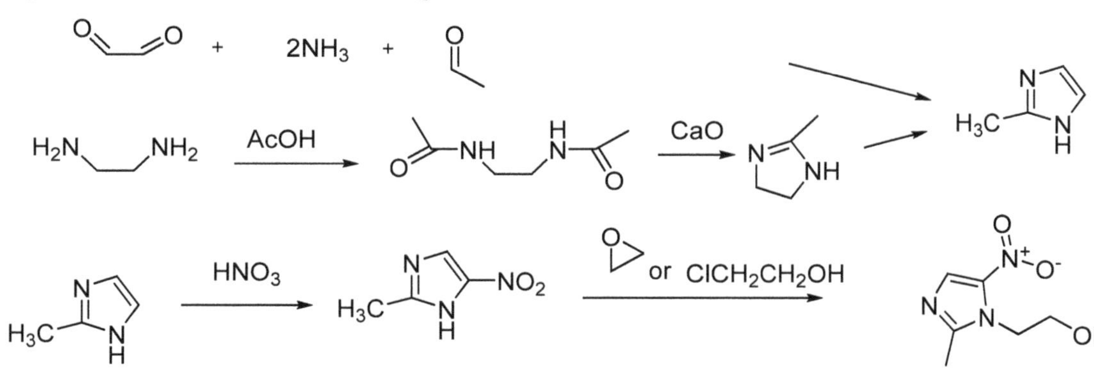

12. Miconazole

(*RS*)-1-(2-(2,4-Dichlorobenzyloxy)-2-(2,4-dichlorophenyl) ethyl)-1*H*-imidazole

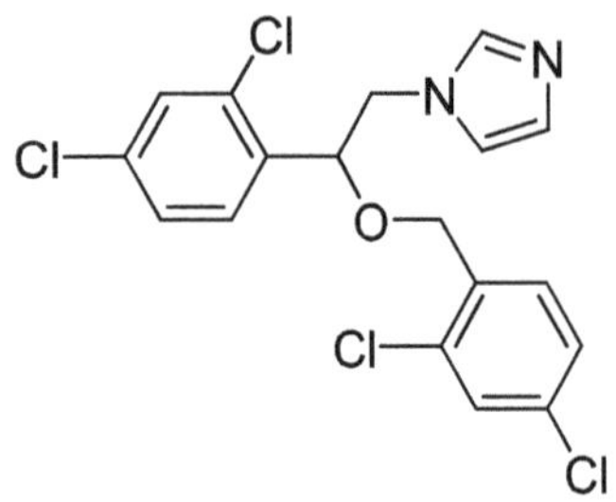

a) Molecular formula: $C_{18}H_{14}Cl_4N_2O$

b) Mol. Wt. 416.12

c) Miconazole was patented in 1968 and approved for medical use in 1971. It is on the WHOs list of essential medicines.

d) Uses: It is a broad-spectrum antifungal agent mainly used as a topical cream against ring worm and yeast infections.

e) Side effects: It is well tolerated medicine. Itching and irritation at the place of application is reported.

f) Mechanism of action: It works by inhibiting the fungal enzyme 14α-sterol demethylase, and reduces the production of ergosterol.

g) Metabolism: It is metabolised in liver. No active metabolites are observed. Excretion is through urine and faeces. Half-life 24hrs

h) Synthesis: 1. Miconazole, 1-[2,4-dichloro-*β*-[(2,4-dichlorobenzyl) oxy] phenethyl]-imidazol, is synthesized from 2,4-dichlorophenacylbromide, which is reacted with imidazole to make 1-(2,4-dichlorobenzoylmethyl)-imidazole[2,4-dichloro-ω-(1-imidazolyl)-acetophenone]. Reduction of the carbonyl group with sodium borohydride gives 1-(2,4-dichlorophenyl)-3-(1-imidazolyl)-ethanol, and the hydroxyl group is alkylated by 2,4-dichlorobenzylbromide employing sodium hydride to make miconazole[50].

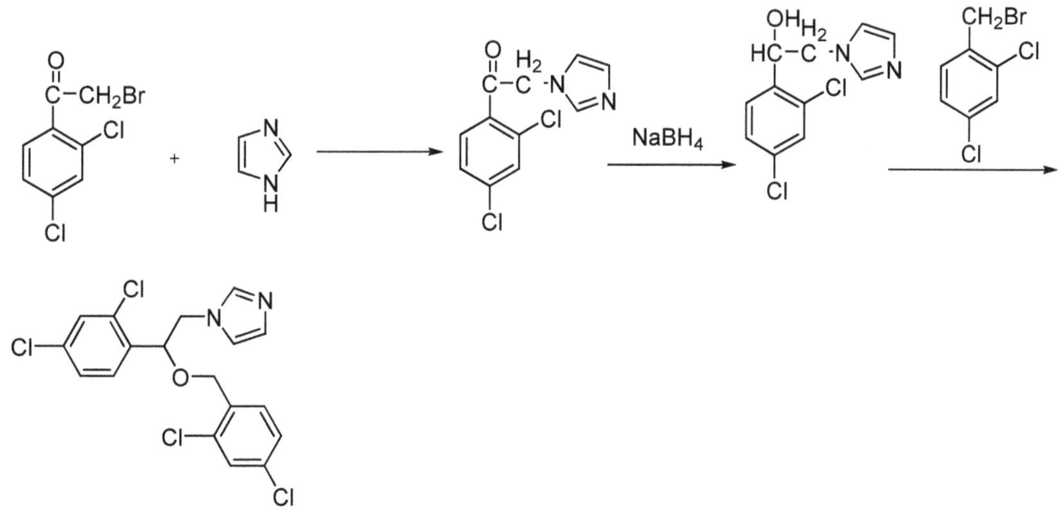

Or

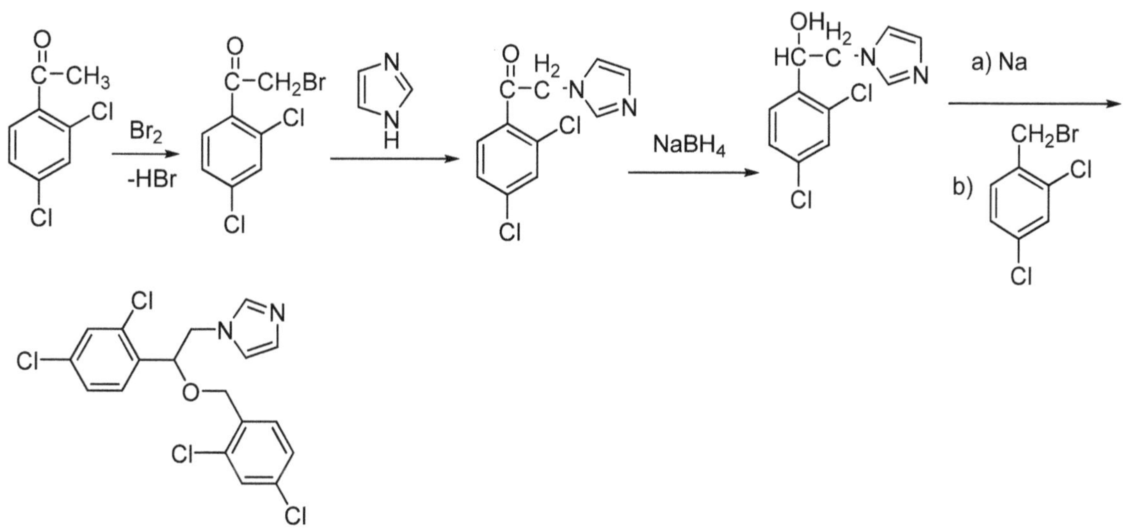

13. Prochlorperazine

2-Chloro-10-[3-(4-methyl-1-piperazinyl) propyl]-10*H*-phenothiazine

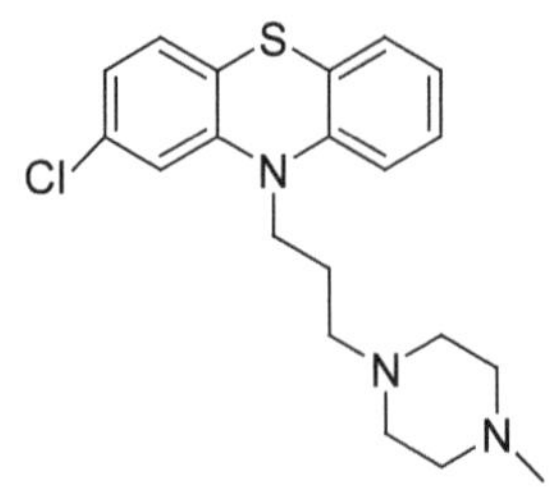

a) Molecular formula: $C_{20}H_{24}ClN_3S$

b) Mol. wt: 373.94 g·mol^{-1}

c) Prochlorperazine, an anti-emetic drug was approved for medical use in 1956, and is one of the most commonly prescribed medication. It belongs to phenothiazine class.

d) Uses: Mainly used for nausea, migraines, psychosis, schizophrenia, and anxiety.

e) Side effects: Sedation, blurry vision, restlessness, and rarely cause high fever, stiff muscles, muscle spasm, irregular pulse, blood pressure, tachycardia, sweating, abnormal heart rhythms.

f) Mechanism of action: Like chlorpromazine this also antagonizes dopaminergic D_2 receptors effecting the central nervous system. This D_2 blockade results in antipsychotic, antiemetic and other effects. It can also block cholinergic and noradrenergic receptors.

g) Metabolism: It is largely metabolized to sulfoxide, 7-hydroxylate and N-desmethylate by cytochrome P450s. N-desmethyl prochlorperazine, prochlorperazine sulfoxide, prochlorperazine-7-hydroxide, prochlorperazine sulfoxide 4-N-oxide are metabolites. It undergoes hepatic metabolism involving hydroxylation, demethylation, oxidation, sulfoxide formation and glucuronic acid conjugation. It is excreted via bile and faeces. Half-life 8-9 hrs.

f) Synthesis: 2-Chlorophenothiazine is alkylated with 1-(3-Chloropropyl)-4-methylpiperazine in the presence of sodamide to give Prochlorperazine. The reaction between 2-Chloro-10-(3-chloropropyl) phenothiazine and 1-methylpiperazine also produces prochlorperazine.

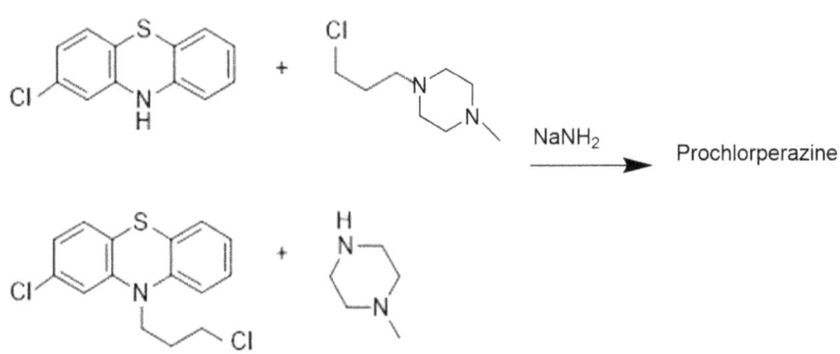

14. Promazine

10-(3-dimethylaminopropyl) phenothiazine

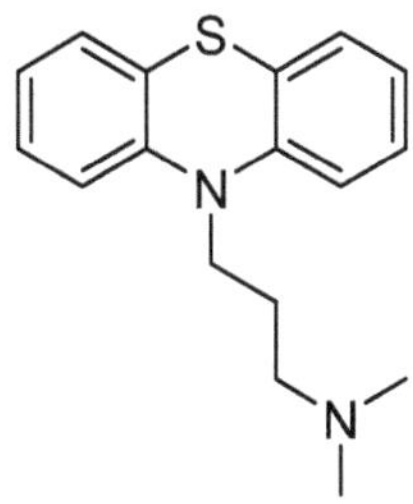

a) **Molecular formula:** C17H20N2S-P

b) **Mol. wt:** 284.42-P

c) Promazine was approved for medical use in the 1950s in USA, and no longer commercially available there.

d) Uses: It is used as tranquilizer in veterinary medicine. It works as antipsychotic. It is a typical antipsychotic phenothiazine class of drug. It has antiemetic and antispasmodic effect also. It is useful in schizophrenia.

e) Side effects: Sedation, agitation, low B.P., fits, weight gain, irregular heart-beat, arrhythmias.

f) Mechanism of action: It works due to antagonism at dopamine and serotonin type 2- receptors (5-HT2) as well as muscarinic receptors H1 and alpha (1)- receptors. It exhibits strong anticholinergic activity by blocking alpha-adrenergic receptors.

g) Metabolism: It metabolizes in liver primarily through N-Desmethyl promazine and promazine-5-sulfoxide. Another important metabolite is 3-hydroxy promazine.

f) Synthesis: 1. It is prepared by the alkylation of phenothiazine with 3-dimethylaminopropylchloride in the presence of sodium amide[51].

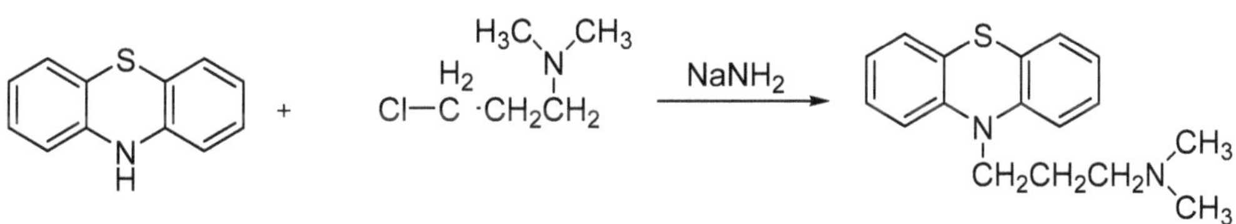

15. Quinacrine

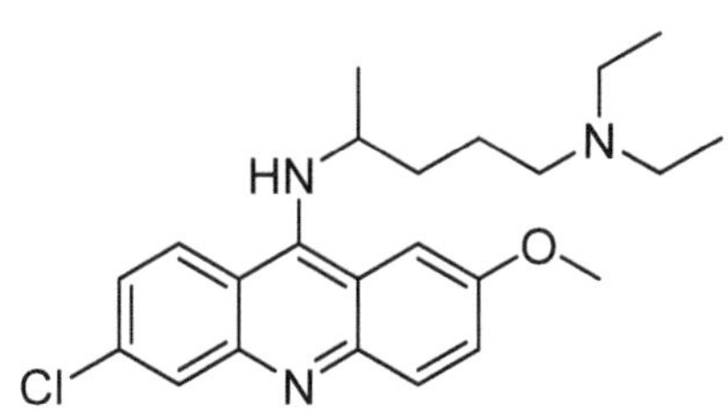

a) Molecular formula: C23H30ClN3O

b) Mol. wt. 399.957

c) Quinacrine, also known as atebrin, atabrine, mepacrine and acrichin, belongs to 9-alkylaminoacridine class. It was developed as a potential antimalarial drug following the success of antimalarials possessing alkyl side chains, like pamaquine. Quinacrine was introduced clinically in 1932. It was the primary drug for prevention and therapy of malaria during World War II. It has been used extensively to treat malaria and multiple ailments over the past several decades. Presently, it is rarely used for treating malaria, but is used to treat amoebiasis.

d) Uses: It is an acridine based chloroquine and mefloquine related compound. Even though initially it is developed as an anti malarial it also acts as antiprotozoal, anthelmintic (for tapeworms), and anti-rheumatic. The compound has many uses. It is also useful in the treatment of lupus erythematosus. It is indicated as a drug against metronidazole resistant giardiasis.

e) Side effects: Headache, yellow skin discoloration, GI upset, and diarrhoea.

f) Mechanism of action: It acts against protozoans and the mechanism is not clear. But it acts against protozoans cell membrane. It also inhibits histamine N-methyl transferase, and succinate oxidation. It binds to DNA and inhibits transcription and translation to RNA. Metabolism: It is absorbed rapidly from GI tract and is mainly metabolised to mono-des methyl quinacrine by CYP- 3A4 / 5 . It has half life 5 to 14 days.

g) Synthesis: Quinacrine, 6-chloro-9-(4-diethylamino-1-methylbutylamino)-2-methoxyacridine, is synthesized from 6,9-dichloro-2-methoxyacridine and 4-diethylamino-1-methylbutylamine. The 6,9-dichloro-2-methoxyacridine is prepared in two steps, from 2,4-dichlorobenzoic acid and *p*-anisidine in the presence of copper dust and potassium carbonate to give 2-(4-methoxyanilino)-4-chlorobenzoic acid, which is further reacted with phosphorus oxychloride to form 6,9-dichloro-2-methoxyacridine[52].

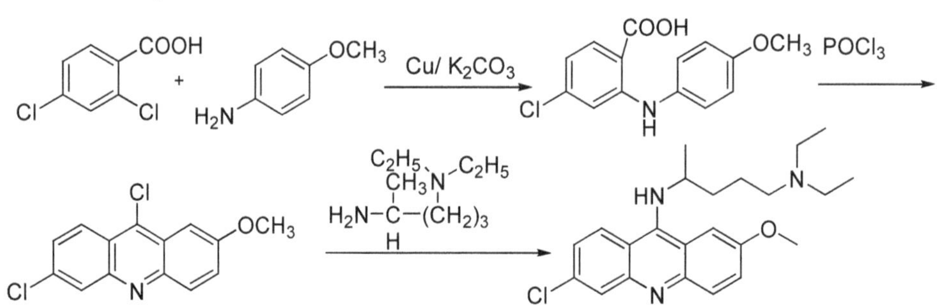

9-Chloroacridine derivative can also be obtained by the reaction of 2,4- dichloro benzoyl chloride, p-anisidine and 4-amino-1-diethyl aminopentane, following Friedel Crafts acylation, amine formation and reductive amination sequence.

16. Quinine

(*R*)-(6-Methoxyquinolin-4-yl) [(1*S*,2*S*,4*S*,5*R*)-5-vinylquinuclidin-2-yl] methanol

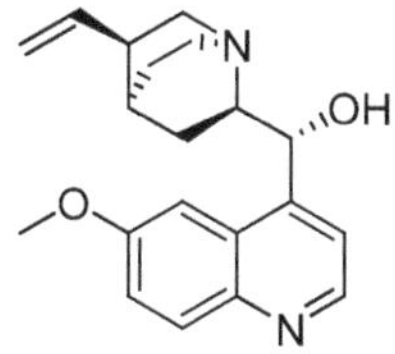

It is isolated from cinchona bark in 1820, and is used chiefly in the treatment of malaria, caused by the plasmodium sp., Earlier, it was also used to treat diphtheria. Quinine, as a bark extract was the only effective remedy for malaria for almost three hundred years between its introduction into western medicine and World War I. Several generations got relief with this. It marked the first successful use of a chemical compound in the treatment of an infectious disease. Quinine was first synthesized in a laboratory in 1944;

a) Molecular formula: $C_{20}H_{24}N_2O_2$

b) Mol. wt: 324.424 $g{\cdot}mol^{-1}$

c) Uses: It is a quinoline based alkaloid, anti-malarial drug, which is no longer used as there are other substances that are equally effective with fewer side effects. It is also used to treat leg cramps, lupus and arthritis.

e) Side effects: nausea, Blurred vision, confusion, diarrhea, tinnitus, fever, fast heartbeat, headache, reddening of skin, swelling, and rarely unusual bleeding.

f) Mechanism of action: It is similar to that of chloroquine. It acts by interfering with the growth and reproduction of the malarial parasites, which inhabit the red blood cells (erythrocytes). It acts as a blood schizonticide (especially against drug resistant falsiparum infections), and gametocide (particularly against P.vivax, P.ovale). It inhibits heme polymerase. It is toxic to malarial parsite and interferes with the ability of the parasite to break down and digest hemoglobin. It is more useful to chloroquine resistant malaria and cerebral malaria. It is effective in preventing transmission of disease.

g) Metabolism: Mainly metabolized by liver to 3- hydroxyl quinine. Excreted via urine. Half-life-18hrs.

h) Synthesis: Initially, in 1944 the first synthesis was achieved by R. B. Woodward and W. E. Doering. Later it was followed by reports of several total syntheses.

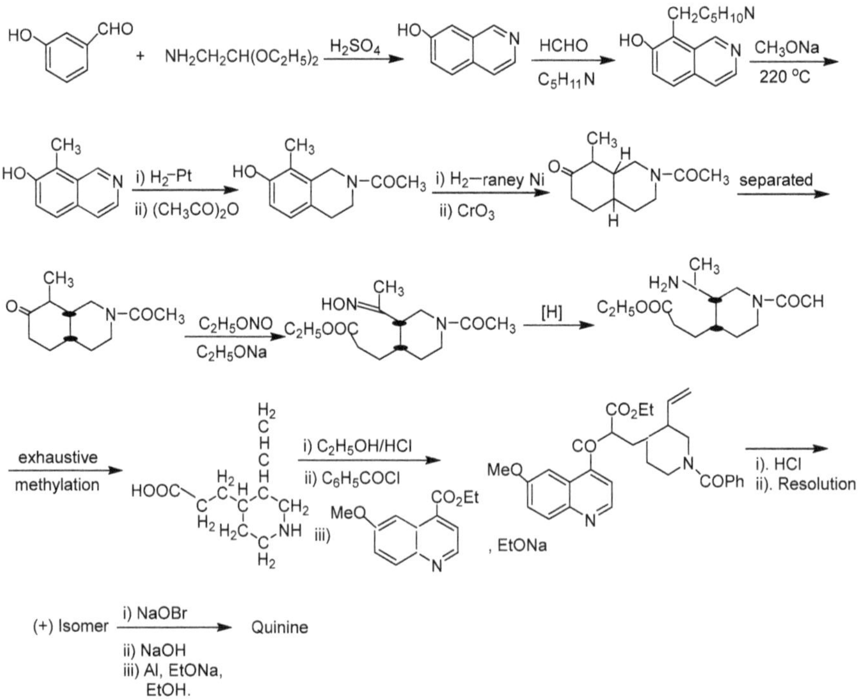

17. Sulfamerazine

4-Amino-*N*-(4-methylpyrimidin-2-yl) benzenesulfonamide

It is a sulfonamide antibacterial.

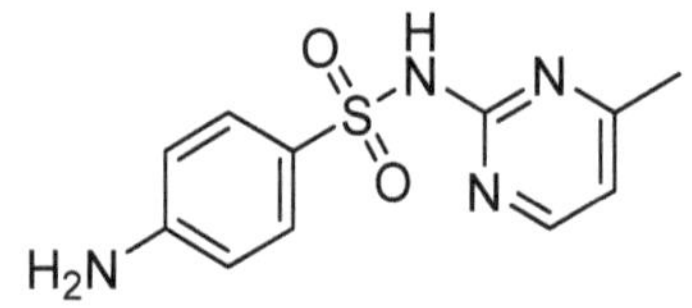

a) Molecular formula: $C_{11}H_{12}N_4O_2S$

b) Mol. wt: 264.30

c) Uses: It is used to treat infections caused by streptococci, gonococci, pneumococci, staphylococci, and also colon bacillus, like bronchitis, prostatitis, pneumonia, enteritis, ulcers and urinary tract infections.

e) Side effects: Nausea, vomiting, diarrhea, anemia, agranulocytosis, thrombocytopenia and hypersensitivity reactions.

f) Mechanism of action: It acts by inhibiting bacterial synthesis of dihydrofolic acid by competing with para-aminobenzoic acid (PABA) for binding to dihydropteroate synthetase leading to decrease in the synthesis of bacterial nucleotides and DNA.

g) Metabolism: It is rapidly absorbed and hydroxylated predominantly at the methyl group of the pyrimidine side chain. N (4)-Acetylsulfamerazine is one of the metabolite.

h) Synthesis: Acetoacetic ester is condensed with guanidine to form 4-methyl-2-aminopyrimidin-6-one. This is converted to 4-methyl-2-amino-6-chloropyrimidine with POCl3. 4-Methyl-2-aminopyrimidine is produced by reducing it with H2/Pd. It is then reacted with 4-acetylaminobenzenesulfonyl chloride to make an acetanilide derivative, which is hydrolysed with base producing sulfamerazine[53].

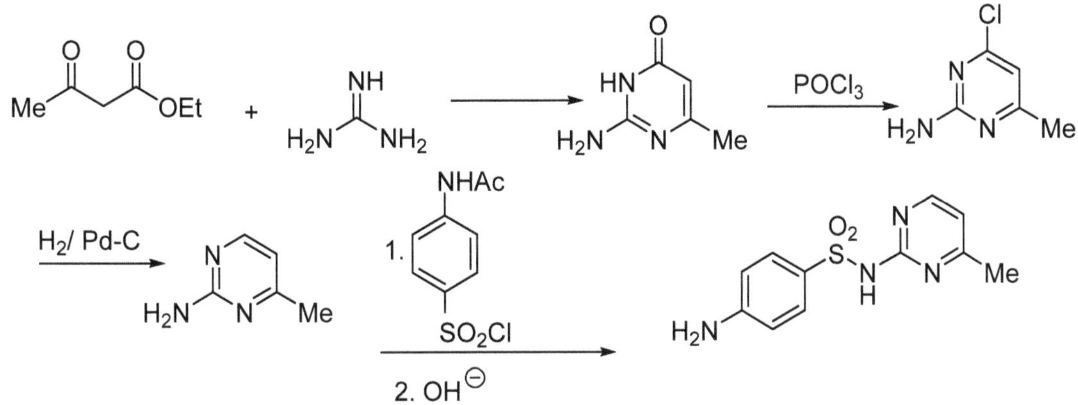

18. Terconazole

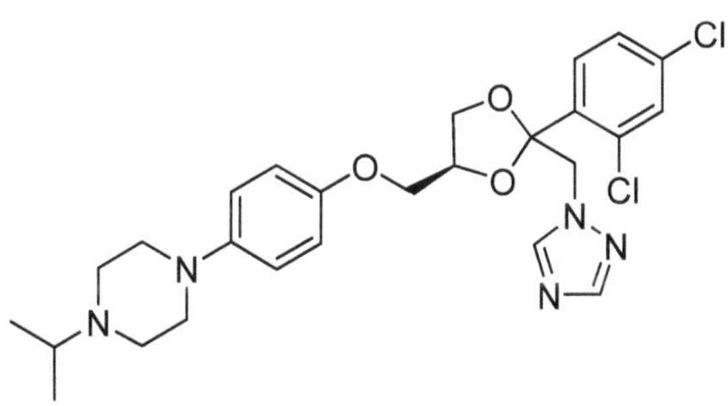

1-[4-[[(2*S*,4*S*)-2-(2,4-Dichlorophenyl)-2-(1,2,4-triazol-1-ylmethyl)-1,3-dioxolan-4-yl] methoxy] phenyl] -4-propan-2-yl-piperazine

a) Molecular formula: C26H31Cl2N5O3

b) Mol. wt: 532.47

c) It is developed by Janssen pharmaceutical in 1983. It was the first triazole based antifungal drug.

d) Uses: Broad spectrum antifungal antimycotic topical agent with triazole ketal structure. It is first line of treatment for candida sp., and effective against dermatomycoses.

e) Side effects: Headache, rashes, itching, but less toxic.

f) Mechanism of action: It binds to the heme iron component of the cytochrome P450 enzyme lanosterol of the fungi (CYP3A4). It works by stopping the biosynthesis of the cell membrane products and transport as well as catabolism. It inhibits morphological changes of the yeast.

g) Metabolism: It is extensive and highly protein bound. Excretion by renal and feacal route. Half-life 6.9 hrs.

h) Synthesis: It is synthesized from 2,4-dichloroacetophenone. It is initially reacted with glycerol in the presence of *p*-toluenesulfonic acid to afford ketal, 2-(2,4-dichlorophenyl)-2-methyl-4-hydroxymethyl-1,3-dioxolane, which on bromination with Br2 and acylation with PhCOCl formed 2-(2,4-dichlorophenyl)-2-bromomethyl-4-benzoyloxymethyl-1,3-dioxolane. This on reaction with 1,2,4-triazole/NaOH gave 2-(2,4-dichlorophenyl)-2-(1H-1,2,4-triazol-1-ylmethyl)-4-hydroxymethyl-1,3-dioxolane. Treating this with CH_3SO_2Cl formed the mesylate. The second fragment, 1-isopropyl-4-(4-hydroxyphenyl)-piperazine is formed from 4-(4-methoxyphenylpiperazine), which on reduction with H2 /Pd/C formed 1-isopropyl-4-(4-methoxyphenyl) piperazine. Treatment with HBr formed 1-isopropyl-4-(4-hydroxyphenyl) piperazine. Finally, mesylate reacted with 1-isopropyl-4-(4-hydroxyphenyl) piperazine provided terconazole[54].

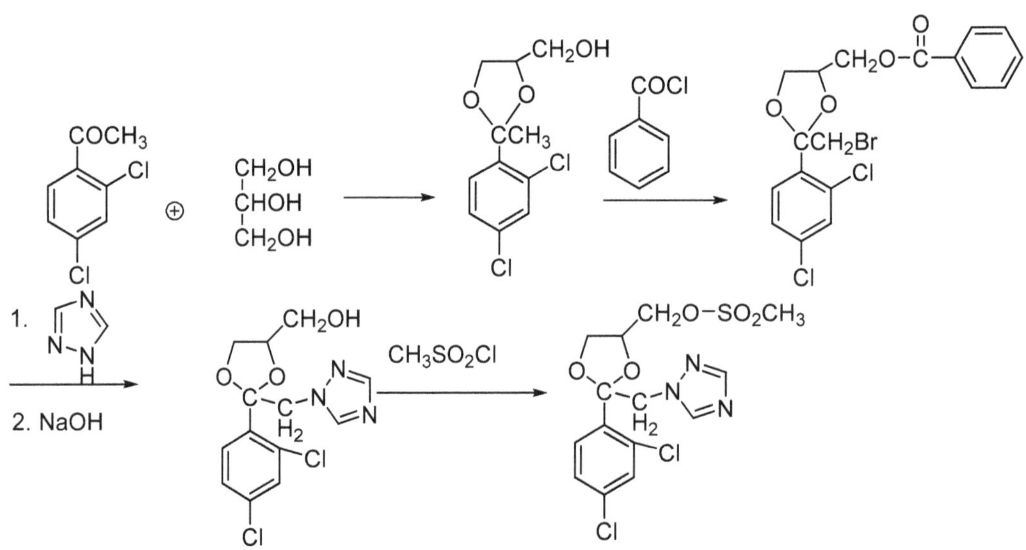

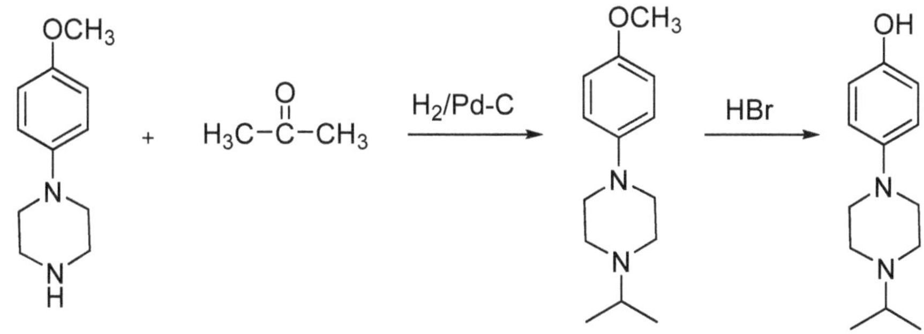

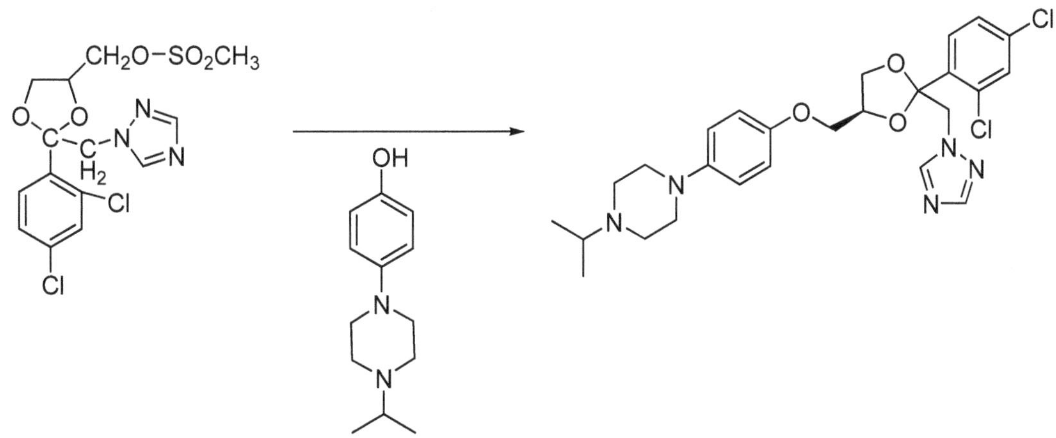

19. Theophylline

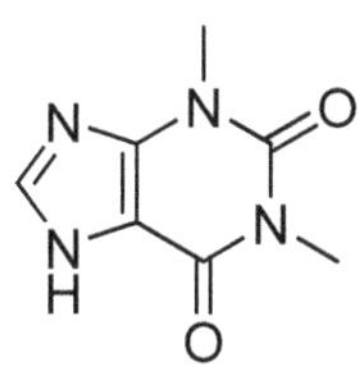

a) Molecular formula: C7 H8 N4 O2

b) Molecular weight: 180.167

c) Theophylline (1,3 Dimethyl Xanthine**)**, was first extracted from tea leaves and chemically identified around 1888 by the German biologist Albrecht Kossel. Seven years later, Emil Fischer and Lorenz Ach described its synthesis from with 1,3-dimethyluric acid. In 1900, Wilhelm Traube proposed an alternative method to synthesize theophylline, known as the Traube purine synthesis. Theophylline's first clinical use as a diuretic came in 1902. It was first reported as an asthma drug 20 years later. It is a competitive nonselective phosphodiesterase inhibitor. Xanthenes belong to a family of compounds containing a purine ring, one of the most important heterocyclic systems found in nature. Three of the most important methylxanthenes are theophylline, theobromine, and caffeine. Methylxanthenes exhibit a similar range of biological activity, and occur in tea, cocoa, and coffee.

d) Uses: It is used in the respiratory diseases like chronic obstructive pulmonary disease- COPD and asthma. It is present in tea, and cocoa. This naturally occurring drug has Xanthine based structure. It has anti-inflammatory CNS stimulating effects. It relaxes bronchial smooth muscles.

e) Side effects: It increases BP, heart rate, renal blood flow, CNS exci, abnormal heart rhythms, insomnia dizziness seizures, Tachyarrhythmias.

f) Mechanism of action: it is a competitive non-selective phosphodisterase inhibitor and also non-selective adenosine receptor antagonist (A1, A2 A3). It also inhibits leucotriene synthesis.

g) Metabolism: It has a good bioavailability and is well distributed. It gets extremely metabolised in liver and undergoes N-demethylation via cytochrome 450/A2. It is excreted by urine. Even though half-life varies 8 hours can be taken as standard for normal adults.

h) Synthesis: 1 *N*, *N*-dimethylurea is reacted with cyanoacetic ether in the presence of acetic anhydride to form cyanoacetylmethylurea. It undergoes cyclization in alkali to 6-amino-1,3-dimethyluracil. On nitrosation with nitric acid, 5-nitroso-6-amino-1,3-dimethyluracil is formed. Reduction of the nitroso group produces 5,6-diamino-1,3-dimethyluracil, which on reaction with formamide gives the desired theophylline[55].

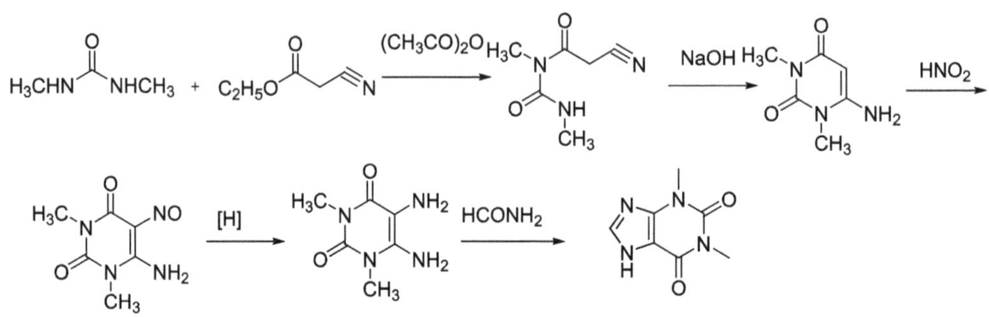

20. Thioguanine

2-Amino-1H-purine-6(7H)-thione

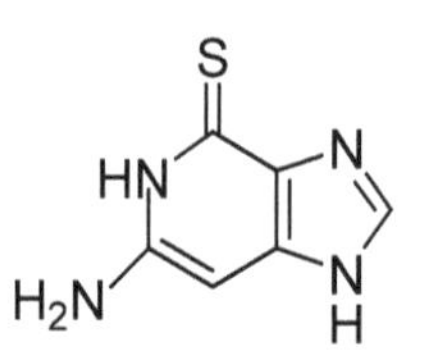

a) Molecular formula: C5H5N5S

b) Mol. wt:167.19

c) It is an antimetabolite and antineoplastic. It has a long history as an effective drug for leukemia. Thioguanine was developed between 1949 and 1951. It is on the WHO's List of Essential Medicines.

d) Uses: It is a purine derivative used to treat acute lymphocytic leukemia, acute myeloid leukemia, chronic myeloid leukemia, Inflammatory bowel disease, ulcerative colitis, and Psoriasis. It is a thio derivative of the naturally occurring purine base guanine.

e) Side Effects: Fever, Chills, Cough, blood in the urine or stools, joint pain, stiffness, swelling, red spots on the skin. It can cause blood dyscrasias/ thrombocytopenia and also hepatic sinusoidal obstruction syndrome (veno-occlusive disease).

f) Mechanism of action: It interferes with purine biosynthesis at different levels. It gets converted to 6-thioguanylic acid (TGMP), which inhibits several purine biosynthetic enzymes. TGMP is converted by phosphorylation to thioguanosine diphosphate (TGDP) and thioguanosine triphosphate (TGTP). 6-TG nucleotides are cytotoxic to cells and also incorporated into DNA and RNA, where they function as fraudulent bases. Eventhough DNA incorporation play important role (S-phase of the cell), primary cause of cytotoxicity is not clear.

g) Metabolism: It has wide variable absorption and half-life (25-240 minutes). Thioguanine undergoes extensive hepatic metabolism to several active and inactive metabolites. It is excreted in the urine.

Thioguanine is converted to thioguanosine monophosphate which is then phosphorylated to thioguanosine diphosphate, which is converted via a thiodeoxyguanosine diphosphate intermediate to thiodeoxyguanosine triphosphate. Thiodeoxyguanosine triphosphate is incorporated into DNA causing cytotoxicity.

h) Synthesis:

1.

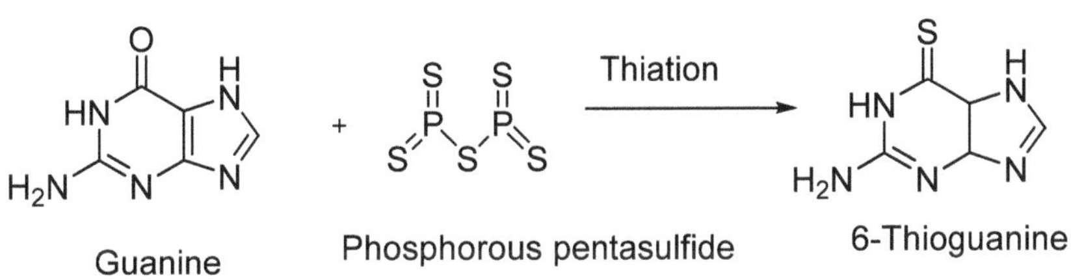

6-Thioguanine can be synthesised through thiation of the guanine with phosphorous pentasulfide, in pyridine.

2. 2-Amino-9H-purine-6-ol is treated with $POCl_3$/Pyridine to form chloro analogue which is treated with NaSCN, followed by hydrolysis to get thioguanine.

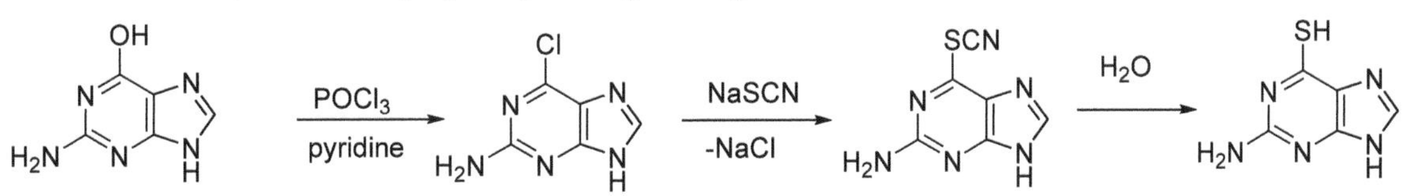

2-Amino-9*H*-purin-6-ol

21. Triamterene

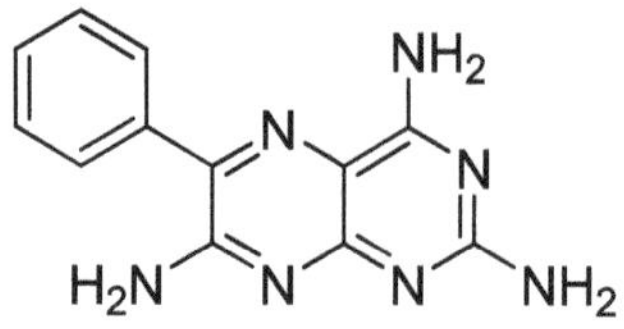

a) Molecular formula: $C_{12}H_{11}N_7$

b) Mol. wt. 253.269

c) Smith Kline and French Laboratories began extensive research to discover potential drugs, as part of a program to discover potassium-sparing diuretics. The first clinical studies were published in 1961. Triamterene was launched as a single agent under the brand Dyrenium in 1964. The combination drug with hydrochlorothiazide, Dyazide, was first approved in the US in 1965., and became most prescribed drug. It is generally given in combination with hydrochlorothiazide for treatment of hypertension (high blood pressure) and edema (water retention)

d) Uses: It is a potassium sparing diuretic prescribed for managing hypertension or swelling. It is used in the treatment of edema. It helps to get rid of excess water in the body.

e) Side effects: Vomiting, nausea, dizziness, diarrhea, fatigue, depletion of sodium, folic acid and calcium, heart palpitations, chills. It may form kidney stones.

f) Mechanism of action: It works by blocking the epithelial sodium channel on the lumen side of the kidney collecting tubule. It is similar to drug Amilioride in action. It decreases potassium excretion. It maintains or increases sodium excretion along with water.

g) Metabolism: It is rapidly absorbed by GI tract with duration of action 12 to 16 hours. It is metabolized via hydroxylation to form 4- hydroxy triamterene which is further transfomed to 4-hydroxy triamterene sulphate by the action of cytosolic sulfotransferases. Metabolites appear greatly in the plasma and urine. It is excreted by the kidney by filtration and tubular secretion. Its half-life is 1.5-2 hours.

h) Synthesis: 1. It is synthesized initially by reacting guanidine with malonodinitrile to give 2,4,6-triaminopyrimidine. This undergoes nitrosation with nitric acid, affording 5-nitroso-2,4,6-triaminopyrimidine. This condenses with benzyl cyanide in the presence of sodium methoxide and cyclizes to triamterene[56].

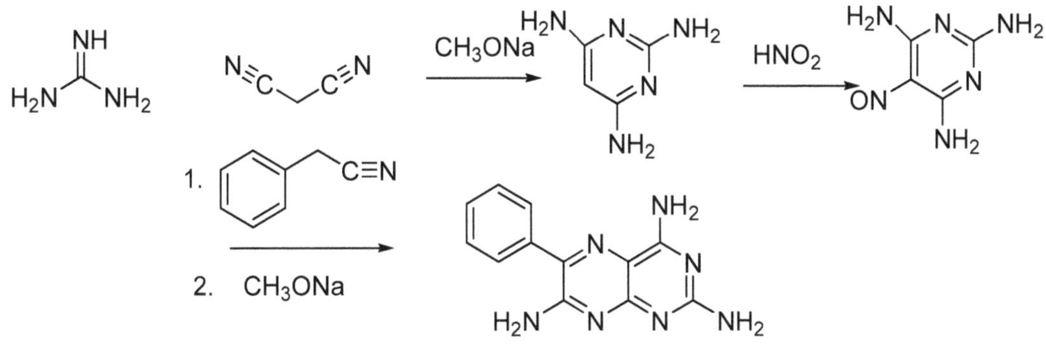

22. Trimethoprim

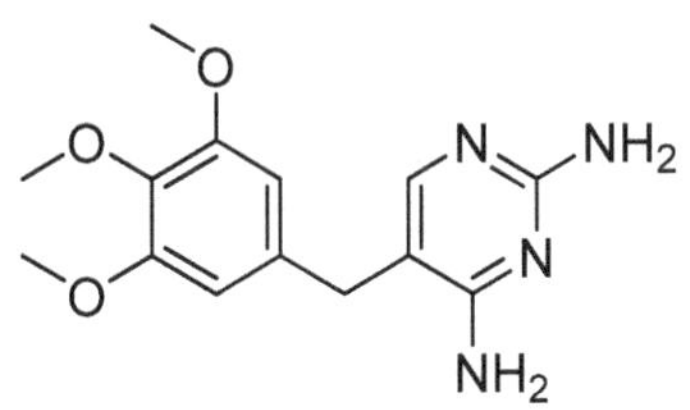

5-(3,4,5-Trimethoxybenzyl) pyrimidine-2,4-diamine

a) Molecular formula: $C_{14}H_{18}N_4O_3$

b) Mol. wt. 290.323

c) Uses: It is a broad spectrum anti-bacterial drug, primarily used in the treatment of urinary tract infections, pneumonia, middle ear infections, travelers' diarrhea and against any susceptible aerobic bacterial infections. Trimethoprim was first used in 1962. It is on the WHO- List of Essential Medicines. The combination of trimethoprim and sulfamethoxazole has significant role in the treatment of various common infections.

d) Side effects: Nausea, vomiting, diarrhea, rashes, itchiness, change in taste, and sun-sensitivity. It can rarely cause thrombocytopenia, hyperkalemia, and megaloblastic anemia.

e) Mechanism of action: Trimethoprim binds to dihydrofolate reductase and inhibits the reduction of dihydrofolic acid (DHF) to tetrahydrofolic acid (THF), a precursor in the thymidine synthesis. This interference inhibits bacterial DNA synthesis.

f) Metabolism: Trimethoprim undergoes oxidative metabolism to a number of metabolites. It undergoes O-demethylation, N-oxide formation, Alpha hydroxyl formylation. It is primarily metabolized in liver and excreted in urine. Half-life is 8- to 10-hour.

g) Synthesis[57]:

1.

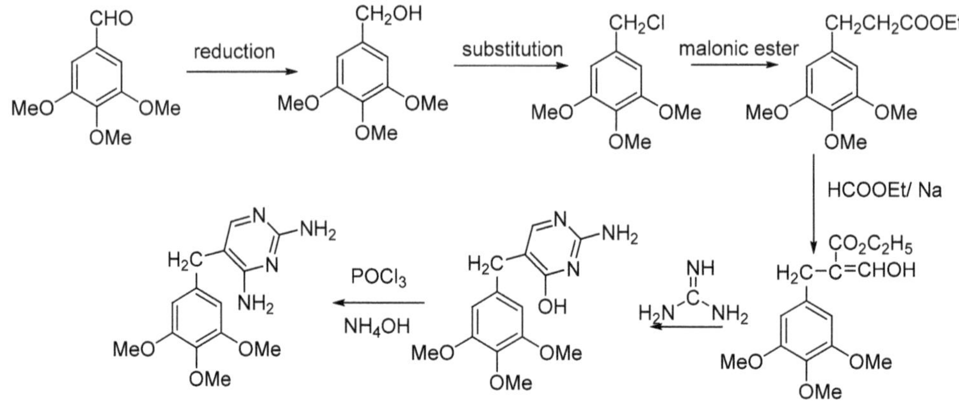

2.

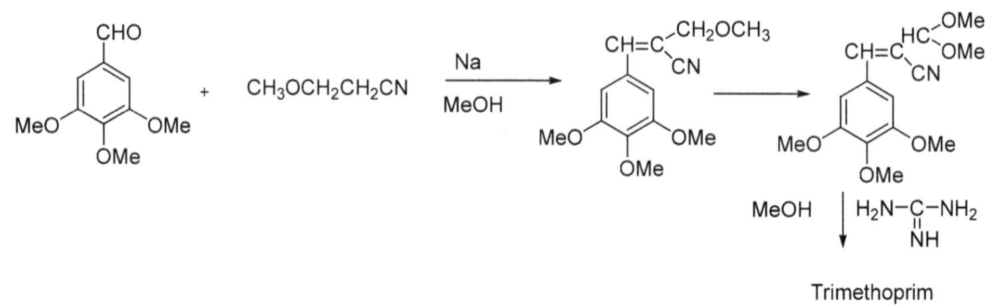

3.

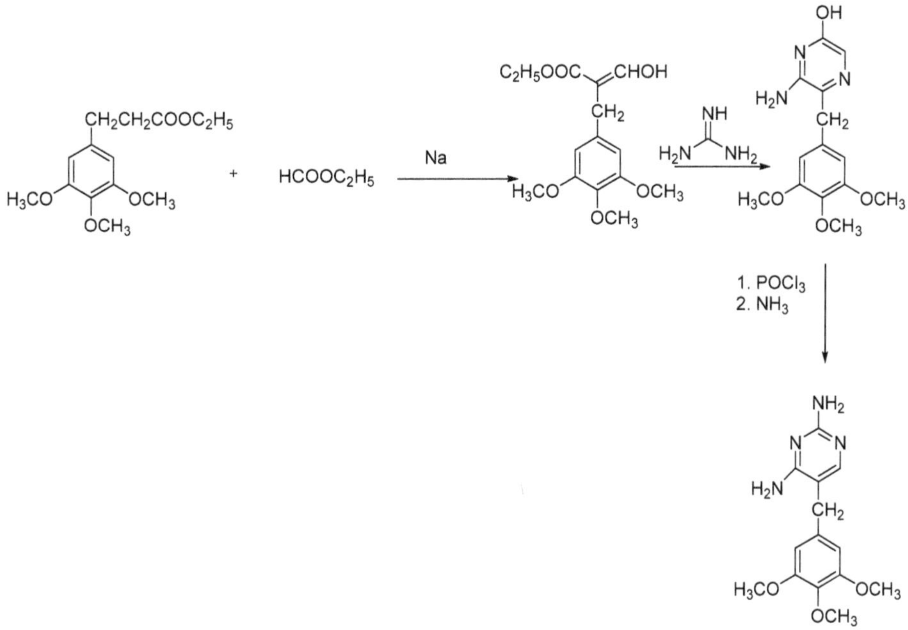
CH2CH2COOC2H5
H3CO
OCH3
OCH3
+
HCOOC2H5
Na
C2H5OOC
CHOH
CH2
H3CO
OCH3
OCH3
NH
H2N
NH2
OH
N
N
H2N
CH2
H3CO
OCH3
OCH3
1. POCl3
2. NH3
NH2
N
N
H2N
CH2
H3CO
OCH3
OCH3

4.

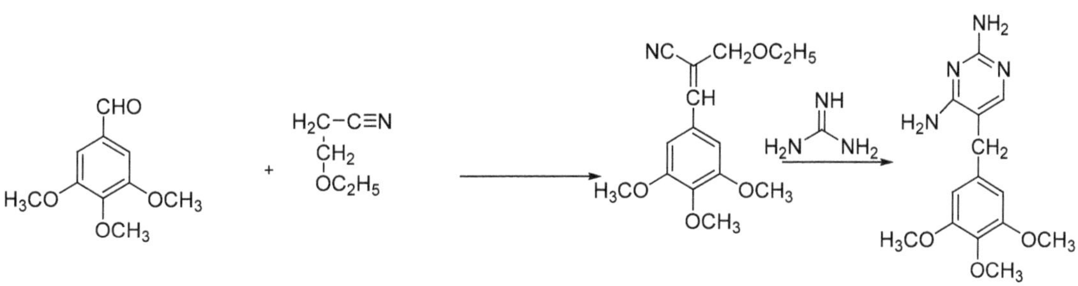
CHO
H3CO
OCH3
OCH3
+
H2C−C≡N
CH2
OC2H5
NC
CH2OC2H5
CH
H3CO
OCH3
OCH3
NH
H2N
NH2
NH2
N
N
H2N
CH2
H3CO
OCH3
OCH3

5.

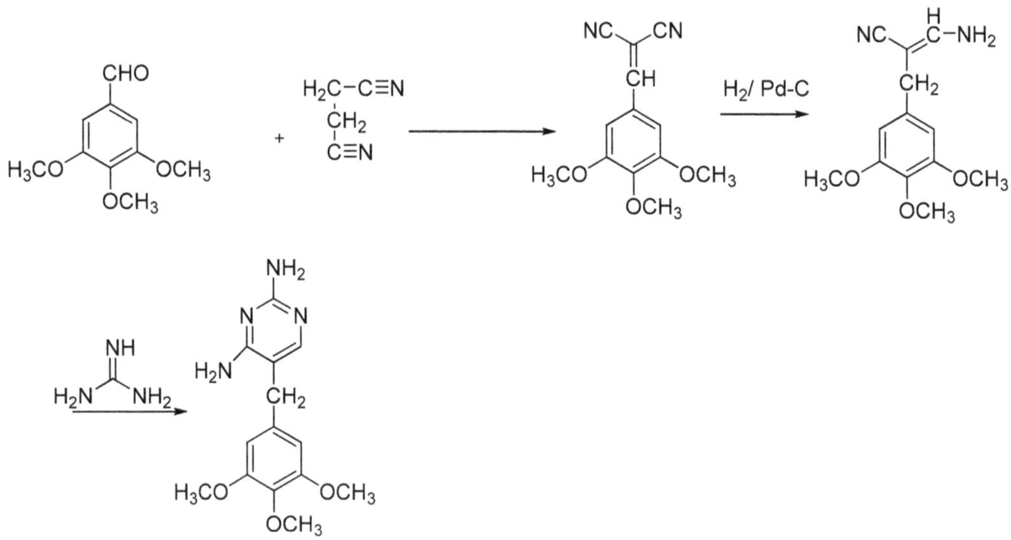

6.

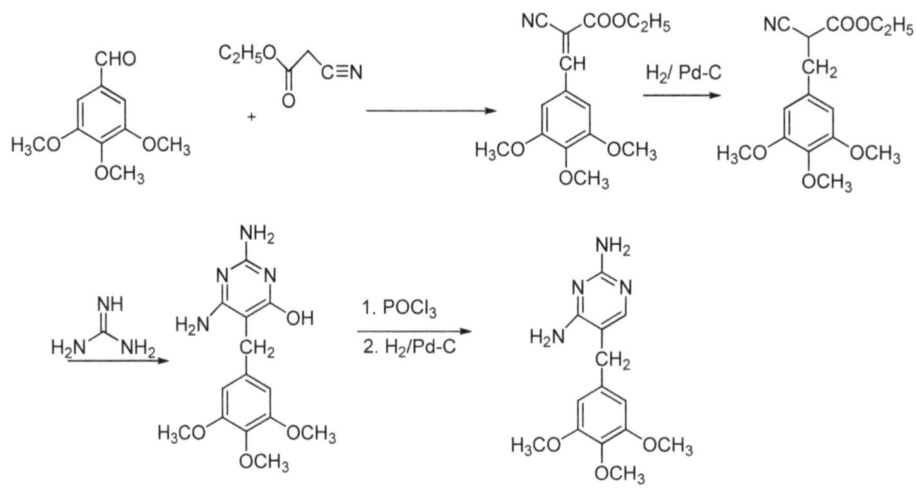

It can be synthesized by different approaches.

The third scheme begins with ethyl ester of 3,4,5-trimethoxydehydrocinnamic acid, which is formylated with ethyl format using sodium as a base to make an enol of the semialdehyde 3′,4′,5′-trimethoxybenzylmalonic ester, which on cyclization with guanidine forms 2-amino-4-hydroxy-5-(3′,4′,5′- trimethoxybenzyl) pyrimidine. Chlorination with $POCl_3$ and amination using ammonia affords trimethoprim.

In the fourth scheme condensation of 3,4,5-trimethoxybenzaldehyde with 3-ethoxy- or 3-anilinopropionitrile gives the corresponding benzylidene derivative, which on cyclization with guanidine gives trimethoprim.

In the fifth scheme 3,4,5-trimethoxybenzaldehyde is condensed with malonic acid dinitrile in a Knoevenagel reaction. This derivative is converted to the enamine by H2Pd/C, which cyclizes with guanidine to form trimethoprim.

In the sixth scheme 3,4,5-trimethoxybenzaldehyde undergoes Knoevenagel condensation with ethyl cyano-acetate, yielding an ylidene derivative. It is reduced with H2Pd/C, giving 3′,4′,5′-trimethoxy-benzylcyanoacetic ester, which on cyclization with guanidine produces trimethoprim.

CHAPTER 5

Synthon Approach and Retrosynthesis Applications

1. Introduction

In practically each organic chemistry department across the globe, chemists synthesize molecules. Formulations, polymer compounds, insecticides, dyestuffs, meals, coloring, flavorings, fragrances, detergents, and disinfecting agents all are created by commercial scientists. Natural products with unknown structures are synthesized by research chemists, as compounds for systematic studies, feasible intermediates in biological and chemical reactions, thousands of promising medications for all individuals that are employed in healthcare practice, as well as molecules that may be beneficial in organic synthesis. This chapter's goal is to discuss with you the disconnection or synthon method towards organic synthesis. Organic chemistry can be a daunting subject, but with the help of the synthon approach and retrosynthesis, it becomes more manageable. The synthon approach involves breaking down complex molecules into synthons, which are simpler building blocks. By doing this, chemists can design efficient and practical synthetic routes to create complex molecules. Retrosynthesis, on the other hand, involves working backward from the desired product to identify possible precursors. The significance of the synthon approach and retrosynthesis in organic chemistry cannot be overstated. These approaches help chemists identify novel synthetic pathways, create new compounds, develop drugs, and synthesize natural products. Understanding these approaches can give researchers and chemists a significant advantage in their work.

History

E. J. Corey developed the synthon technique in the 1960s, which established the principle of synthons as imaginary components for retrosynthetic examination. Synthons are functional group arrangements that can be isolated from their target compound. This method revolutionized the process of synthesis by allowing the organized separation of complicated compounds into smaller building components, allowing for the easier design of routes. Depending upon the synthon technique, retrosynthesis has now found widespread use in the manufacturing of naturally derived goods, medicines, and various other organic molecules. It has evolved into a key method for building effective and synergistic organic chemistry procedures.

Synthon approach

The synthon method is a highly effective analytical tool. It is a method of analysis to organic synthesis that involves the target molecule being disassembled into fragments by a sequence of logical disconnections in order to get the most feasible and most probably starting materials (i.e., synthons or building blocks) for the target molecule. In the synthon approach complex organic molecules are broken down into manageable parts. The synthon approach is a strategy that involves designing a synthetic equivalent of a target molecule's key functional group. This synthetic equivalent can be used to design a synthetic path backward from the target molecule of interest. Choosing a synthetic substitute for the crucial functional group found in the target molecule is the first and most important step in creating a synthon. The synthon should be easily accessible, stable, and adaptable in terms of synthesis. Following the decision, we determine the first components needed to construct the synthon. After simplification, the synthon should be developed so that we might readily obtain readily available starting materials. A methodical strategy is used to break down the synthon into simpler or commercially accessible chemical entities using the chosen starting components. The synthon approach is a reliable and efficient strategy for building complex molecules. It is popular in natural product synthesis, drug development, and total synthesis of complex molecules. With the synthon approach, it is possible to break down complex molecules into simpler, more accessible parts and achieve a theoretical understanding of chemical reactions and processes.

Retrosynthesis

Retro means "backward" and synthesis means "the process of merging simpler reactions to generate a chemical compound/molecule. Retrosynthesis is ideal for identifying and comparing alternative synthetic pathways in a rational and easy manner. At each level of the study, a collection of data may be used to check whether the aspect is already present in the available research (Fig.5.1).

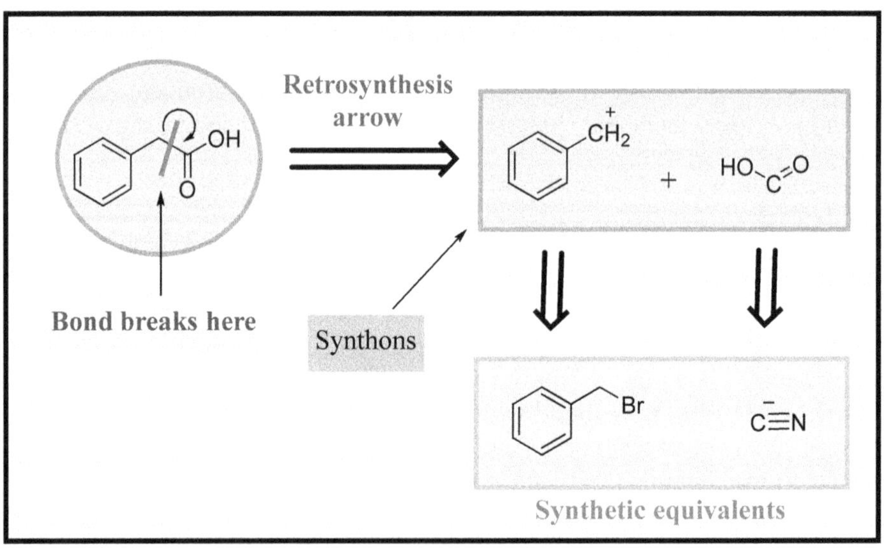

Figure: 5.1 Retrosynthesis approach.

Retrosynthesis is the planning process that chemists use to design or invent complex molecules. It helps to break down a compound into simpler starting materials, which can be sources of chemical building blocks. It is not a trial-and-error process; it requires extensive knowledge of organic chemistry, chemical reactivity and reaction mechanisms. The importance of retrosynthesis in organic chemistry cannot be overemphasized. It allows chemists to plan the most direct, efficient and feasible way to construct a target molecule. It also helps in the identification of potential reaction intermediates and by-products that could pose a challenge during the synthesis process. Retrosynthesis analysis involves a step-by-step approach, starting from the target molecule and working backward to the precursor materials. Each step should be evaluated for feasibility, availability of reagents, functionality, and selectivity. This methodical approach helps to optimize the synthetic route, minimize waste and reduce the need for expensive reagents. Retrosynthesis is not just theoretical; it has practical applications in the synthesis of natural products, drug design and total synthesis of complex molecules. With retrosynthesis, chemists can create custom molecules for specialized applications, such as catalysts, polymers, and electronic materials. Since its conception, retrosynthesis has contributed immensely to the advancement of organic chemistry.

Applications of Synthon Approach and Retrosynthesis

The synthon approach and retrosynthesis reveal their remarkable impact in numerous scientific domains, particularly in the realm of organic chemistry. This approach has found significance in the synthesis of natural products, drug synthesis, and the total synthesis of complex molecules. The synthon approach can effectively simplify the process of creating complex molecules. By deconstructing the target molecule into simpler fragments, we can choose a synthetic strategy to yield the required product easily. Natural product synthesis is the most fruitful application of retrosynthesis. In recent times, drug synthesis has also utilised this approach. The challenge arises when dealing with highly complex natural products as they require extensive modifications that demand knowledge of the subtleties of chemical reactions. When it comes to drug synthesis, for instance, the retrosynthetic approach can be applied to select the building blocks, and the synthon approach can simplify the complex molecules synthesis. Finally, the total synthesis of complex molecules and their intermediate structures has offered several exciting challenges, and the synthon approach has proved to be very useful here. The synthon approach and retrosynthesis have also been used extensively in peptide and carbohydrate synthesis. Those were some of the applications of synthon and retrosynthesis in the world of organic chemistry.

Advantages and Limitations of Synthon Approach and Retrosynthesis

Retrosynthesis evaluation is an approach for tackling difficulties in organic synthesis management. This is accomplished by converting the desired compound into simpler precursor molecules independent of possible reagent reactivity/interaction. The same procedure is used to investigate each precursor component.

Advantages of Synthon Approach and Retrosynthesis: The synthone approach and retrosynthesis have revolutionized organic chemistry, making it easier and more efficient to synthesize complex molecules. The biggest advantage of this approach is that it simplifies the synthesis process by breaking down the target molecule into smaller and easily available synthons. This way, the synthesis can be performed using readily available building blocks. This approach enables scientists to use the same synthons for different molecules, thus reducing the number of steps in the synthesis process. Additionally, this approach is useful in predicting the stability, stereochemistry, and reactivity of the intermediate building blocks.

Limitations of Synthon Approach and Retrosynthesis: Despite its advantages, the synthon approach and retrosynthesis have some limitations. The approach assumes that all building blocks are accessible from a commercially available set of compounds, which is not always true, and there may be a requirement for an additional set of reactions. Also, the approach requires knowledge of the properties of starting materials and intermediate compounds, making the process time-consuming and complex. Furthermore, the approach is bound by the limitations of the available reagents and functional groups, limiting its application to specific domains of chemistry. Overall, the synthon approach and retrosynthesis have enabled scientists to make complex organic molecules more efficiently and quickly. While it has some limitations, it still remains one of the most useful tools in organic chemistry synthesis.

With an optimistic outlook, we can envision a promising future for the Synthon Approach and Retrosynthesis. Their potential applications span across various fields, including drug discovery and catalysis, promising remarkable advancements. As cutting-edge research persists, these approaches will undoubtedly push the limits, resulting in exhilarating breakthroughs.

Retrosynthesis

Retrosynthesis can be a tricky word to wrap your head around, but it's actually a really useful tool for chemists. The process involves breaking down intricate molecules into smaller, more straightforward components that can serve as initial building blocks. The technique has been around for quite a while, but it wasn't until the 1970s that it really caught on. Retrosynthesis is important because it allows chemists to plan out how they're going to make a molecule before they even start working. This saves a lot of time and money, and it also makes the process more environmentally friendly. Additionally, there is an undeniable fascination in being able to analyze a complex molecule and possess the knowledge to deconstruct it into its fundamental elements. So, that's retrosynthesis in a nutshell. It might take a bit of practice to get the hang of it, but once you do, it can really streamline your work as a chemist.

Principles of Retrosynthesis

Retrosynthetic analysis (retrosynthesis) is a technique for planning synthesis, especially of complex organic molecules, whereby the complex target molecule (TM) is reduced into a sequence of progressively simpler structures along a pathway which ultimately leads to the identification of a simple or commercial. Retrosynthesis is an essential tool used by chemists to plan the synthesis of complex and natural products. This article will provide an in-depth understanding of the principles of retrosynthesis, including terminologies and advantages. Retrosynthesis follows strict principles that guide the disconnection of bonds within the target molecule. The first principle is bond disconnection, where chemists identify bonds to break to achieve retrosynthesis. This process follows strategic bond disconnection, where the molecule's functionality guides the bond's disconnection, keeping the intermediates stable throughout synthesis. Finally, the synthon approach is used to identify the reaction's building blocks and their respective synthon equivalents used during retrosynthesis. Bond disconnection involves identifying the breakdown patterns of a complex molecule and grouping them into smaller fragments. Every fragment defines a unique synthesis path towards reaching the target. Strategic bond disconnection involves identifying the available reagents and catalysts to develop a workable strategy towards total molecule synthesis. Synthon approach constitutes finding fragments that represent easily accessible synthons and reacting these as building blocks to yield the required complex molecule. In summary, retrosynthesis approaches molecule synthesis by first identifying the target bond disconnection pattern, followed by a strategic bond disconnection that outlines a synthesis strategy. Finally, the synthon approach is adopted where the reaction's building blocks are identified and matched with their equivalents for synthesis.

Guidelines for Molecule Dissection Chemists use different guidelines when dissecting a molecule into its available precursors for retrosynthesis. Firstly, identifying key functional groups is critical, and every stable group is preserved during synthesis. Secondly, the molecule's dissection path begins from the target molecule to the available starting materials, finally leading to the reactants. Finally, stereochemistry is critical, and preserving the original configuration ensures the final synthetic molecule's success. It is not ideal for complex molecules that feature several dependencies. The process assumes ideal conditions and may sometimes over-rely on retrosynthetic software. Additionally, the methodology has limitations as it's labor-intensive and costly, making it impractical when dealing with a large number of concurrent syntheses. In conclusion, retrosynthesis is a valuable tool for chemists in planning complex molecule synthesis. The process follows strict principles and terminologies and presents numerous advantages when planning molecule synthesis, making it an ideal methodology for small and industrious molecule synthesis.

Terminologies in Retrosynthesis

Retrosynthesis involves breaking down a molecule into a smaller, simpler starting material through a series of retrosynthetic steps. Retrosynthesis has several terminologies essential for complete comprehension. The disconnection approach is employed to cleave the target bond; the transform approach, where existing functional groups are transformed into a new molecule, yielding the target molecule. The retrosynthetic tree is designed as a decision tree, highlighting the different pathways of synthesizing a target molecule from readily available precursors or starting materials. Retrosynthesis presents numerous benefits, making it an ideal method of planning molecule synthesis. Notably, it's time-saving, as chemists can synthesize complex molecules in fewer steps, utilizing readily available precursors. Additionally, retrosynthesis is cost-effective and environmentally friendly. The process eliminates the need for specialized equipment, saving on industrial infrastructure expenses. Finally, the process is easily scalable, making it suited for industrial-level molecule synthesis. The process's overall goal is to identify the best synthetic route for producing a target molecule, taking-into account cost, time, and environmental impact. Some essential terms to know in retrosynthesis include the disconnection approach, transform approach, and retrosynthetic tree. In the disconnection approach, the target molecule's bonds are disconnected to yield a set of simpler precursor molecules that could produce the target molecule through reversible chemical reactions. This approach favors modifying known reactions to produce new molecules, the basis of synthetic organic chemistry. In the transform approach, the target molecule is modified by exchanging functional groups or altering bond configurations in a series of steps that lead to simpler intermediate molecules. Eventually, these intermediates could synthesize the target molecule through irreversible chemical reactions. The retrosynthetic tree is similar to a family tree, beginning with the target molecule branching backward to simpler synthesized precursor molecules that ultimately trace back to commercially available starting materials. It is a graphical representation of the disconnection approach and helps to simplify the synthetic route to a target molecule. Retrosynthesis is a disconnection approach that provides guidelines for molecule dissection and offers many advantages, including time-saving and cost-effectiveness. However, it's not without its limitations in challenging complex molecule synthesis, assuming ideal conditions and with over-reliance on retrosynthetic software. Understanding these retrosynthesis terminologies is essential for chemists to analyze the synthesis of complex molecules and improve the efficiency of chemical production.

Advantages of Retrosynthesis

First and foremost, retrosynthesis saves time. By planning backward, chemists can streamline the entire synthetic pathway, thereby reducing the trial-and-error approach of traditional synthesis methods. In addition to saving time, retrosynthesis is also cost-effective. By identifying feasible and alternative methods for a given synthetic pathway, chemists can eliminate unnecessary steps, thereby reducing the cost of reagents, solvents and equipment. Furthermore, retrosynthesis is environmentally friendly. The process minimizes the generation of waste by limiting the number of reaction steps and optimizing stoichiometry. By minimizing the resources required for synthesis, we can reduce the environmental impact of our work. Last but not least, retrosynthesis is easily scalable. With a pre-planned synthetic pathway, chemists can easily replicate the synthesis at a larger scale. This not only saves time and resources but also ensures consistent product quality. In conclusion, retrosynthesis is a powerful tool that saves time, cuts costs, is environmentally friendly, and easily scalable. By adopting a strategic approach and using retrosynthesis in our work, we can optimize our synthesis processes while minimizing environmental impact.

Guidelines for Molecule Dissection

Retrosynthesis is all about molecule dissection, and its principles, terminology and advantages are well-known to us at this point. So, let's talk about guidelines for Molecule Dissection. The first step is to identify the key functional groups present in the target molecule. It is important to break down the molecule into its individual functional groups to ensure we have a clear understanding of what is required to make the product. Once the functional groups are identified, dissect the molecule from the target molecule to an available starting material. We can take advantage of various sources like chemical catalogues and patents to access the starting material. Devising enzymes and reagents to modify the starting material to make the target molecule is one way to go about. During dissection, it is important to keep track of stereochemistry. If not done properly, the final product may have an incorrect stereochemistry, changing its physical and chemical properties. This can be done by understanding the chemical reactions that we are using to link different functional groups. To summarise, molecule dissection may seem like a simple process, but it involves many critical steps.

It is important to understand the starting material availability and the feasibility of modifying the starting material to produce the yield required. Careful analysis of functional groups and stereochemistry is a must. Now that we have a clear understanding of guidelines for molecule dissection, let's see how limitations may impact the retrosynthesis process.

Functional Group Interconversion and Addition

Functional Group Interconversion (FGI) is the process of converting one functional group into another during retrosynthetic analysis. FGI mostly involves oxidation, reduction, and substitution. It is applicable where we do not have a real and workable reaction reverse to a disconnection. Example- In designing a synthesis of local anesthetic benzocaine we know that esters are made from alcohols and acids so we can write a C-O disconnection.

Organic synthesis refers to the process of constructing complex molecules from simpler ones. This process is essential in the production of drugs, materials, and polymers. Functional Group Interconversion (FGI) and Functional Group Addition (FGA) are crucial processes in organic synthesis. In this article, we will explore the fundamentals of these processes and their applications in organic synthesis. FGI is the process of converting one functional group to another. This process is important in the synthesis of complex molecules. For example, converting a carbonyl group to an alcohol group is useful in the synthesis of ethanol from acetaldehyde. FGI reactions can be classified into four types: nucleophilic substitution, electrophilic substitution, reduction, and oxidation. Nucleophilic substitution is the replacement of a leaving group with a nucleophile. For example, the reaction of an alcohol with a hydrogen halide yields an alkyl halide. Electrophilic substitution is the replacement of an aromatic hydrogen with an electrophile. For example, nitration is an electrophilic substitution reaction that yields nitroaromatics. Reduction is the process of converting a functional group to a lower oxidation state. For example, the reduction of an alkyne to an alkene is useful in the synthesis of alkenes. Oxidation is the process of converting a functional group to a higher oxidation state. For example, the oxidation of a primary alcohol yields an aldehyde. FGI reactions have numerous applications in organic synthesis. For example, these reactions can be used to manipulate the properties of complex molecules, or to convert one functional group into another so that it can be further modified. In contrast to FGI, FGA involves the addition of a functional group to a molecule. The addition can occur to a double or triple bond, or it can occur to a heteroatom. FGA reactions can be classified into nucleophilic addition, electrophilic addition, and radical addition. Nucleophilic addition is the addition of a nucleophile to a carbonyl group. For example, the addition of a Grignard reagent to a carbonyl group yields an alcohol. Electrophilic addition is the addition of an electrophile to a double bond. For example, the addition of hydrogen halides to alkenes yields alkyl halides. Radical addition is the addition of a radical to an unsaturated bond. For example, the addition of a halogen radical to an alkene yields a halogenated alkane. Differences Between FGI and FGA the key difference between FGI and FGA is that FGI involves the conversion of one functional group to another, while FGA involves the addition of a functional group to a molecule. FGI can be used to modify complex molecules, while FGA can be used to introduce new functional groups into a molecule. In FGI, the starting material must contain the functional group being converted. In contrast, FGA requires the starting material to have a carbon-carbon unsaturated bond or a heteroatom. Applications of FGI and FGA in Organic Synthesis FGI and FGA reactions have numerous applications in organic synthesis. For example, these reactions can be used to modify the properties of complex molecules or to introduce new functionality into a molecule. FGA, in particular, is useful in the production of pharmaceuticals and other complex molecules. One advantage of using FGI and FGA in synthesis is that these reactions can be carried out under mild conditions, thus minimizing unwanted side reactions. Challenges and Future Prospects for FGI and FGA Despite their usefulness in organic synthesis, FGI and FGA reactions have some limitations and drawbacks. For example, these reactions can be difficult to control, and the process can be slow or inefficient. However, ongoing research is focused on addressing these challenges and improving the efficiency of these reactions. Future developments in FGI and FGA research will likely involve the discovery of new catalysts and reaction conditions, as well as advancements in green chemistry. In conclusion, FGI and FGA reactions are critical processes in organic synthesis. These reactions can be used to modify the properties of complex molecules or to introduce new functionality into a molecule. Despite their limitations, ongoing research is aimed at improving these reactions and developing new applications for them in organic synthesis.

Functional Group Addition (FGA)

The addition of functional groups such as double bonds or carbonyl groups can serve to direct reactivity to specific locations of a molecule and allow disconnection based on dependable reactions. This can significantly simplify a synthesis.

Organic chemistry is a fascinating subject that involves the synthesis and analysis of organic compounds. Functional Group Interconversion (FGI) and Functional Group Addition (FGA) are two critical concepts in organic chemistry that are widely used in organic synthesis. Functional Group Addition (FGA): FGA refers to the addition of a functional group to a carbon atom in an organic molecule. This process results in the formation of a new functional group and often leads to the formation of a new compound. Definition of FGA: FGA involves the addition of a new functional group to an existing molecule. The process involves breaking a bond in the existing molecule and adding a new group to one of the resulting fragments. This results in the formation of a new compound with a different functional group. Types of FGA: There are several types of FGA, including nucleophile addition, electrophile addition, radical addition, and carbene addition. Nucleophile addition involves the addition of a nucleophile to a molecule, while electrophile addition involves the addition of an electrophile to a molecule. Radical addition involves the addition of a free radical to a molecule, while carbene addition involves the addition of a carbene to a molecule. Examples of FGA reactions: One example of an FGA reaction is the addition of a halogen to an alkene. This process involves the addition of a halogen (such as chlorine or bromine) to a carbon-carbon double bond, resulting in the formation of a dihalide. Another example is the addition of water to an alkene, which forms an alcohol.

FGI and FGA: The key difference between FGI and FGA is that FGI involves the conversion of one functional group to another, while FGA involves the addition of a functional group to an existing molecule. FGI is often used in the production of new compounds, while FGA is used to modify existing compounds.

Applications of FGI and FGA in Organic Synthesis: FGI and FGA are widely used in organic synthesis, as they allow chemists to create new compounds with specific functional groups. Using FGI and FGA, chemists can experiment with different functional groups to create compounds with specific properties. For example, FGI can be used to convert an alcohol to a ketone, while FGA can be used to add a halogen to an alkene.

Challenges and Future Prospects for FGI and FGA: Despite their many benefits, FGI and FGA also have some limitations. One challenge is that the reactions can be difficult to control, leading to unwanted side products. Another challenge is that the reactions can be expensive and time-consuming. However, researchers are exploring new methods to overcome these challenges and improve the efficiency of FGI and FGA reactions. Conclusion: FGI and FGA are two essential concepts in organic chemistry. FGI allows chemists to convert one functional group to another, while FGA allows chemists to add a new functional group to an existing molecule. These processes are widely used in organic synthesis and have many applications in the production of new compounds with specific properties. Despite some challenges, FGI and FGA are likely to remain critical concepts in organic chemistry for years to come.

Differences Between FGI and FGA

Functional Group Interconversion (FGI) and Functional Group Addition (FGA) are two important conversion mechanisms in organic synthesis. FGI involves changing one functional group into another, while FGA refers to the addition of a new functional group to a molecule. Although the two mechanisms may seem similar, they have key differences. FGI is associated with interconverting one functional group to another, either through substitution or elimination reactions. In FGA, a new functional group is introduced onto an existing molecule via addition reactions. FGI conversions mostly take place on carbon atoms, while FGA can occur on any atom in a molecule. Both mechanisms, however, require careful selection of reagents, solvents, and reaction conditions for optimal outcomes. The key difference between FGI and FGA is that FGI involves replacing a functional group with another, whereas FGA adds a new functional group without removing any existing entity. This difference has significant implications for the reactions' outcomes, as the functional groups' position can affect molecular properties such as reactivity, solubility, and melting point. In summary, FGI and FGA are two essential mechanisms in organic synthesis. While FGI involves converting one functional group into another, FGA adds a new functional group without removing any substituents. Understanding the differences between the two mechanisms is crucial when selecting the appropriate mechanism for a specific synthesis or reaction.

Applications of FGI and FGA in Organic Synthesis

Are you ready to dive deep into the world of functional group interconversion and addition? Hold on tight as we explore how these reactions bring about changes in organic molecules. One of the most significant applications of functional group interconversion (FGI) and functional group addition (FGA) is in organic synthesis. The combination of these reactions offers several advantages compared to traditional synthetic methods. Advantages of using FGI and FGA in synthesis One of the significant advantages of FGI and FGA reactions is the broad range of functional groups that can be interconverted or added to a molecule. These reactions can be used to introduce heteroatoms such as nitrogen or oxygen into a hydrocarbon chain, allowing for the synthesis of complex structures. Moreover, FGI and FGA reactions are mild and selective, making it possible to perform the desired transformations without disturbing the rest of the molecule. These reactions also occur under ambient conditions, making them efficient and convenient. Examples of synthesis reactions using FGI and FGA One of the most notable examples of FGI in organic synthesis is the conversion of a carbonyl group to an alcohol. This reaction is useful in the synthesis of diols and triols, which are essential in various chemical processes. FGA finds its application in the synthesis of alkenes and alkynes. For example, the hydroboration of an alkene leads to the addition of borane, followed by oxidation to yield an alcohol or an ether. FGI and FGA have also been extensively used for the synthesis of natural products such as alkaloids and terpenes. These reactions offer a versatile approach to achieve the desired functionalization pattern, making them an indispensable tool in synthetic organic chemistry. Limitations and drawbacks of FGI and FGA Despite the numerous advantages of FGI and FGA reactions, there are some limitations that must be considered. These reactions are often sensitive to the steric and electronic nature of the substrate, making it challenging to achieve the desired product selectively. Moreover, some FGI and FGA reactions require highly reactive intermediates, making them potentially hazardous. Therefore, special care and attention must be given when carrying out such reactions. Emerging trends and future developments in FGI and FGA research the development of new and selective catalysts for FGI and FGA reactions is an area of active research. Nanoparticle catalysts and metal organic frameworks have been shown to enhance the reaction rate and selectivity of FGI and FGA reactions, making them promising alternatives to traditional catalysts. Furthermore, with the growing significance of green chemistry, the development of FGI and FGA reactions that use renewable feedstocks and produce minimal waste is being pursued aggressively. In conclusion, FGI and FGA reactions have revolutionized the synthesis of organic compounds, offering an efficient and versatile approach to achieving complex functionalization patterns. With the continued development of new catalysts and more sustainable methods, these reactions are poised to play an even more critical role in the future of synthetic organic chemistry.

Challenges and Future Prospects for FGI and FGA

As with any scientific process, these methods are not without limitations. For one, the selectivity between reactive functional groups can be low, leading to unwanted side reactions. Additionally, certain substrates may require harsh or specialized reaction conditions, making scaling up a challenge. So, while FGI and FGA have demonstrated significant potential in synthetic applications, there is still work to be done to optimize their integration into industrial processes. But fear not, research on FGI and FGA continues to evolve and improve. For example, there has been a growing interest in using photochemistry to drive FGA reactions, which could increase the specificity of the reaction, and reduce the need for harsh reaction conditions. Furthermore, emerging applications of FGI and FGA in the development of functional materials and biologically active compounds are providing new opportunities to apply these techniques. So, while there are certainly challenges to overcome in the practical implementation of FGI and FGA, the ever-evolving research landscape offers hope that these methods will continue to become increasingly versatile and accessible to both academic and industry researchers.

Functional group interconversion (FGI) and functional group addition (FGA) play a crucial role in organic synthesis. With FGI, chemists can transform one functional group into another while FGA allows them to add new functional groups to a molecule. Understanding the difference between these two reactions is crucial. While FGI involves the breaking and forming of new bonds, FGA only involves the addition of new bonds. Despite their limitations, FGI and FGA have significant advantages in organic synthesis. They allow for the creation of complex molecules from simple starting materials. In conclusion, FGI and FGA are essential tools for synthetic chemists, and continued research will lead to more efficient and sustainable methods for organic synthesis

C-X disconnection

The C-X disconnection approach is mainly applicable to a carbon chain attached to any of the heteroatoms like O, N, or S. Here, a bond joins the heteroatom (X) to the rest of the molecule like a C-O, C-N, or C-S group. This point is a good point to initiate a disconnection (Fig.5.2).

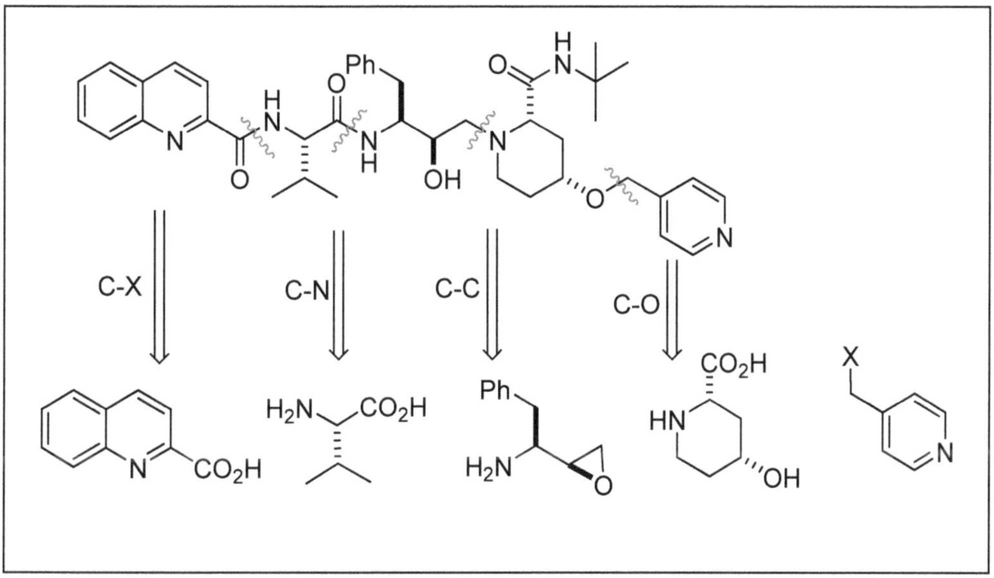

Figure: 5.2 Example Of C-X Disconnection.

C-C disconnections – alcohols-

Alcohols, also known as hydroxy compounds, are an important functional group in organic chemistry. They have a hydroxyl (-OH) group attached to a carbon atom, making them polar compounds. And, due to their reactivity, alcohols are used in various industrial applications such as solvents, fuels, and pharmaceuticals. One way to form alcohols is through C-C disconnections. C-C disconnections refer to the formation of a carbon-carbon bond, followed by the introduction of a functional group. In the case of alcohols, C-C disconnections are used to form a C-O bond. There are several ways to perform C-C disconnections to form alcohols, including:

1. Grignard reagents - Grignard reagents are important organometallic compounds that can react with carbonyl compounds to form alcohols through C-C bond formation.
2. Reduction of carbonyl compounds - Aldehydes and ketones can be reduced by $NaBH_4$ or $LiAlH_4$ to form primary and secondary alcohols, respectively.
3. Hydroboration-oxidation - This reaction involves the addition of borane to alkenes, followed by oxidation with hydrogen peroxide to form alcohols.
4. Wohl-Ziegler reaction - This reaction uses 1,3-dimethylbarbituric acid to form dialkyl malonates, which undergo intramolecular cyclization to form alcohols.
5. Corey-Chaykovsky reaction - This reaction involves the formation of sulfonium ylides, which react with carbonyl compounds to form epoxides that can be opened to form alcohols.
6. Oxy-Mercuration-Demercuration reaction - This reaction involves the addition of mercuric acetate to alkenes, followed by reduction with sodium borohydride to form alcohols.

In summary, C-C disconnections are an important strategy for the formation of alcohols. By forming a carbon-carbon bond, followed by the introduction of a hydroxy group, alcohols can be synthesized in an efficient and selective way. Different reagents and conditions can be used to perform C-C disconnections, providing a versatile toolkit for organic synthesis. Overall, alcohols are important functional groups in organic chemistry with numerous industrial applications. C-C disconnections provide a great strategy for their formation, with different methods available to achieve this goal.

Synthesis of alcoholic compounds by 1,2 C-C disconnections

This reaction involves cleavage and formation of C-C bonds in a single step making synthesis quicker and more efficient. The mechanism of 1,2 C-C disconnections involves the breaking of a bond between two adjacent carbon atoms followed by the reformation of the bond between the same atoms but with the opposite orientation. This rearrangement can be applied to various types of disconnections such as aldol, retro-aldol, and 1,2-cyclohexadienyl systems. In Aldol disconnections, an α-carbon of a carbonyl compound is cleaved along with a β-hydrogen, which yields an enolate. Retro-Aldol disconnections involve the reverse of this reaction. In 1,2-cyclohexadienyl systems, a cyclic diene is subjected to heat that leads to the cleavage of two adjacent carbon-carbon bonds and the subsequent formation of a highly reactive carbene intermediate (Fig.5.3).

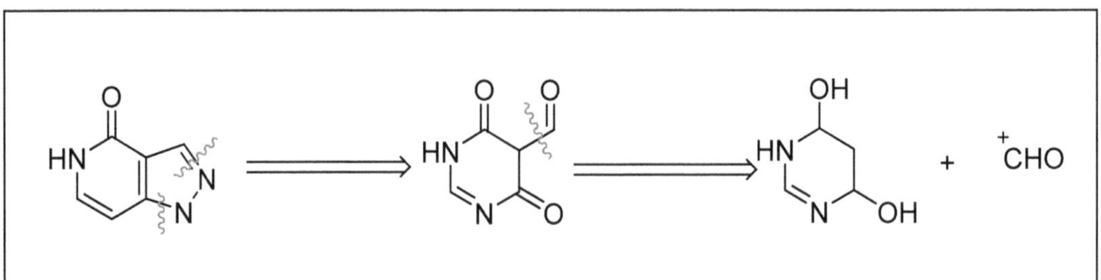

Figure: 5.3 Example Of C-C Disconnection.

Synthesis of Alcohols via 1,2 C-C Disconnections

Synthesizing alcohols via 1,2 C-C disconnections is a highly effective technique. One way to achieve this is through the use of 1,2-cyclohexadienyl systems - a simple and effective method. These systems act as precursors to fulvenes, which then undergo electrocyclic ring opening, followed by stereoselective protonation, to produce alcohols. Another way to achieve this synthesis is through metal-catalyzed cross-coupling reactions. This involves coupling two different molecules through the use of a metal catalyst, forming a new molecule that contains both of the original molecules' components. This method is particularly useful in producing complex, functionalized alcohols. Electrocyclic reactions are also used in the synthesis of alcohols via 1,2 C-C disconnections. These reactions rely on the ability to control the stereochemistry of a reaction to form the desired product. By selectively breaking bonds within a molecule, desired stereochemistry can be achieved. While these methods have limitations, such as difficulty in controlling regio- and stereoselectivity, they have proved to be valuable tools in organic synthesis. New and improved methods for synthesizing alcohols via 1,2 C-C disconnections continue to be developed, providing exciting possibilities for future research and development. Weighing the benefits and limitations, there's no denying the efficiency of 1,2 C-C disconnections in the synthesis of alcoholic compounds. On the upside, it offers simplified methods and high selectivity while boasting low toxicity; however, the challenge is that it requires high computational power and is highly dependent on the structure of the reactants.

Recent Advancements: Alcohols produced via asymmetric 1,2-C-C disconnections proved to be highly useful in drug synthesis.

Any compound bearing an alcoholic group can also be disconnected at the C-C bond next to the adjacent bond to the oxygen atom. The retrosynthetic analysis in Figure 10 shows the C-C disconnection.

Carbonyl compounds; 1,2-, 1,3-, 1,4-, 1,5-, 1,6-difunctionalized compounds

Carbonyl compounds are molecules containing the carbonyl group, C=O. In addition, acetaldehyde (CH_3CHO) has been shown to be abundant in the atmosphere and also released from the combustion and photooxidation of hydrocarbons.

Strategies for Synthesis of Three, Four, Five and Six-Membered Ring

Before we get into the nitty-gritty of it, let's figure out what synthesis even means. Simply put, synthesis is the process of creating something new from existing elements. In the world of chemistry, this means building new molecules from smaller building blocks. It allows chemists to create new compounds with unique properties that can be used in a variety of industries, from pharmaceuticals to materials science. However, it's not always a walk in the park. Synthesis can be a long and tedious process and often requires a lot of trial and error before you get the desired result. Now, let's talk about some common challenges that chemists may face during synthesis. It's not uncommon for reactions to yield unexpected products, or for yields to be lower than expected due to side reactions. Plus, some reactions require very specific conditions to occur, making them difficult to carry out on a large scale. But fear not, for there are always new strategies being developed to tackle these challenges head-on. Now that we've got the basics out of the way, let's dive into some specific strategies for the synthesis of three, four, five, and six-membered rings.

Strategies for Synthesis of Three-Membered Rings

In the realm of chemistry, synthesis involves the creation of new compounds, and it is crucial to advancing the field of science. While synthesis is an exciting field, it also comes with its fair share of challenges. One of the most common problems faced during synthesis is the creation of impurities or unintended products. However, with the right strategies, these challenges can be mitigated. Now, let's dive into the specific strategies for synthesizing various ring sizes. Three-membered rings are the smallest and most strained cyclic compounds known to chemists. Despite this, they are essential building blocks for many naturally occurring and synthetic compounds. There are a few distinct strategies for their synthesis, including cyclic acylation, ring-closing alkyne metathesis, and cycloaddition reactions. In cyclic acylation, dicarbonyl compounds react with organic halides to produce three-membered rings. On the other hand, ring-closing alkyne metathesis involves the reaction of an alkyne with an alkenyl-substituted carboxylic acid to form the desired three-membered ring. Finally, cycloaddition reactions involve the formation of two new carbon-carbon bonds to create a cyclic compound. Each of these strategies has its advantages and disadvantages, and it is up to the chemist to determine which one is suitable for their specific use case. While three-membered rings may be small, they play a vital role in many natural products and synthetic compounds. The task of synthesizing them may seem daunting at first, but with the right strategy and techniques, their formation becomes quite simple. Conclusion: The synthesis of three-membered, four-membered, five-membered, and six-membered rings is essential to the advancements being made in the field of chemistry and science as a whole. By using the strategies discussed above, the synthesis of each sized ring can be achieved with relative ease. It is crucial to select the right strategy based on the specific use case and chemistry involved. The future of ring synthesis is an exciting one, and we look forward to seeing how chemists and scientists alike continue to innovate in this area (Fig.5.4).

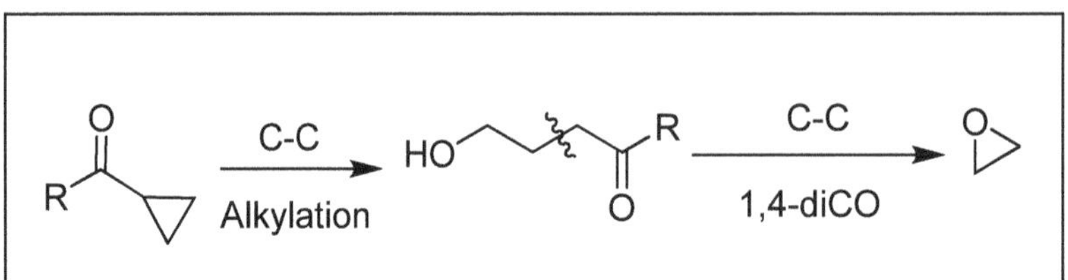

Figure: 5.4 Ring cyclization of three-member ring.

Strategies for Synthesis of Four-Membered Rings

From creating new medicines to developing innovative technologies, synthesis serves as the foundation of many scientific endeavors. While synthesis is critical, it can also be challenging. Synthetic chemists face numerous obstacles, including finding the right reaction conditions, optimizing yields, and dealing with complex starting materials. However, these challenges pale in comparison to the satisfaction of successfully synthesizing a new molecule. Strategies for Four-membered rings, also known as cyclobutanes, are small but essential molecules that exhibit a range of biological and chemical properties. Fortunately, several synthetic strategies can be used to generate these molecules. One approach involves the formation of cyclobutanes through [2+2] cycloaddition. This process involves two alkenes reacting to form a four-membered ring. While this strategy can be effective, it often suffers from low yields and limited substrate scope. Another approach is the Olefin Metathesis approach. This method involves the use of transition metal catalysts to break and reform carbon-carbon double bonds, resulting in the formation of a four-membered ring. This approach has gained popularity due to its high selectivity, mild reaction conditions, and broad substrate scope. A third strategy utilizes reactions involving transition metal catalysis, such as palladium-catalyzed cross-coupling reactions and ruthenium-catalyzed ring-closing reactions. These reactions are effective at generating complex four-membered rings and can be optimized to achieve high yields. In conclusion: Synthesizing four-membered rings is challenging, but there are several effective strategies available. From [2+2] cycloadditions to olefin metathesis, chemists have many tools at their disposal to create these important molecules. By choosing the right approach and optimizing reaction conditions, synthetic chemists can overcome the challenges of ring synthesis and unlock new opportunities in science and technology (Fig.5.5).

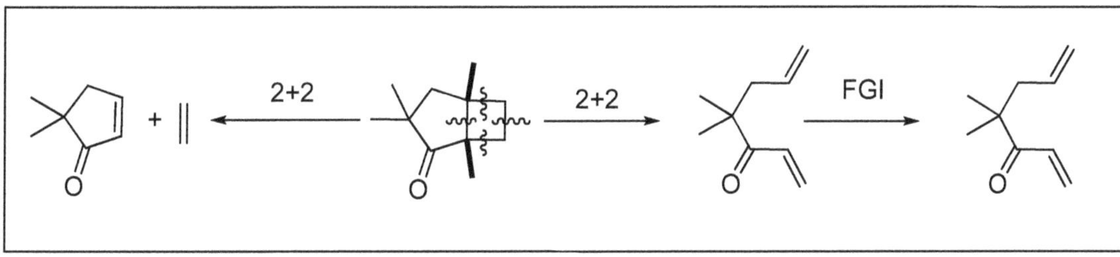

Figure: 5.5 Ring Cyclization of Four Membered Rings.

Strategies for Synthesis of Five-Membered Rings

It is essential in various fields of chemistry, including drug discovery, materials science, and natural product synthesis. However, synthesizing complex molecules can be challenging due to the unique structures of the molecules. Therefore, it requires a precise and strategic approach to overcome those barriers efficiently. Strategies for Synthesis of Five-Membered Rings: In the previous sections, we discussed the strategies for synthesizing three, four, and six-membered rings. The five-membered ring is known as the "golden mean" of chemistry, and its synthesis is notably crucial because of its structural and functional diversity. The following are the strategies used for synthesizing five-membered rings:

Cycloaddition reactions using 1,3-dipoles: Cycloaddition reactions are among the most efficient and versatile methods for the synthesis of five-membered rings. This method involves adding nucleophilic and electrophilic reactants known as 1,3-dipoles to give the desired product. The reaction is usually stereoselective, and it yields a single product, making it an attractive strategy for synthesizing five-membered rings. Formation of cyclopentanes using the acyl anion strategy: This approach involves using acyl anion chemistry to construct carbon-carbon bonds that form the cyclopentane core. The acyl anion acts as a nucleophile and attacks an electrophilic compound, forming a new bond. The reaction is generally efficient and selective, making it a viable strategy for synthesizing five-membered rings.

Ring expansion/closing reactions: Ring expansion/closing reactions deal with the functionalization of the strained or unstrained cyclic systems, and it involves the manipulation of the cyclic system. The formation of five-membered rings via ring expansion usually involves using carbene intermediates. On the other hand, the ring closing strategy utilizes elimination reactions, which involves the removal of a leaving group from a functionalized small ring to yield a more massive ring.

Choosing the right strategy is essential for synthesizing complex molecules. In the case of five-membered ring synthesis, the strategies mentioned above are some of the most efficient methods. However, it's essential to note that there are other strategies for synthesizing five-membered rings, and researchers continue to explore new methods. With this continuous research, the field of ring synthesis is expected to expand and form more diverse molecules in the future (Fig.5.6).

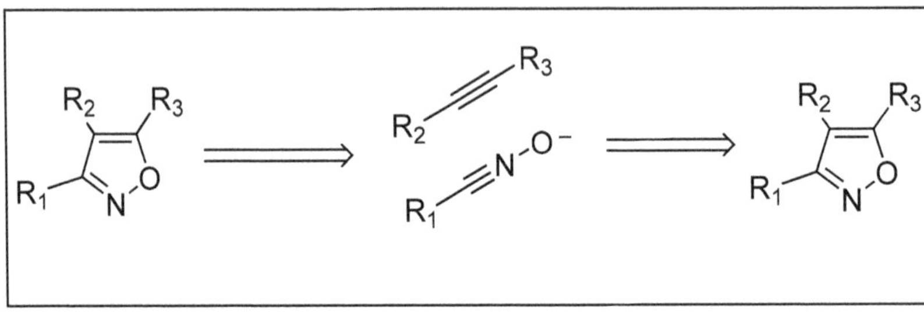

Figure: 5.6 Synthesis of Five Member Oxygen and Nitrogen Containing Rings.

Strategies for Synthesis of Six-Membered Rings

The first is cyclocondensation reactions involving ketenes. This method involves the reaction of ketenes with 1,3-diketones in the presence of a catalyst such as silver or sodium ethoxide to form cyclohexenones. The cyclohexenones formed can then be further reacted with different reagents to form the desired benzene ring system. Another effective method is ring-closing metathesis reactions for the formation of medium-sized carbocycles. Here, we use ruthenium-based catalysts to trigger the reaction of two olefinic compounds to close the ring. Unlike the methods discussed earlier, this approach can be used to realize medium-sized rings with precise control over the stereochemical geometry of the newly formed bond. Finally, we have the classic Friedel–Crafts reactions that can be used to synthesize benzene rings. This method involves the reaction of an arene with an alkyl halide or alkyl benzene in the presence of a lewis acid to form a new carbon-carbon bond. This is a versatile method that can be used to synthesize a variety of substituted and unsubstituted benzene ring systems. While each strategy has its own advantages and disadvantages, the choice of which method to use depends on several factors such as the size of the ring, the desired stereochemistry, and the available starting material. Some of the other strategies discussed earlier, such as cycloaddition reactions using 1,3-dipoles and cycloalkenation reactions may also be applicable in the synthesis of six-membered rings. In conclusion, the field of ring synthesis has come a long way, and with continued research, we can expect to see even more innovative strategies being developed in the future. As a synthetic chemist, the key to success lies in selecting the right strategy based on the specific requirements of the target compound.

First and foremost, the success of any ring synthesis reaction depends heavily on choosing the right strategy. From cyclic acylation to ring-closing alkyne metathesis, there are a variety of options available depending on the ring size and desired composition. Secondly, the field of ring synthesis is constantly evolving, with new techniques and strategies being developed all the time. Who knows what the future holds for the synthesis of three, four, five, and six-membered rings? The possibilities are endless. In conclusion, we hope that this brief overview has given you a taste of this fascinating field, and perhaps even inspired you to delve deeper into the exciting world of ring synthesis.

Conclusion

In summary, the synthon approach and retrosynthesis are two essential concepts in organic chemistry that have transformed the way chemists design and synthesize complex molecules. The synthon approach provides a step-by-step method for designing synthetic building blocks, while retrosynthesis offers a systematic way to break down complex molecules into simpler compounds. The applications of these concepts are vast and include the synthesis of natural products, drug development, and total synthesis of complex molecules. However, it is important to note the limitations of these approaches, such as their reliance on heuristic rules and the complexity of certain target molecules. Despite these limitations, the future prospects of synthon approach and retrosynthesis are promising, given the increasing demand for sustainable and efficient chemical synthesis methods. Overall, understanding and applying these concepts is crucial for advancing the field of organic chemistry (Fig.5.7).

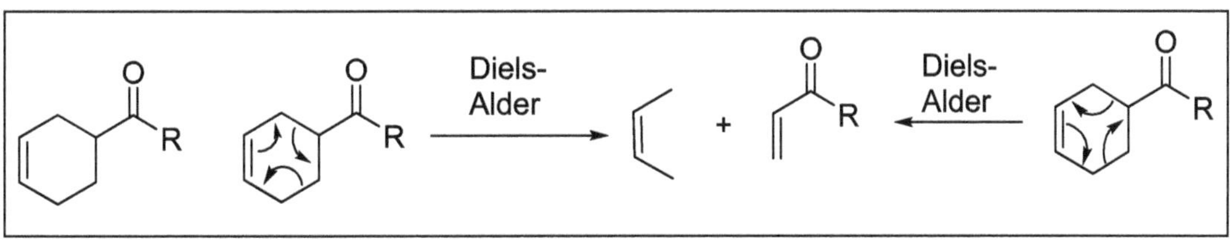

Figure: 5.7 Ring cyclization of the six-membered ring.

References

1. George A. Olah, Qi Wang, Nirupam J. Trivedi, G. K. Surya Prakash, Synthesis, 1991(9): 739-740.
2. M. A. Goodman, M. R. Detty, *Synlett*, 2006, 1100-1104.
3. Ping Zhang, Mei Yang, Xiaoping Lu, Pingfang Han, Yanru Wang, Ultrasonics, 2006, 44, 393-395.
4. Akira Tsubouchi, Miki Itoh, Kotaro Onishi, Takeshi Takeda, *Synthesis*, 2004, 1504-1508.
5. Tsuyoshi Mita, Yuki Higuchi, Yoshihiro Sato, Org. Lett., 2014, 16, 1, 14-17.
6. Azusa Kondoh, Kohei Aita, Sho Ishikawa, Masahiro Terada, *Org. Lett.* 2020, 22, 5, 2105–2110.
7. Javier E. Horta, J. Chem. Educ. 2011, 88, 7, 1014–1015.
8. Green Chemistry: Environmentally Benign Reactions, V.K. Ahluwalia.
9. Jennifer R. Shell, Kathleen A. Poole, Thomas F. Guetzloff, J. Chem. Educ., 2011, 88(10), 1439-1441.
10. G. Sivaprasad, R. Rajesh, P.T. Perumal., Tetrahedron Lett., 2006., 1783-1785.
11. Janeeka Jayram and Vineet Jeena, Heterocycles, 2016, 92(12), .2213-2224.
12. Organic Syntheses; Collective Volume 1, p 272.
13. Organic Syntheses; Collective Volume 4, p 652.
14. Organic Syntheses; Collective Volume 6, p 648.
15. *Ikawa, M.; Stahmann, M. A.; Link, K. P. J. Am. Chem. Soc.,1944, 66 (6): 902.*
16. H. Surya Prakash Rao, S. Jothilingam., J. Chem. Sci., 2005, 117, (4), 323–328.
17. Salvatore. D. Lepore, Yuanjun He, J. Org. Chem., 2003,68,8261-8263.
18. Theodore Cohen, Albert G. Dietz Jr., Jane R. Miser., J. Org. Chem., 1977, 42, 12, 2053-2058.
19. Martin Anker Nielsen, Micheal Kim Nielsen, Thomas Pittelkow, Org. Proc. Res. Dev. 2004, 8, 6, 1059-1064.
20. Maier, T. M.; Sandl, S.; Shenderovich, I. G.; Jacobi von Wangelin, A.; Weigand, J. J.; Wolf, R. Chem. Eur. J. 2019, 1, 238.
21. Vyvyan, J.R., Tetrahedron Letters 1999, 40 (27): 4947–4949.
22. W.-J. Liu, Y.-X. Xie, Y. Liang, J.-H. Li, Synthesis, 2006, 860-864.
23. J. Huang, X. Du, K.V. Hecke, E.V.Van der Eycken, O.P. Pereshivko, V.A. Peshkov., Eur.J. Org. Chem., 2017, (30), 4379-4388
24. S. Kumar, K. Mukhesh, K. Harjai, V. Singh., Tetrahedron Lett., 2019., 2019, 60, (1), 8-12.
25. Zhong-Zheng Zhou, Wei Huang, Feng-Quinji, Ming Wu Ding, Guang-Fu-Yang., Heteroatom Chemistry., 2007,18, 381-389.
26. Bhavna Kaveti, Sandra C. Ramírez-López, Rocío Gámez Montaño, Tetrahedron Lett., 2018, 59, (49), 4355-4358.
27. Razvan. C. CIOC., Eelco Ruijter, Romano. V.A. Orru., Green Chemistry, 2014. 6.

28. Younis Baqui and Christa E. Muller., Org. Lett., 2007, 9, 7, 1271-1274.
29. T. Gupton etal., Tetrahedron, 2008, 64(22), 5246-5253.
30. Greene, T.W.; Wutts, P.G.M., Protecting groups in organic synthesis., John Wiley & Sons.
31. Seijas, J. A.; Vazquez-Tato, M. P.; Martinez, M. M.; Rodriguez-Parga, J. Green Chem. 2002, 4, 390-391.
32. Chundawat TS, Sharma N, Kumari P, Bhagat S. Synlett. 2016;27(3):404-408.
33. Sonar J, Pardeshi S, Dokhe S, Pawar R, Kharat K, Zine A, Matsagar B, Wu K, Thore S. SN Applied Sciences. 2019; 1(9):1-7.
34. Khorramabadi-zad A, Azadmanesh M, Mohammadi S., South African Journal of Chemistry. 2013; 66:244-247.
35. Murthy SN, Madhav B, Nageswar YVD. Tetrahedron Letters. 2010; 51(40):5252-5257.
36. J.L.Chiara, Comprehensive Organic Functional Group Transformations II2, 2005, 709-852.
37. J. Clayden, Lithium Compounds in Organic Synthesis, ed., R. Luisi and V. Capriati, Wiley-VCH, 2014, Ch 13,.375-394.
38. Waldau, E.; Pütter, R. Angew. Chem., Int. Ed. Engl. 1972, 11, 826.
39. Lulu Wang, Minjie Liu, Meifen Jiang, Li Wan, Weijian Li, Dang Cheng, Fener Chen, Chemistry – A European Journal, 2022, 10, DOI:10.1002/chem.202201420.
40. R.S. Vardanyan, V.H. Hruby, Synthesis of Essential Drugs, 2006, 69-82.
41. R.S. Vardanyan, V.H. Hruby, Synthesis of Essential Drugs, 2006, 389-418.
42. Ambatkar MP, Rathi LG, Rokde VV, Danao KR, Mahajan UN, Der Pharma Chemica, 2018, 10(S1): 29-31.
43. R.Vardanyan,Victor Hruby, Synthesis of Best-Seller Drugs, Chapter 3, Analgesics, 2016, Pages 15-64.
44. R.S. Vardanyan, V.J. Hruby, 83-101, Synthesis of Essential Drugs, Elsevier, 2006.559,582.
45. R. S. Vardayan, V.J. Hruby, Synthesis of Essential Drugs, Elsevier, 2006, 83-101.
46. Schmolka SJ, Zimmer H (1984). Synthesis. 1984 (1): 29–31.
47. R.S. Vardanyan, V.J. Hruby, Synthesis of Essential Drugs, 2006, 535-547.
48. R.S.VardanyanV.J. Hruby, Synthesis of Essential Drugs, 2006,19-55.
49. R.S. Vardanyan, V.J. Hruby, 559-582, Synthesis of Essential Drugs, 2006.
50. R.S. Vardanyan, V.J. Hruby, Synthesis of Essential Drugs, 2006, 535-547.
51. R.S. Vardanyan, V.J. Hruby, Synthesis of Essential Drugs, Elsevier, 2006, 83-101.
52. R.S.Vardanyan, V.J.Hruby, Synthesis of Essential Drugs, 2006, 559-582.
53. R.S.Vardanyan, V.J.Hruby, Synthesis of Essential Drugs, 2006, 499-523.
54. R.S. Vardanyan, V.J. Hruby, Synthesis of Essential Drugs, 2006, 2006, 535-547.
55. R.S. Vardanyan, V.J. Hruby, Synthesis of Essential Drugs, 2006, 2006, 311-321.
56. R.S. Vardanyan, V.J. Hruby, Synthesis of Essential Drugs, 2006, 2006, 277-293.
57. R.S. Vardanyan, V.J. Hruby, Synthesis of Essential Drugs, 2006, 2006, 499-523.

www.ingramcontent.com/pod-product-compliance
Ingram Content Group UK Ltd.
Pitfield, Milton Keynes, MK11 3LW, UK
UKHW061536190726
13845UKWH00006B/127